Manual of
Clinical
Emergency Psychiatry

Manual of
Clinical
Emergency Psychiatry

Edited by

James Randolph Hillard, M.D.

*Professor and Chairman, Department of Psychiatry,
and Executive Director of Psychiatric Emergency Services,
University of Cincinnati College of Medicine,
Cincinnati, Ohio*

American
Psychiatric
Press, Inc.

1400 K Street, N.W.
Washington, DC 20005

Copyright © 1990 American Psychiatric Press, Inc.
ALL RIGHTS RESERVED
Manufactured in the United States of America
First Edition
94 93 92 91 90 5 4 3 2 1

Library of Congress Cataloging-in-Publication Data

Manual of clinical emergency psychiatry/edited by James Randolph Hillard—1st ed.
    p.   cm.
  Includes bibliographic references.
  ISBN 0-88048-285-0 (alk. paper)
  1. Psychiatric emergencies.   I. Hillard, James Randolph, 1951-

  [DNLM: 1. Emergencies. 2. Mental Disorders—diagnosis. 3. Mental Disorders—therapy. 4. Mental Health Services. WM 100 M2945]
RC480.6.M34   1989
616.89′025—dc2O
DNLM/DLC
for Library of Congress   89-18112
                                                                        CIP

CONTENTS

PART I   GENERAL PRINCIPLES OF EMERGENCY DIAGNOSIS AND TREATMENT

PART II   SPECIFIC PROBLEMS

PART III SPECIAL POPULATIONS

List of Tables

List of Figures

List of Appendixes

Contributors

Gail A. Barker, M.D.
Assistant Professor of Psychiatry
University of Cincinnati
Cincinnati, Ohio

Paulette Gillig, M.D., Ph.D.
Assistant Professor of Psychiatry
University of Cincinnati
Cincinnati, Ohio

James Randolph Hillard, M.D.
Professor and Chairman
Department of Psychiatry
Executive Director of Psychiatric Emergency Services
University of Cincinnati College of Medicine
Cincinnati, Ohio

George W. Lackemann, M.D.
Assistant Professor of Psychiatry
University of Cincinnati
Cincinnati, Ohio

Kevin Merigian, M.D.
Assistant Professor of Emergency Medicine
University of Cincinnati
Cincinnati, Ohio

Joseph Parks, M.D.
Assistant Professor of Psychiatry
University of Cincinnati
Cincinnati, Ohio

Terry Perlin, Ph.D.
Professor of Interdisciplinary Studies
Miami University
Oxford, Ohio

Douglas Puryear, M.D.
Associate Clinical Professor
University of Texas Southwestern Medical College
Director of Psychiatric Emergency Services
Parkland Hospital
Dallas, Texas

Marcia Slomowitz, M.D.
Associate Clinical Professor of Psychiatry
University of Cincinnati
Cincinnati, Ohio

Ole Thienhaus, M.D.
Associate Professor of Psychiatry
University of Cincinnati
Cincinnati, Ohio

Lawson R. Wulsin, M.D.
Assistant Professor of Psychiatry
University of Cincinnati
Cincinnati, Ohio

Preface

Emergency psychiatry is about caring for people who need help *right now*. It is about deciding what help to give and about making sure that help is really given. The movement to deinstitutionalize chronic psychiatric patients, along with the movement toward briefer inpatient and outpatient therapies, has led to a greater demand for emergency psychiatric services. Improved psychopharmacology and improved community treatment resources have led to increased ability to meet emergency demands. The increased demand and increased resources, however, have made the tasks of emergency decision making more complicated.

Nowhere else in psychiatry is it as important to make a rapid biopsychosocial assessment and to decide rapidly on which level or levels to intervene. What is an adequate medical evaluation for the patient? Is this a psychological problem to treat now or to refer elsewhere? Is this primarily a problem of mental illness or primarily a problem of poverty and homelessness? Do I deprive these patients of their liberty or do I release them at the risk of their safety? This manual is designed to provide a framework for answering these questions and many others like them that an emergency clinician must deal with every day.

The manual is designed to provide comprehensive and internally consistent guidelines for emergency psychiatric assessment and treatment. The approach is designed to be practical and prescriptive but not dogmatic. For some important clinical issues in emergency psychiatry, as in the rest of medicine, there is not unanimous agreement among respectable practitioners. Rather than glossing over these issues, we have highlighted them as areas of "controversy" by shading them in the text. For each such controversy, we present the range of current professional opinion, along with a statement of and rationale for our recommended approach to the issue.

Like other American Psychiatric Press Clinical Manuals, this volume provides more discussion and depth than a Concise Guide, but is not meant to be a textbook of psychiatry. Each chapter emphasizes the aspects of a given disorder or technique or population that are unique to an emergency setting. The book can be read cover to cover as a companion to starting emergency psychiatry, or individual chapters can be read in random sequence as the problems they deal with are encountered.

The book is geared primarily toward psychiatrists but should also be useful to other mental health professionals and to physicians in other specialties. The special problems of psychiatric emergency services receive attention, but the principles discussed are applicable to acute mental health care rendered in any setting.

The manual has three main sections. The first outlines general principles of emergency diagnosis and treatment. The second discusses specific clinical problems. The third discusses the care of specific clinical populations with special needs. Each chapter includes up-to-date references, and some chapters suggest readings for those who want to study a topic further. DSM-III-R criteria are used throughout.

This book was made possible by the help of many people. I thank Mel Fariello and Carol Hamilton for preparation of the manuscript and Audrey Rothenberg for many types of ongoing assistance; Gail Barker, David Garver, Paulette Gillig, Marshall Ginsburg, Gary Harris, Mark Mills, Grace Nadolny, and Harold Woodward for critically reviewing chapters before publication; and the contributors for their willingness to modify their chapters on the basis of such critical reviews. I am grateful to the staff of the University of Cincinnati Psychiatric Emergency Service for having taught me a lot about both the technical and human aspects of emergency psychiatry. Finally, I must thank my wife, Paula Hillard, for her support and material assistance through my long period of obsession with this project.

PART I

GENERAL PRINCIPLES OF EMERGENCY DIAGNOSIS AND TREATMENT

Chapter 1

History and Mental Status Assessment

J.R. Hillard, M.D.

Emergency psychiatric practice begins with triage and assessment of the patient. These functions must occur in a safe environment and must yield a data base adequate for planning appropriate treatment and referral. Throughout the process, there must be a continuing search for possible medical illness and possible patient dangerousness. This chapter and the one that follows outline an approach to emergency assessment and triage.

BEFORE EXAMINING THE PATIENT

Emergency evaluations usually involve patients who are in acute distress and who are not well known to the examiner. Clinicians must never forget that this is a potentially dangerous state of affairs. Whether emergency evaluations are performed in an emergency room setting, a mental health center, or another site, the site should be equipped with 1) rooms that the clinician will not be easily trapped in, 2) a procedure to screen for weapons, 3) ways to call for help, 4) adequate available

---

Shaded sections indicate areas of legitimate diversity of professional opinion in the literature. See Preface for further discussion.

personnel to aid a staff member if attacked, and 5) procedures to involve police if needed.

TRIAGE

Once a patient requests an emergency evaluation from a facility that offers such a service, the facility has some responsibility for that patient. Professional liability might occur if such a patient were to leave before being seen and commit suicide. Within minutes of a patient's arrival, the following issues need to be assessed:

- Is this an acute medical or surgical rather than psychiatric emergency?
- Is this patient at acute risk for assaulting staff or other patients?
- Should this patient be allowed to leave should he or she want to?
- Does this patient need to be seen right away or can he or she safely wait for awhile?
- Does this patient need to be seen at all?

Assessment of orientation and level of consciousness, measurement of vital signs, and a history of current medications and illnesses will screen out nearly all patients requiring acute medical or surgical intervention (see Chapter 2). It is most important at this stage to avoid false negatives (i.e., missing pathology). Indications for immediate medical evaluation include elevated temperature, difficulty breathing, markedly elevated blood pressure, or obtundation (i.e., decreased level of consciousness such that arousal is difficult, and patient, when aroused, is confused) (Strub and Black 1985).

Acute risk of assaultiveness is difficult to predict (see Chapter 11), but patients with acute drug or alcohol intoxication with a history of recent violence, with loud or abusive behavior, or with acute paranoia need to be regarded as at high risk for assault. These patients should, if possible, be removed from the general waiting room and allowed to wait in a quiet, low-stimulation area. If threatening behavior does not decrease in such an environment, seclusion or restraint needs to be considered. Triage should also involve screening for weapons (see Chapter 11). At a minimum, this should involve asking each patient about weapons and arranging for them to be stored during the patient's visit. All emergency settings should have a procedure for searching selected individuals. Some settings may require an airport-style metal detector staffed by security personnel to screen everyone entering the area.

All states have laws that allow for the involuntary treatment of patients at imminent risk of harm to themselves or others due to mental illness. If there is reason to believe that a patient meets the state involuntary treatment statute, then the patient should be detained long enough for further assessment. If such a patient tries to leave before complete assessment, there is probably less liability for unnecessarily detaining him or her for some reasonable time than for inappropriate release (see Chapter 6).

All patients who present as psychiatric emergencies are, of course, better off being seen sooner than later, but most can wait an hour or more without any ill effects. Patients who are acutely agitated, psychotic, or suicidal or who have realistic needs to be somewhere else soon (e.g., to pick up children from school) tolerate waiting poorly, and their evaluations should be expedited or rescheduled.

Some patients show up in psychiatric emergency facilities but have really come to the wrong place. These patients should be offered a full evaluation if they wish it but may be encouraged to go directly to other appropriate agencies. Examples include patients without psychiatric symptoms who are seeking food or housing or patients seeking scheduled outpatient therapy.

ASSESSMENT

The emergency psychiatric assessment is designed to elucidate the biological, psychological, and social problems and resources of a patient. The assessment must allow the following decisions to be made:

- Should the patient be referred to inpatient treatment or outpatient treatment or should the patient be treated in the emergency setting?
- If to be treated as an outpatient, to which of the available resources should the patient be referred?
- If to be treated as an inpatient, to which facility should the patient be admitted and should he or she be admitted involuntarily?
- Do medical problems need further evaluation? (See Chapter 2.)
- Does the patient need help from outside the mental health system, e.g., from other social agencies?

In addition, the assessment should inspire trust and hope that treatment can be useful. If this sort of trust and hope have not been established, the patient is unlikely to complete whatever referral is made. As discussed in Chapter 4, the diagnostic and treatment functions of the interview are inseparably linked with one another.

Psychiatric History

Most patients who request emergency psychiatric evaluation are capable of cooperating with a more or less standard psychiatric interview. Table 1-1 lists the components of the psychiatric history as usually recorded, with areas of particular importance to emergency psychiatric evaluations highlighted. The following guidelines are appropriate in emergency evaluations just as they are in nonemergency evaluations:

- Start with what is worrying the patient most. The patient should ordinarily be allowed to talk with minimal interruption for at least 5 minutes. Even when a patient's greatest concern is not what seems to be the greatest source of medical concern, it is important to let the patient know that you are interested enough to listen. For example, a patient may have auditory hallucinations but may be most concerned with the anticholinergic side effects of his or her medication. The former is certainly a more medically worrisome symptom; but if the latter do not receive appropriate attention, the patient will not feel understood and will likely be noncompliant with treatment.
- Move from open-ended questions (e.g., "What brought you here?") to close-ended questions (e.g., "Have you been having trouble with hearing voices?"). For each problem the patient mentions, open-ended questions should ordinarily be asked first (e.g., "Tell me some more about your drinking"), followed by more specific requests for information (e.g., "So, about how long have you been drinking that much every day?").
- The interview must clarify what particular problems brought this particular person to this particular place at this particular time.
- Ask for specific examples (e.g., "What are some examples of 'tricks,' or 'mean things,' that people have been doing to you lately?") and ask the patient to define more specifically terms they use (e.g., "Tell me some more about what 'depression' means to you").
- Help the patient to establish a chronology of symptoms (e.g., "How long have you been sleeping as poorly as you are now?" "When did you start losing weight?" "What was going on in your life when all this started?" "How long has it been as bad as it is now?").
- Do not be so intent on collecting data that you fail to follow up on emotional reactions from the patient. Use empathic responses to establish rapport with the patient and to help him or her feel understood.
- Pay attention to the close of the interview. Let the patient know when

Table 1-1. Outline of psychiatric history for use in emergency evaluations

- Identifying data
  - Age, race, sex, marital status
- Chief complaint
  - According to patient
  - According to whoever decided that patient needed help (if not decided primarily by patient)
- Sources of information and estimate of their reliability
- Present history
  - Symptoms
  - Onset
  - Precipitating factors
  - Current treatment
- Past psychiatric history
  - Previous symptoms and diagnoses
  - Previous treatment
- Medical history
  - Present medical illness
  - Important past medical illness
- Present living situation
  - Where does patient live?
  - Whom does patient live with?
  - How does patient support himself or herself?
  - Does patient have medical insurance?
- Social history
  - Educational
    How far did patient go in school?
    Was patient in special classes?
  - Occupational
  - Marital
  - Military (i.e., is patient eligible for Veterans Administration services?)
- Family history of psychiatric disorders

the interview is almost over, giving him or her a chance to share some last-minute data. Share your preliminary formulation with the patient and make sure that he or she understands your recommendations.

Modifications of the standard interview. The emergency interview differs from the first outpatient or inpatient interview in several ways. Unlike interviews in other settings where decisions can be delayed, the emergency interview must lead to an immediate plan of action. Patients with emergency presentations may be more anxious and uncooperative than those routinely evaluated in other settings. In addition, emergency evaluations are likely to occur in less controlled environments with multiple interruptions and with intrusion of multiple outside agencies.

The need to make an immediate decision leads to the following modifications of the all-purpose interview:

- There must be more focus on the history of the present illness and on current living conditions, usually at the expense of extensive past history, developmental history, and family history, although aspects of each of these may be quite relevant to a given case. Current living situation is particularly relevant to immediate treatment planning in that, for example, a patient who would ordinarily be sent home with an outpatient referral may need to be dealt with quite differently if homeless. Precipitating conditions as well as presenting symptoms are extremely important to explore. The question, *Why now?*, is always critical, both in terms of why did this problem develop now and why did this person seek treatment now.
- Treatment expectations, both conscious and unconscious, must be elucidated—those of the patient and those of everybody else involved in the case (e.g., family members, friends, therapists, ministers). Sometime after establishing a relationship with the patient, it is often worthwhile to ask explicitly, "What do you think might help?" or "What sort of treatment have you been thinking we might recommend?" Realistically, psychiatric emergency patients know less what to expect from mental health treatment than do patients seen in most other settings. Related issues to clarify are, Who felt the patient needed help? Who identified the problem as psychiatric (McKinnon and Michels 1971)? The answers to these questions can help the clinician to present treatment recommendations to patient and family members in a way that is acceptable to them.
- The interview must be more directive. After a patient has been allowed to describe the problem on his or her own, specific questions need to be asked to allow appropriate decision making. It is not possible to wait over several interviews for the patient to bring up information about living situation, suicide fantasies, or substance abuse.
- Medical problems need more of a focus than in most psychiatric interviews in that emergency patients probably are less likely than others to have had an adequate medical assessment and in that medical problems may be more likely to cause acute presentations.

● Assessment of baseline level of function is very important. A 40-year-old patient with new onset of delusions requires a very different evaluation and disposition than does a 40-year-old patient with exactly the same symptoms, but who has had them for years. Often it is necessary to get collateral information from other sources (e.g., family members) to establish the baseline for comparison.

The need to rapidly assess anxious or uncooperative patients also necessitates modifications of usual interview techniques.

● Reassurance must be more freely given. Emergency psychiatric patients may never have talked to a psychiatrist before and may not know what to expect. They are often extremely anxious and may expect to end up in the hospital from *One Flew Over the Cuckoo's Nest*. They are likely to feel ashamed that they have had to ask for help. They may feel that they are "going crazy," whatever that means to them, or they may be afraid that they are going to die, literally. Specific reassurance (e.g., "I don't think that you are crazy" or "that would be a lot for anyone to handle") is often appropriate.

● A therapist's silence must be used very sparingly. Silence is very useful in many psychiatric interview situations as a way of keeping the responsibility for the interview on the patient. It is always anxiety provoking for the patient, however, and may be quite counterproductive with patients already feeling very anxious and helpless.

● At times, it may be necessary to give medication before an interview can be completed. Chapter 3 discusses the use of neuroleptics, benzodiazepines, and amobarbital sodium for this purpose. Such premedication may be needed for patients with acute psychosis, catatonia, mutism, or extreme agitation.

● The interview approach must be kept flexible. Some patients brought for evaluation will be so intoxicated, confused, or uncooperative that a standard interview will be impossible or, at best, unproductive. For such patients, an extended triage with referral, usually inpatient, for more definitive evaluation is all that can be hoped for. Extremely heavy patient volume may also necessitate, at times, an extended triage rather than a definitive assessment approach.

The environments in which emergency psychiatric interviews take place are less controlled than those where most mental health evaluations occur. Any environment set up for easy accessibility of new cases will fail to provide optimum protection from interruption. Interruption should be minimized, but needs to be expected both by the therapist and by the patient. It is reasonable to let patients know that ongoing therapy will be different in this regard.

Emergency settings may also involve multiple interviews of the same patient within a short period of time. The same patient may, for example, be interviewed by a triage nurse, a social worker, and a physician. Before coming to the psychiatric facility, the patient may have been interviewed by a primary-care doctor, by a case manager, or by various other individuals. It is usually best to ask the patient to tell in his or her own words what the problem is, because secondary sources are not always reliable. If there are discrepancies between what the patient says and what others have said about him or her, the patient should usually be asked to clarify these.

If a patient has been brought in with documents requesting involuntary admission, it is often useful to read these to him or her and to ask for his or her version of events. When family and patient disagree about recent behavior, it is often useful to interview the patient and family together. However, for highly agitated patients or for patients with a history of violence toward family members, such an approach is usually to be avoided.

Considerations in Interviewing Acute Versus Chronic Patients

Patients seeking emergency psychiatric help tend to be bimodally distributed in terms of their experience with mental health services. Many are making their first contacts with the mental health system and have no idea what to expect. Many others have been in "the system" for years and are very familiar with what it has to offer. Each group calls for a different sort of interview.

Patients with no previous mental health contact have special needs. They may be reluctant to admit pathology. They may be confused about what is happening to them. They usually know that they need "help," but they may have only a vague idea what sort of help it is that they need. Interviews with such new patients need to make it as easy as possible for the patient to admit pathology and must include a fairly extensive review of symptoms with reference to possible psychiatric syndromes. For example, if a patient describes depressed mood and has failed to respond to an open-ended question about other symptoms, each specific depressive symptom should be asked about. New patients also need a lot of help completing referrals because they may not have come to terms with their illness and because they may have inaccurate expectations of treatment. Preparing such patients for what to expect from treatment and giving them a feeling of being listened to and understood are among the most important benefits an emergency service can bestow.

Chronic patients often know their patterns of symptoms quite well and often know the treatment system quite well. It is possible to get a meaningful response from a chronic patient to a question like, "Have you been having any trouble with being paranoid lately?" Such a question should be followed up with a request for specific examples. The patient is often in treatment with somebody else, and it is always essential to gather information about what is going on in the patient's relationship with the primary therapist.

Interviewing Relatives

Gathering information from patients' relatives is extremely important under emergency circumstances but poses many difficult problems. It is important because patients often are unable to give complete histories and because families are often the people best able to provide information about the patient's baseline level of functioning. Problems posed by such interviews involve confidentiality issues, issues related to conflict between patient and family, and issues related to family members' levels of stress.

Confidentiality is discussed at more length in Chapter 6. Confidentiality considerations are extremely important but must, at times, be compromised to protect the patient or others from physical harm. For example, if there is reason to believe that a patient may be an appropriate subject for involuntary treatment and the only way to verify this is by contacting a family member, the family member needs to be interviewed, even if the patient objects. It is always best to gain a patient's consent to contact family, but absolute confidentiality should never be promised.

At times, it is difficult to determine which family member is most appropriately to be regarded as "the patient." A particularly common situation where this can come up is with an abusive husband who brings his wife in for treatment due to her "being crazy."

Family members of the mentally ill have a lot to deal with, and many have had bad experiences with mental health professionals. Family members generally want help with their relatives and generally do not want to be treated like patients themselves. On the other hand, they should be given the chance to talk about their feelings and should be offered help when appropriate, either professional or, where available, through a support group for families, such as those operated by the Alliance for the Mentally Ill.

Obtaining Old Records

Old records from your own institution should be routinely requested and reviewed. There are potentially serious medicolegal, as well as clinical, consequences if this practice is not followed. Current outpatient therapists or case managers should ordinarily be contacted. The hospital where a patient has most recently been admitted also can often provide useful information but is often unwilling to do so by phone, even with the patient's verbal permission.

Mental Status Examination

The mental status examination is generally divided into two parts—observational and psychometric. The observational part is conducted concurrently with the collection of psychiatric history but is generally reported separately. It systematically records observations about the patient that are obtained while interviewing him or her. The psychometric part of the examination records the patient's responses to specific tests of cognitive function.

Observational component.   The mental status examination may be recorded as illustrated in Table 1-2. In emergency psychiatry, the mental status examination is particularly important to document because the next time a patient is seen, it may be by a different examiner who will need to assess baseline level of functioning, without having seen the patient before. Some aspects of the examination that are particularly important to record are 1) evidence of adequacy of self-care, 2) suicidal or homicidal ideation, and 3) evidence of hallucinations or delusions.

As noted above, new patients often have trouble admitting psychiatric symptoms and often need encouragement to talk about them. Tables 1-3 through 1-6 suggest progressions of questions that may be asked to make it easier for patients to admit suicidal or homicidal ideation, psychotic symptoms, or substance abuse. The chapters in this book on each of these specific problems suggest ways to follow up on positive screening questions. Questions along these lines should be folded into the course of the interview when patients spontaneously mention material related to

Table 1-2. Outline of mental status examination for use in emergency evaluations

---

● Appearance and behavior
  • General appearance: evidence of appropriate self-care, apparent age, peculiarity of dress, physical defects
  • Motor behavior: psychomotor agitation or retardation, stereotyped activities, gait, posture, tremor, facial expression
  • Behavior toward interviewer: cooperative, suspicious, angry, threatening

● Mood and affect
  • What patient says mood has been like lately
  • Range of affect as observed
  • Appropriateness of affect

● Characteristics of speech
  • Quality: tone, loudness, flow, tempo, difficulty in word finding, neologisms
  • Quantity: pressure of speech, monosyllabic responses
  • Organization: loose associations, circumstantiality, flight of ideas, vagueness

● Thought content
  • Suicidal ideation
  • Violent or homicidal ideation
  • Hallucinations
  • Delusions
  • Preoccupations

● Cognitive functions
  • Level of consciousness: alert, lethargic, stuporous
  • Orientative: time, place, person
  • Memory: immediate, recent, remote
  • Attention and concentration
  • Construction
  • Higher cortical functions
    General information
    Calculation
    Abstract thinking
    Reasoning and judgment
    Insight

---

them rather than held to the end of the interview and asked as a group.

Psychometric component.   The psychometric component of a mental status examination involves asking specific questions in specific ways to gather standardized information about cognitive functioning. Just as physicians in emergency medicine seldom do a complete physical examination, emergency mental health professionals seldom do a com-

Table 1-3. Suicide screening questions arranged from easiest to admit to most specific

---

0. It sounds as though you have been feeling pretty bad lately?
1. Have you ever felt things are so bad that it is difficult to go on?
2. Has the thought of suicide crossed your mind?
3. Have you thought about how you might do it?
4. Do you have the means to carry out that plan?
5. Do you think that you could go through with it?

Table 1-4. Violence screening questions arranged from easiest to admit to most specific

---

0. It sounds as though you have been pretty angry lately?
1. Have you had the impulse to hurt somebody?
2. Have you been concerned that you might lose control of your impulse?
3. Have you ever lost control and hurt somebody?
4. Do you think you might hurt somebody sometime soon?

Table 1-5. Psychosis screening questions arranged from easiest to admit to most specific

---

0. Have you been having any trouble with your thoughts or feelings?
   Has anything strange happened to you lately?
   Did you ever feel especially important in some way or that you had power to do things that other people couldn't do?*
1. Have you been afraid that you were losing your mind or something?
   Has anything happened to you that has seemed so strange that other people have had a hard time believing it?
2. Did it ever seem that people were talking about you or taking special notice of you?*
   What about anyone going out of their way to hurt you?*
   Did you ever hear things that other people couldn't hear, such as noises or the voices of people whispering or talking?*
   Did you ever have visions that other people couldn't see?*
   Have you ever smelled things that other people couldn't smell?*
3. Have you had any trouble with hearing voices or anything like that?
   Have you had any trouble with people putting thoughts into your head or taking them out or controlling your actions or anything like that?
   Have you been concerned that people were plotting against you?

---

* These questions are modified from the psychotic screening section of the Structured Clinical Interview for DSM-III-R (Spitzer et al. 1986).

Table 1-6. Substance abuse screening questions arranged from easiest to admit to most specific

---

0. Do you drink alcohol at all?
   Are you taking any kind of medication?
1. How often do you drink? When was your last drink?
   Have you even taken any kind of drugs to get high, to sleep better, or to change your mood?*
2. Do you use alcohol (drugs) pretty much every day?
3. Have you ever had a drinking problem?
   Have you ever had problems related to your use of drugs?
4. Have you ever had the shakes when you have stopped drinking?
   Have you ever had trouble withdrawing from a drug?

---

* Modified from the Structured Clinical Interview for DSM-III-R (Spitzer et al. 1986).

plete mental status examination. Emergency physical and mental status examinations need to be targeted to the particular patient being examined. Table 1-7 lists some commonly used tests of cognitive status.

It would be quite unusual for any emergency psychiatric patient to be asked all of these questions. Some patients do not need to be asked any of them. Some systemic assessment of cognitive status should be made in any case where either the form or content of the psychiatric history indicates the possibility of an organic brain syndrome. If a patient shows difficulties with speech, memory, attention, or orientation, these should be assessed more systemically. Even if the form of the patient's responses gives no indication of problems in these areas, they should be systemically assessed if the patient is elderly or gives a history of confusion, extensive substance abuse, or major recent physical illness. A reasonable screening battery would include naming and repetition, orientation, memory for three words, serial 3s or 7s, copying figures, and a couple of similarities. These tests are best integrated into the interview as much as possible (e.g., "Have you been having any trouble with your memory?" "Is it OK if I ask you some memory questions?" "Do you remember what month it is?").

General intelligence level is a significant confounding factor in many tests of cognitive function (Nelson et al. 1986), particularly those of general information, vocabulary, similarities, judgment, and insight. These tests should, therefore, be interpreted in light of what is expectable, given a patient's level of intelligence as inferred from level of education.

Asking patients to copy drawings and shapes may be a useful adjunct in some cases. Arguably, such exercises test nondominant hemispheric

Table 1-7. Commonly used tests of mental status

- Aphasic screening
  - Naming objects and parts of objects
  - Following one- to three-step commands involving right and left extremities
  - Repetition of short phrases such as "no ifs ands or buts"
- Orientation
  - Month, year, about what day of month
  - Name of "this place" where examination is occurring
  - Do you remember my name? names of others in room? of self?
- Memory
  - Remember three unrelated items (e.g., a street address, a color, and an object such as a baseball) immediately and after 5 minutes
  - Ability to repeat back a story with some details in it
- Attention—concentration
  - Serial 7s (start with 100 and take away 7 and take 7 away from that and keep going). Serial 3s (start with 30, etc.) may be more satisfactory with lower-IQ populations.
  - Digit span forward: "I am going to say some numbers (one digit per second) then you say them back to me."
  - Digit span backward: 5 forward and 3 backward is probably acceptable for most emergency populations.
- Construction
  - Copy pictures of a cross, a triangle, a square, intersecting figures, etc.
  - Draw a clock face with the numbers
- Higher cortical functions
  - General information: name the last several presidents, large cities, etc.
  - Calculations: simple addition, subtraction, multiplication, or division
  - Abstraction: similarities (e.g., What is similar about beer and wine, cat and mouse?), proverbs
  - Reasoning and judgment (What would you do if you saw a fire in a movie theater? If you found a stamped, addressed letter by a mailbox? etc.)

---

functioning, whereas most other mental status examination items test primarily the dominant hemisphere (Strub and Black 1985).

Formal mental status inventories. A number of short tests of cognitive function have been developed to aid in detection of organic brain syndromes. These include the Mini-Mental State Exam (Folstein et al. 1975; Teng and Chui 1987), the cognitive-capacity screening examination (Jacobs et al. 1977), and others (Baker 1989; Nelson et al. 1986). All have been shown to have some ability to discriminate "organic" from "nonorganic" patients, and their wider use has been recommended. The main question about all of these is their incremental validity, i.e., how much they add to our ability to discriminate organic brain syndrome from functional psychiatric disorders over and above our ability to do so on the basis of an ordinary examination. So far there have been few studies addressing this question, and those that have been done do not suggest that such minitests add very much (Webster et al. 1984). We do not recommend any of them as essential clinical instruments at this time but feel that any of them would be a reasonable adjunct to a mental status examination. Similar comments apply to the use of depression checklists in emergency settings.

DOCUMENTATION

- One to two pages of documentation is adequate for most emergency mental health contacts.
- Documentation should be detailed in terms of present history and living situation, but may be more general in terms of past history (e.g., "patient has a history of multiple admission for exacerbations of chronic psychosis, the most recent admission was 6 months ago at this hospital").
- If there is any question of suicide or violence risk, the history and mental status relevant to these issues need more detailed documentation (see Chapters 8 and 11).
- All contacts with family members, therapists, or others should be noted and telephone numbers should generally be recorded.
- Information related to the disposition decision should be recorded. Information that did not have a bearing on the disposition decision can generally be omitted or can be referred to nonspecifically.
- Mental status examination should routinely be recorded, but may be abbreviated (e.g., "An appropriately dressed man appearing his stated age. Full range of affect. No hallucinations or delusions. No current suicidal or violent ideation. Cognition grossly intact.").

REFERENCES

Baker FM: Screening tests for cognitive impairment. Hosp Community Psychiatry 40:339–340, 1989

Folstein MF, Folstein SE, McHugh PR: Mini-Mental State. J Psychiatr Res 12:189–198, 1975

Jacobs JW, Bernhard MR, Delgado A, et al: Screening for organic mental syndromes in the medically ill. Ann Intern Med 86:40–46, 1977

McKinnon RA, Michels R: The emergency patient, in The Psychiatric Interview in Clinical Practice. Edited by McKinnon RA, Michels R. Philadelphia, PA, WB Saunders, 1971, pp 401–427

Nelson A, Fogel BS, Faust D: Bedside cognitive screening instruments: a critical assessment. J Nerv Ment Dis 174:73–83, 1986

Spitzer RL, Williams JB, Gibbon M: Structured Clinical Interview for DSM-III-R—Patient Version (SCID-P 10/1/86). New York State Psychiatric Institute, Biometrics Research Department, 722 West 168th St, New York, NY 10032

Strub RL, Black FW: The Mental Status Examination in Neurology, 2nd Edition. Philadelphia, PA, FA Davis, 1985, p 30

Teng EL, Chui HC: The modified Mini-Mental State (3 MS) examination. J Clin Psychiatry 48:314–318, 1987

Webster JS, Scott RR, Nunn B, et al: A brief neuropsychological screening procedure that assesses left and right hemispheric function. J Clin Psychol 40:237–240, 1984

Chapter 2

Physical and Laboratory Assessment

O. Thienhaus, M.D.

PHYSICAL EXAMINATION

When psychiatric patients are admitted to the hospital, they receive a full physical examination as a matter of course—like any other inpatient. Outside the hospital ward, however, physicals play a less consistent role in clinical psychiatry. Systematic studies have repeatedly shown that only a small minority of psychiatrists ever physically examine outpatients (McIntyre and Romano 1977; Patterson 1978).

In the interdisciplinary setting of a psychiatric emergency room, the questions arise which patients, if any, should receive a physical examination when they come in, which professional should perform those physicals, and how comprehensive physicals in the emergency room ought to be. This chapter will discuss these questions, present divergent opinions reflecting the controversy in the field, and describe our own policies as one possible way of pragmatically resolving the issue. This chapter will also make recommendations for the medical evaluations of psychiatric emergencies treated in non–emergency room settings.

Do Physicals Belong in the Psychiatric Emergency Room?

Surveys have shown that independent of presenting mental status changes, physical illness is more common among psychiatric patients than among nonpsychiatric comparison groups (Davies 1965; Koranyi 1979). Various authors have presented convincing data suggesting that in a substantial percentage of psychiatric patients who come to a hospital, physical illness is not only coexistent with mental symptoms, but has a causative relationship to the psychiatric presentation (Hall et al. 1978; Hall et al. 1981; Muecke and Krueger 1981).

Physical factors can be associated with any kind of mental symptomatology (Hall et al. 1981). Current nosological classifications such as DSM-III-R (American Psychiatric Association 1987) or the ICD-9-CM system reflect the phenomenological heterogeneity of organically induced mental illness. DSM-III-R, for instance, provides the diagnostic categories of organic hallucinosis, organic delusional disorder, organic anxiety disorder, organic mood disorder, and organic personality disorder. These diagnoses can capture conditions as diverse as cimetidine-induced auditory hallucinations, hypothyroid depression, or the personality changes of a patient with a brain tumor.

A number of physical conditions causing acute mental status changes are summarized in Table 2-1. This list, which follows an outline developed by Anderson (1980, 1987), is obviously not complete. It is meant to highlight relatively common conditions in which failure to consider the physical problem will be hazardous. The need to detect such conditions clearly necessitates physical assessment of patients who present as psychiatric emergencies.

Clearly, psychiatrists need to know the limits of their skills. They should be ready to request a medical or surgical consultation to confirm or disconfirm a suspected finding. An example concerns ophthalmoscopic examination. The mere suspicion of abnormal appearance suggests that a colleague be called in who has more ongoing experience in performing fundoscopic examinations, in order to rule out papilledema or acute vascular lesions.

A common argument against physical examinations in psychiatric emergency settings is the time constraint. Psychiatrists' time is in short supply in the emergency room, and performance of physicals can be delegated only to a limited degree (see below). But a basic physical examination (Tables 2-2 and 2-3), when done by a practiced professional, need not be unduly time-consuming unless positive findings necessitate more extensive assessment. Often, part of the examination is already on record and only requires review by the attending psychiatrist.

Patients who refuse to be examined pose a problem. If, in our clinical judgment, omission of physical evaluation poses a risk to the safety or

Table 2-1. Immediately life-threatening conditions that may present with psychiatric symptoms

Physical problem	Signs and alerting symptoms	Acute laboratory evaluation
Meningitis or encephalitis	Fever, seizures, headaches, stiff neck	White blood cell count
Adrenergic deliria due to • Sedative-hypnotic • Withdrawal • Hypoglycemia • Thyrotoxicosis • Stimulant intoxication	Tachycardia; hypertension; diaphoresis; tremor; dilated, but reactive pupils	Toxic screen; blood sugar
Hypertensive encephalopathy or intracranial hemorrhage	Hypertension, headache, stiff neck, abnormal fundi	
Low cerebral oxygenation due to cardiovascular or pulmonary conditions	Cyanosis, signs of labored breathing, signs of congestive heart failure	Arterial blood gasses
Anticholinergic poisonings	Fixed dilated pupils, tachycardia, fever, dry mucous membranes	
Wernicke's encephalopathy	Nystagmus and acute confusion in alcoholic patients	

continued

Table 2-1. Immediately life-threatening conditions that may present with psychiatric symptoms (*continued*)

Physical problem	Signs and alerting symptoms	Acute laboratory evaluation
Postictal state	History of seizure disorder, confusion, often an abnormal neurologic exam	Anticonvulsant levels
Subdural hematoma	History of (recent) head injury, focal neurologic signs, papilledema	
Hyper- or hypothermia	Altered body temperature	
Subacute bacterial endocarditis	New heart murmur	
Hepatic failure	Jaundice, in some cases a palpable liver	Liver function tests
Uremia		Renal profile (electrolytes)

Table 2-2. Basic physical status examination

- Vital signs
  Blood pressure
  Pulse rate
  Temperature
  Respiratory rate

- General appearance
  Nutritional status and hydration
  Discoloration of skin, mucosae, sclerae
  Signs of trauma, especially head injury

- Neck
  Range of motion, stiffness
  Palpation of thyroid

- Heart and lungs
  Inspection and auscultation

- Abdomen
  Inspection, palpation, and auscultation

- Feet
  Inspection

Table 2-3. Concise neurological status examination

- Level of alertness

- Eyes
  Pupil size, equality, and responsiveness to light
  Ocular movements, nystagmus, exophthalmos

- Motor status
  Deep tendon reflexes—knees and ankles
  Gross motor strength

- Cerebellar function
  Gait
  Coordination

- Suck, snout, grasp, and Babinski reflexes

- Hands
  Tremor, asterixis, chorea

life of the patient (see, for instance, examples in Table 2-1), do we advocate performing the physical, including laboratory work as indicated, against a patient's will? In that case, we proceed even if the patient has to be restrained for the purpose (see Chapter 6). Obviously, the physical examination of uncooperative patients yields less information than that of compliant ones.

Who Should Be Physically Examined?

The question of who should be physically examined is controversial. One extreme position holds that every patient who presents to a psychiatric emergency service should, as a matter of principle, receive a physical examination. This stance has the advantage of being straightforward and logically consistent. However, it has the disadvantage of being impractical. Even though physical problems do play a significant role in psychiatric emergency practice, in terms of relative frequency, the primary presenting problem in most cases is a function of psychological and situational distress. Physical examination might unnecessarily deflect the focus of attention of both patient and clinician from the actual problem, delaying the psychodiagnostic and therapeutic process.

A specific and comprehensive policy definitively identifying which patients should be physically examined is, in our opinion, not feasible. Indeed, such a policy could lead to complex legal problems if a patient who in fact needed physical assessment failed to receive it because the psychiatrist adhered to policy criteria that did not fit the patient in question. Instead of a policy, we suggest certain general guidelines, leaving, by necessity, the ultimate decision to the attending psychiatrist on site.

- We recommend that for general screening purposes, every patient's vital signs (pulse, blood pressure, respiratory rate, and temperature) be measured and recorded. In addition, we recommend a screening medical history for all patients (at a minimum, "Do you have any kind of medical problems that you know about? Are you taking any kind of medication or drugs?").
- A physical examination is recommended
  - When one or more vital signs are outside normal limits (on repeated assessments)
  - For patients whose mental status suggests the differential diagnosis of delirium (see Chapter 12)

- For patients with active medical problems, by history, that may be unstable
- For geriatric patients who have a new, acute onset of mental status symptoms or an acute change in previously existing psychopathology (see Chapter 25)
- When in doubt, do a physical. It is safer to do a physical that turns out to be noncontributory than to omit one that would have been diagnostically important. Obviously, a physical examination does not guarantee that causative conditions are detected. However, failure to physically examine a patient with an underlying organic disorder will almost certainly result in misdiagnosis and, subsequently, misdirected disposition from the emergency service.

How Extensive Should the Physical Be?

A person who goes to the surgical emergency room because of a broken wrist will typically not receive a full-fledged physical examination including fundoscopy and rectal palpation. The means will fit the ends. In the case of psychiatric patients, the questions we want answered by a physical primarily concern the possibility of systemic or neurologic pathology impacting on mental status. Thus, we recommend that the psychiatrist obtain vital signs, examine lungs, heart, and abdomen (Table 2-2), and perform a concise neurological status examination (Table 2-3). Specific findings may direct the examiner toward additional areas of inquiry, require subsequent laboratory tests, or suggest the patient be seen by a consultant. Fluctuating level of consciousness or other fluctuating symptoms may necessitate repeated examinations.

How Comprehensive Should the Assessment Be When Evaluating Psychiatric Emergencies in Nonhospital Settings?

Every setting that provides psychiatric care needs to have facilities available for the screening physical assessment outlined above. If the screening suggests the need for further assessment, a protocol for transfer of the patient to another facility or for medical consultation should be activated.

Who Performs Physicals?

Nurses typically obtain blood pressure, pulse, respiratory rate, and temperature (vital signs) from patients, but the remainder of the physical examination is largely the physician's responsibility. The physician in charge in the psychiatric emergency service is the attending psychiatrist. This person is thus responsible for obtaining the physical, whether he or she performs it himself or herself or delegates it to another physician, a physician's assistant, or a nurse clinician under his or her supervision.

Frequently, a physical—more or less comprehensive—is on record when the patient is referred from medicine or surgery. In such a case, it is the responsibility of the psychiatrist in charge to review the physical status record. "Medically clear" is a problematic term, as Weissberg (1979) has demonstrated. We rarely find what we are not looking for. Certainly, the psychiatric physician needs to take into account colleagues' findings when undertaking the diagnostic assessment. However, the psychiatrist's specific expertise makes it possible to interpret physical data in the context of mental status changes observed. Conversely, a particular mental status presentation can lead the psychiatrist to complement the original examination in order to rule out a contributing physical factor that was not elicited in the original assessment. In addition, physical as well as mental status can fluctuate over time, leading in some cases to a need for repeated examinations.

LABORATORY TESTS

Laboratory tests and radiological studies should be understood and used as extensions of the patient's clinical evaluation, which in turn includes both physical and mental status examination.

Complete blood count, renal panel, blood sugar, urinalysis, electroencephalogram, and toxicological analysis of blood and urine can be considered basic laboratory studies and are often initiated from the psychiatric emergency room. Other tests, such as liver function tests, can be ordered, but in many centers, results will not be available before the patient must leave the emergency setting.

Laboratory tests can be ordered at little or no expense of time and effort by the psychiatrist, and therefore may occasionally be used as a substitute for a physical examination. This is not good practice. Specific laboratory studies should be ordered if the history or physical examination suggest a particular problem, and the laboratory test is expected to confirm or disconfirm the suspected pathology. Which particular studies are indicated depends on the clinical leads derived from history and physical. For example, a psychotic patient with excessive water drinking certainly needs a check of electrolytes (Illowsky and Kirch 1988), as does a bulimic patient with frequent vomiting or a patient taking thiazide diuretics without potassium supplements.

Similarly, a mental status change in a patient who is known to be diabetic should always be reason for immediate checks of blood glucose, ketones, electrolytes, and osmolarity (renal panel). Table 2-1 includes some particularly compelling situations in which laboratory studies are needed. Any such listing must necessarily be incomplete. In addition to the basic laboratory studies mentioned, numerous other tests are also available on an emergency basis, e.g., arterial blood gasses, skull films and other X rays, computed tomographic scans, and lumbar puncture. We have found that, in general, these tests are ordered by nonpsychiatric consultants after our clinically founded suspicion of a major medical problem has led to referral of the patient for emergency intervention by other specialists.

Toxicological Screens

Toxicological screens are now a widely available diagnostic test in most emergency departments. Several types of screens can be distinguished. General qualitative tests serve to rule out or demonstrate presence of one or more substance classes. For example, we frequently order a toxic screen for benzodiazepines and/or barbiturates. These studies are expedient and relatively inexpensive. "Comprehensive" toxic screens for 100–200 substances or more are also available. Their value may, however, be compromised in a given institution because of a high rate of false-positive results or a slow turnaround time (e.g., results may not be back within 24 hours or more). Alternatively, the emergency room physician can request a qualitative screen for a particular substance, such as phencyclidine (PCP) or methaqualone (Quaalude). Finally, there are quantitative assays that provide serum or plasma concentrations of the substances requested. Quantitative assays are more costly and time-consuming.

Toxicological screening of blood and urine samples applies in three situations:

- Immediate past history indicates that the patient has been exposed to poisonous substances, either accidentally or with suicidal intent (or possibly with homicidal intent by someone else). Examples are carbon monoxide levels or salicylate levels. (Chapter 9 discusses more thoroughly the evaluation and treatment of overdose.)
- History and/or physical examination and mental status support the suspicion that the patient may have abused street drugs and/or alco-

hol. The alcohol Breathalyzer test is the most simply used toxic screen available. Stimulants and sedative-hypnotics can be reliably detected by toxic screen, lysergic acid diethylamide (LSD) and PCP less reliably so. Cannabis may be detected for a long time after acute intoxication. (Chapter 15 discusses further the use of toxic screens in the evaluation of substance abuse.)

- A patient is on prescribed medication, and history, physical, and mental status (or any one of these components by itself) indicate the possibility of drug levels outside established therapeutic limits. Digitalis, diphenhydantoin, carbamazepine, theophylline, heterocyclic antidepressants, and lithium are all substances that can cause multiple neuropsychiatric symptoms. It should be remembered that the concentration of carrier protein in geriatric or malnourished patients may be reduced. In those cases, seemingly therapeutic blood levels can in fact reflect excessive amounts of unbound, i.e., active, drug.

The appropriateness of ordering a toxicology screen is predicated on clinical data. Like other laboratory studies, the toxic screen is invaluable as an additional source of information to arrive at a diagnosis. At one point, toxic screens were reported to be underutilized (Lundberg et al. 1974). It is unclear what the utilization pattern is today. Rational use presupposes judicious clinical judgment on the part of the physician ordering the test.

CONCLUSION

Throughout this chapter, reference has been made to the clinician's judgment. The physician who legally signs off on the dispositional decision in the emergency department is considered accountable for the adequacy of a patient's comprehensive clinical assessment. It is this physician's decision to what degree to rely on recorded data, whether to expand the physical data base by requesting consultations or laboratory services, or whether it is safe to abridge or omit a physical evaluation. No detailed policy can replace professional judgment, which is a function of training, experience, and knowledge.

REFERENCES

American Psychiatric Association: Diagnostic and Statistical Manual of Mental Disorders, 3rd Edition, Revised. Washington, DC, American Psychiatric Association, 1987

Anderson WH: The physical examination in office practice. Am J Psychiatry 137:1188–1192, 1980

Anderson WH: The emergency room, in Massachusetts General Hospital Handbook of General Hospital Psychiatry, 2nd Edition. Edited by Hackett TP, Casson NH. Littleton, MA, PSG Publishing, 1987, pp 419–437

Davies DH: Physical illness in psychiatric outpatients. Br J Psychiatry 111:27–33, 1965

Hall RCW, Popkin MK, Devaul RA, et al: Physical illness presenting as psychiatric disease. Arch Gen Psychiatry 35:1315–1320, 1978

Hall RCW, Gardner ER, Popkin MK, et al: Unrecognized physical illness prompting psychiatric admission: a prospective study. Am J Psychiatry 138:629–635, 1981

Illowsky BP, Kirch DG: Polydipsia and hyponatremia in psychiatric patients. Am J Psychiatry 145:675–683, 1988

Koranyi EK: Morbidity and rate of undiagnosed physical illness in a psychiatric clinic population. Arch Gen Psychiatry 36:414–419, 1979

Lundberg GD, Malberg CB, Pantlick VA: Frequency of clinical toxicology test-ordering and results in a large urban general hospital. Clin Chem 20:121–125, 1974

McIntyre J, Romano J: Is there a stethoscope in the house (and is it used)? Arch Gen Psychiatry 34:1147–1151, 1977

Muecke LN, Krueger DW: Physical findings in a psychiatric outpatient clinic. Am J Psychiatry 138:1241–1242, 1981

Patterson CW: Psychiatrists and physical examinations: a survey. Am J Psychiatry 135:967–968, 1978

Weissberg MP: Emergency room medical clearance: an educational problem. Am J Psychiatry 136:787–790, 1979

Chapter 3

Biological Treatment Principles

J.R. Hillard, M.D.

This chapter will discuss some general principles of medication use in an emergency setting, including detailed discussion of the use of antipsychotics and benzodiazepines, the most often initiated drugs in such settings. Considerations involved in the emergency use of other specific medications will also briefly be addressed.

GENERAL PRINCIPLES

- Communicate with the ongoing therapist. Optimally, medication should always be prescribed by the physician working with a patient on an ongoing basis. When this is not possible, communication with the ongoing therapist is always indicated. When such communication is not possible, only small supplies of medication should be prescribed.
- If a patient is doing fairly well, do not change the medication. Even if the medication regimen is not what the emergency physician would choose, it should probably be continued and concerns com-

---

Shaded sections indicate areas of legitimate diversity of professional opinion in the literature. See Preface for further discussion.

municated to the ongoing physician rather than attempting to change a long-term regimen on a short-term basis. An exception, of course, would be a case in which the emergency physician considers the ongoing medication to be so unacceptable as to constitute malpractice (e.g., long-term high-dose amphetamines for weight loss). In such a case, it would be unethical to continue the regimen.

- Be careful with medications that can be abused or that are medically dangerous when taken in overdose. Benzodiazepines and tricyclics should ordinarily not be prescribed in more than 2-week quantities from an emergency service. For patients who are very suicidal or on very high doses, even a 1-week supply of tricyclics may be risky, in that 1 g of amitriptyline may be potentially fatal for a patient weighing 50 kg (Frommer et al. 1987).

- Avoid prescribing narcotics. Narcotics for pain should be prescribed by the physician treating the condition causing the pain. Narcotics for treatment of withdrawal should ordinarily be prescribed only at a licensed detoxification center. Refilling "lost" narcotic prescriptions almost always means prescribing drugs for abuse or for resale on the streets.

- Discourage use of the emergency service as an alternative to ongoing treatment. It is acceptable to write prescriptions for patients from time to time when they have missed a clinic appointment, but not to do so repetitively.

- Do not expect too much benefit acutely. It is widely recognized that tricyclic antidepressants do not have an immediate onset of action, but, in fact, neither do antipsychotics for most patients, nor do most other psychotropics.

- Do not get too fancy. An emergency situation is not the situation for trying complicated or experimental regimens. Patients will have trouble complying with them and physicians will have trouble evaluating the results.

- Ascertain what other medications the patient may be taking and which illnesses the patient may have. A medical history and, in many cases, a physical examination (see Chapter 2) is called for before initiation of medication.

- Nonpharmacologic interventions are generally preferable.

- Write out in longhand the number of units to be dispensed (e.g., Disp: #10 [ten]) to guard against prescription alteration.

ANTIPSYCHOTIC MEDICATION

Indications

The paramount indications for antipsychotic medications are

- Acute treatment of psychotic states of any etiology
- Maintenance of symptomatic remission in patients with chronic schizophrenia and related disorders

The efficacy for these indications is proven by an enormous number of studies. Antipsychotics can also be effective for the acute treatment of agitated states not due to schizophrenia (Clinton et al. 1987). Antipsychotics can be useful for maintenance treatment of some patients with borderline personality disorder (Gunderson 1986) and in some cases of mental retardation with behavior disorder and dementia with behavior disorder (Schatzberg and Cole 1986). They have been used in maintenance treatment for some patients with chronic symptoms of anxiety or depression, but such usage should probably be avoided.

Patients with new onset of psychotic symptoms generally deserve an inpatient evaluation rather than initiation of antipsychotics from the emergency room. Patients who have previously benefited from antipsychotics can generally be restarted on them safely from the emergency room.

Patients with recent exacerbation of behavior disorders associated with borderline personality disorder, mental retardation, or dementia should have a comprehensive biopsychosocial evaluation before medications are begun. At times, it is acceptable to start antipsychotics from an emergency room for these conditions if good outpatient follow-up is available.

Contraindications

Known allergy to a specific drug is certainly a contraindication to use of that agent or agents of the same class (e.g., phenothiazines or butyrophenones). However, the vast majority of patients who report being "allergic" to a specific antipsychotic, such as haloperidol, will prove on further questioning merely to have suffered a severe dystonic reaction to it. A history of neuroleptic malignant syndrome (see below) should be a contraindication to the outpatient initiation of any antipsychotic. Pregnancy is a relative contraindication to any medication, and inpatient evaluation is indicated for most pregnant women requiring antipsychotics (Nurnberg and Prudic 1984).

Complications

Extrapyramidal syndrome. All antipsychotic drugs are capable of producing the extrapyramidal side effects of dystonia, akathisia, and akinesia. Any patient can suffer an extrapyramidal reaction, but patients early in their course of treatment are the most at risk. Younger patients (less than 40 years old) (Moleman et al. 1986), blacks, and males may all be at higher risk for an extrapyramidal syndrome.

An acute dystonic reaction can be rapidly treated with 1 or 2 mg of benztropine mesylate im, which should generally be followed with a prescription for 1 mg of benztropine po bid. Intravenous administration of 1–2 mg of benztropine or 25–50 mg of diphenhydramine may be indicated in more severe dystonic reactions and may lead to a faster onset of action.

Akathisia, an extremely unpleasant motor restlessness, responds less well than dystonia. It may need to be treated by a change in antipsychotic drug or dosage. Some recent literature suggests that centrally acting beta-blockers, such as propranolol, may be useful for some patients with refractory akathisia (Dupuis et al. 1987), and use of an empirical dosage of 20 mg twice daily or 10 mg po tid may be appropriate to try on an emergency basis with appropriate follow-up.

Autonomic side effects. Anticholinergic side effects include the unpleasant symptoms of dry mouth, visual blurring, constipation, and retrograde ejaculation. Sedation is a related side effect of all antipsychotic medications. More serious side effects, which are especially likely to occur in the elderly, are orthostatic hypotension, urine retention, and, occasionally, bowel stasis or delirium. If these symptoms occur in a patient who has been taking maintenance anticholinergic medication along with an antipsychotic, the former can usually be stopped without precipitation of an extrapyramidal syndrome, or the patient can be switched to a different antipsychotic medication.

Prophylactic anticholinergics. Most patients on antipsychotic medication can manage without anticholinergic drugs, and many patients on anticholinergics develop the side effects mentioned above. Given these facts and the general wisdom of avoiding unnecessary medication, it is easy to understand why many authors have taken a dim view of routine prescription of anticholinergics with antipsychotics.

On the other hand, acute dystonic reactions are common adverse side effects of certain drugs and with certain classes of patients. Furthermore, an acute dystonic reaction can be terrifying, humiliating, and painful for a patient. If patients are in an inpatient setting, they can get immediate treatment for an extrapyramidal syndrome. But if they are in the community, it will take considerable time and expense to get treated, and the likely outcome is that they will stop taking the medication and, forever after, will tell people that they are allergic to it.

We recommend prophylactic anticholinergic medication for patients started or restarted on a high-potency neuroleptic from the emergency or outpatient setting unless they have previously been on the same neuroleptic dosage and have not needed anticholinergics (Winslow et al. 1986). I generally recommend that after the patient has been on the medications for 3–4 weeks, their ongoing physician attempt to taper the anticholinergic. After that interval, the patient should have a better appreciation of the value of the neuroleptic and will be less likely to develop an extrapyramidal syndrome.

Neuroleptic malignant syndrome. This is a potentially life-threatening condition, characterized by extreme extrapyramidal syndrome, elevated temperature, and elevated blood levels of the muscle enzyme creatine phosphokinase and, at times, is accompanied by tachycardia, abnormal blood pressure, tachypnea, altered consciousness, diaphoresis, and leukocytosis. Estimates of the prevalence of neuroleptic malignant syndrome have varied widely. Some authors have reported it in 1.4–2.4% of inpatients taking neuroleptics (Addonizio et al. 1986), whereas others have found it in less than 0.1% (Gelenberg et al. 1988). Those who have reported the highest prevalence have, not surprisingly, been those who have used the lowest threshold for diagnosis (i.e., $37.2°C$ = elevated temperature) (Addonizio et al. 1986). Others authors have pointed out that patients on neuroleptics are liable to get febrile illnesses just like everybody else and that extrapyramidal symptoms plus elevated temperature do not uniformly indicate a specific neuroleptic malignant syndrome. There is evidence that neuroleptic malignant syndrome, however defined, is more associated with rapidly increased or unusually high doses of high-potency neuroleptics (Rosebush and Stewart 1989), lending one more rationale to a conservative neuroleptic dosing strategy. Our recommendations for treatment of patients who have elevated temperature and extrapyramidal symptoms are similar to those proposed by Levinson and Simpson (1986). Patients with mild extrapyramidal symptoms without impairment of breathing, swallowing, or mobility and with temperatures below 39.4°C should be assumed to have a nonneuroleptic cause for fever, and that cause should be investigated. Patients with moderate to severe extrapyramidal symptoms and temperatures and vital functions as outlined above should receive 1–2 standard doses of anticholinergics before discontinuation of neuroleptics is considered. For patients with impairment of vital functions or with an unexplained temperature greater than 39.4°C with new hypertension or with obtundation, inpatient medical evaluation is indicated.

Tardive dyskinesia.   Patients are seldom seen on an emergency basis for the chief complaint of tardive dyskinesia, but patients seen on an emergency basis often suffer from tardive dyskinesia. Often the diagnosis is first made in an emergency room because patients are seen there after running out of, or discontinuing, antipsychotic medication. While the patient is being seen in an outpatient aftercare setting, symptoms of tardive dyskinesia may be largely suppressed by continued medication, and symptoms may emerge only after the medication is stopped. Tardive dyskinesia is easy to miss, especially when it involves choreiform movement of the extremities rather than the "classic" buccal/oral movements (Weiden et al. 1987). Any patient who has been on neuroleptics for more than 6 months should be observed carefully for abnormal and/or involuntary movements of mouth, face, trunk, or extremities.

Tardive dyskinesia may be recognized under numerous different circumstances, each requiring a different response.

- If the patient is currently taking neuroleptic medication, the medication should be continued. The patient's ongoing physician should be informed of the possibility of tardive dyskinesia. The American Psychiatric Association task force recommends that "at earliest sign of dyskinesia [the clinician should] lower the dose, change to a less potent agent, or, ideally, stop treatment" (Task Force on Late Neurological Effects of Antipsychotic Drugs 1980, p. 1172). This decision, however, needs to be made in the context of an ongoing treatment relationship and not on a one-time emergency basis. A few more weeks on medication is less likely to have bad long-term consequences than is a precipitous change in regimen.

● If the patient is off medication and relatively asymptomatic in terms of psychosis, medication should not be restarted, but the patient should be referred for ongoing outpatient treatment.

● If the patient, either on or off medication, has developed significant psychotic symptoms, restarting or increasing neuroleptic dosage is acceptable on an acute basis, in consultation with the patient's source of long-term care.

Choice of Medication

As noted above, neuroleptic side effects are unavoidable, but the physician does have some choice of which side effects a given patient will have to tolerate. Table 3-1 summarizes characteristics of commonly used antipsychotic agents. In general, it is best to let the patient choose the particular agent that he or she has had the best experience with in the past.

Some patients who have been repeatedly noncompliant with oral medication do better on long-acting intramuscular forms (i.e., fluphenazine decanoate or enanthate or haloperidol decanoate). When starting patients on any of these medications, it is best to give them a 3- to 7-day supply of oral preparation of the same drug to take until the long-acting form has started working.

For use in "rapid tranquilization," long-acting forms are clearly contraindicated because they do not control symptoms until several days after administration. All of the high-potency short-acting antipsychotics are acceptable for this indication. Low-potency antipsychotics like chlorpromazine are less satisfactory due to their high incidence of orthostatic hypotension when given in moderate dosage. As discussed below, benzodiazepines are a reasonable alternative to antipsychotics for rapid tranquilization.

Dosage

Because antipsychotic medications can be given in high doses without a high level of acute side effects, it is tempting to give extremely high doses to extremely agitated patients. Such an approach was the treatment of choice in emergency services as recently as 10 years ago. This dosing initially seemed to be supported by flexible-dose clinical trials (e.g., giving 10 mg of haloperidol im every 30 minutes until a patient quieted down or went to sleep). Subsequently, predetermined fixed-dose

Table 3-1. Antipsychotic drug characteristics

				Side effects	
				Sedative and	
Generic name	Brand name	Approximate equivalent dosage (mg)	Injectable?	anticholinergic	Extrapyramidal
acetophenazine	Tindal	25	No	+	+ +
chlorpromazine	Thorazine*	100	Yes	+ +	+ +
chlorprothixene	Taractan	50	Yes	+ + +	+
droperidol	Inapsine	2	Yes†	+	+ +
fluphenazine decanoate	Prolixin Decanoate*	1 cc/month = 400 mg/day	Yes†	+	+ + +
fluphenazine HCl	Prolixin, Permitil*	1.2	Yes	+	+ + +
haloperidol	Haldol*	2	Yes	+	+ + +
haloperidol decanoate	Haldol Decanoate	1 cc/month = 200 mg/day	Yes†	+	+ + +
loxapine	Loxitane	2	Yes	+ +	+ + +
mesoridazine	Serentil	55	Yes	+ +	+ +
molindone	Moban	10	No	+ +	+ + + +
perphenazine	Trilafon*	10	Yes	+	+ + +
pimozide	Orap	2	No	+	+
piperacetazine	Quide	10	No	+	+ + +
prochlorperazine	Compazine*	15	Yes	+ + +	+
thioridazine	Mellaril*	100	No	+ + +	
thiothixene	Navane*	5	Yes	+	+ + +
trifluoperazine	Stelazine*	3	Yes	+	+ + +

Note. + = least severe. + + + = most severe. †Not available in oral form.
*Available in generic form.

trials (e.g., giving one dose of 10 mg of haloperidol and observing the patient for improvement) have uniformly failed to support routine use of doses equivalent to more than 10 or 15 mg of haloperidol, and, in fact, there is some evidence for decreased acute effectiveness at doses higher than this (Baldessarini et al. 1988). It has been determined that time elapsed is more closely related to effect than is dosage administered. In addition, there has been no experimental support for using an initially high loading dose of medication to achieve a more rapid response over the next few days (Baldessarini et al. 1988).

Over a period of hours, antipsychotics can generally lead to decreased agitation and hostility in psychotic patients and, for that matter, in patients who are agitated or hostile for other reasons (Lerner et al. 1979). Generally, hallucinations and delusions respond more slowly, over a period of days to weeks (Baldessarini et al. 1988). When a patient with acute auditory hallucinations receives an appropriate dose of an antipsychotic drug and is observed for a few hours, the patient is likely to report that the voices are "not as loud" or "not as frightening" or "not as frequent" or "easier to ignore," but he or she is unlikely to report them to be totally gone.

Route of Administration

Intramuscular antipsychotics have a faster onset of action than oral preparations, but not a great deal faster. A good response, as defined above, usually takes 1.5–2 hours after intramuscular medication and about 2–2.5 hours after oral administration (Dubin et al. 1985). Intravenous antipsychotics probably have a still faster onset of action and are probably safe (Menza et al. 1987). Droperidol, a butyrophenone similar to haloperidol, which is not marketed for psychiatric indications, may produce even better tranquilization responses when administered intravenously than does haloperidol (Resnick and Burton 1984). On the other hand, the definite difficulty of starting an intravenous line on an acutely combative patient may not be offset by the possible advantage of faster onset of action. Oral concentrate is preferable to pills because it is easier to make sure that the patient has swallowed it. We generally recommend acute administration of antipsychotic medication either in intramuscular or oral concentrate form as preferred by the patient.

ALTERNATIVES TO ANTIPSYCHOTICS

Physical Restraints

Physical restraints are a safe, effective, and humane treatment when applied appropriately (see Chapter 11). Unlike "chemical restraints," physical restraints are immediately effective, can be discontinued immediately should they prove unnecessary, and can be removed in a stepwise fashion (i.e., four-point restraints reduced to two-point restraints). The first response in managing a patient who is so agitated as to be unexaminable should ordinarily be an attempt at verbal intervention (see Chapter 11), followed by physical restraint if verbal interventions have been ineffective.

Benzodiazepines

The main alternative medications to antipsychotics for acute treatment of agitated or psychotic states are benzodiazepines (Baldessarini et al. 1988; Lenox et al. 1986; Lerner et al. 1979). As noted above, those symptoms most likely to respond to antipsychotic medication over a period of hours are not hallucinations or delusions, but agitation and hostility, symptoms for which benzodiazepines are definitely indicated (Baldessarini et al. 1988). Two milligrams of lorazepam is roughly comparable in quieting effect to 10 mg of haloperidol, administered either orally or intramuscularly. Choice of benzodiazepine and route of administration will be discussed later in this chapter. Table 3-2 compares lorazepam with haloperidol for acute treatment of psychosis and agitation. The question of paradoxical hostility will be addressed below.

Table 3-2. Comparison of intramuscular lorazepam and intramuscular haloperidol for acute treatment of agitation

	Lorazepam	Haloperidol
Safe, even for the medically ill	Yes*	Yes
Minimal hypotension	Yes	Yes
No major drug interactions	Yes†	Yes
Controls agitation	Yes	Yes
Specific for psychosis	No	Yes
Extrapyramidal reactions	No	Yes
Paradoxical hostility	Possibly	No
Respiratory depression	Possibly*	No

*Respiratory depression possible with high or repeated doses.
†Some additive effect with other sedatives.

We recommend that if an agitated patient is clearly hallucinating or delusional or if the patient has a known history of past psychosis responsive to antipsychotics, then antipsychotics should be the first line of treatment. Antipsychotics should also be the first-line drugs in patients with agitation due to acute sedative-hypnotic intoxication and perhaps in elderly patients. Under other circumstances, benzodiazepines should probably be the first-line drug. If a patient initially treated with a benzodiazepine subsequently turns out to have had a response to a neuroleptic in the past, a neuroleptic can be added. If a patient initially treated with a neuroleptic remains agitated, a benzodiazepine may be added. This combination has an additive sedative effect but has been shown to be safe even in shockingly high doses, e.g., 10 mg of haloperidol plus 10 mg of lorazepam iv every 60 minutes for up to 2 weeks (Adams 1984). Please note that I am not recommending such a regimen. Figure 3-1 is a flow sheet for a recommended approach to rapid tranquilization.

Indications. Benzodiazepines are indicated for the short term (up to 2 weeks) treatment of anxiety or insomnia (Adams 1984; Chapters 17 and 20). As noted above, they are useful in the acute treatment of agitation, including psychotic agitation, and in some cases of catatonia (Greenfeld et al. 1987). Their long-term use for any indication is controversial (Tyrer and Murphy 1987). The use of alprazolam in treating panic disorder and depression is the long-term indication with the most experimental support (Warner et al. 1988).

When a patient is facing a severe but time-limited stressor, benzodiazepines can be a useful adjunct to treatment if the patient understands that they will be used only in the short term. Special considerations for their use in grief reactions and panic disorder will be discussed in Chapters 11 and 17. Benzodiazepines are also useful in the treatment of alcohol withdrawal syndrome, as discussed in Chapter 14. Intravenous diazepam (5–10 mg administered at no more than 5 mg/minute) is the treatment of choice for status epilepticus, and injectable diazepam should be kept ready should such use be required.

Contraindications. Benzodiazepines should not be used by pregnant or lactating women. Teratogenicity has not been definitely proven, but the evidence is disturbing, and risks outweigh benefits (Laegrid et al. 1987).

Complications. The main complications of benzodiazepines are habituation and dependence. At doses greater than the equivalent of 40

Figure 3-1. Recommended approach for rapid tranquilization.

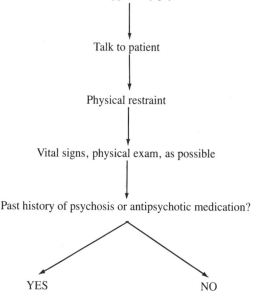

Patient presents agitated, hostile, apparently psychotic, and uninterviewable

↓

Talk to patient

↓

Physical restraint

↓

Vital signs, physical exam, as possible

↓

Past history of psychosis or antipsychotic medication?

YES

- 5–10 mg haloperidol im or po
- If still agitated in 2 hours, consider 2 mg lorazepam
- If hospitalized, no anticholinergics
- If not hospitalized, consider anticholinergics

NO

- Elderly or with a history of adverse reaction to benzodiazepines, use haloperidol, otherwise:
  - 2 mg lorazepam im or po
  - If still agitated in 30 minutes, repeat, up to twice
  - If psychotic, consider 5 or 10 mg haloperidol

mg of diazepam per day for a period of over 8 months, a withdrawal syndrome similar to delirium tremens but more protracted can result (Owen and Tyrer 1983). At lower doses, around the equivalent to 15 mg of diazepam per day, a withdrawal syndrome characterized by anxiety, insomnia, and headaches and, in some cases, by persistent tinnitis, involuntary movements, paresthesia, perceptual changes, or confusion has been well documented (Busto et al. 1986). Benzodiazepines have a low abuse potential compared with cocaine or opiates, but benzodiazepine abuse is by no means rare, and benzodiazepine abusers frequently come to emergency services seeking more pills.

A second reported complication of benzodiazepines is "paradoxical aggression" or "disinhibition." Some patients without a history of aggressive behavior have been reported to get violent when taking lorazepam or other benzodiazepines, even in some cases after a single dose (Gardiner and Cowdry 1985). Such reactions are apparently rare (Dietch and Jennings 1988), but caution is appropriate in prescribing benzodiazepines to "calm down" patients who already have a history of recent violence or aggression. Another sedative-hypnotic, alcohol, has certainly been implicated in disinhibiting aggressive behavior. So, it is plausible that benzodiazepines could too. A single dose of haloperidol may be preferable to lorazepam for quieting down agitated, acutely intoxicated patients, who may already be at greater risk for disinhibited behavior.

Amnesia due to large doses of benzodiazepines can be a significant problem and is reason to warn patients against taking more than the prescribed amount. In elderly patients, amnesia and disorientation may be particularly severe; therefore, much lower doses of benzodiazepines are advised for this group (Plasky et al. 1988).

Refilling prescriptions. The hard-line position is that benzodiazepine prescriptions should only be given by a patient's ongoing physician. The soft-line position is that the drugs do not have much abuse potential and are not very dangerous in overdoses and may, therefore, be refilled from time to time. We recommend splitting the difference on this one. As always, it is best to try to contact the ongoing therapist before renewing any prescription. If the ongoing therapist cannot be contacted, prescribing a few days of pills will probably not cause that much of a problem—once. This sort of flexibility is particularly necessary when dealing with patients who have been on high doses (e.g., alprazolam for panic) for long periods.

Choice of agent dosage and route of administration. Table 3-3 compares characteristics of currently available benzodiazepines. In elderly or debilitated patients, relatively shorter-acting medications at lower doses are probably preferable, even though they may be more likely to be associated with amnesia (Mac et al. 1985).

Intramuscular administration of lorazepam or midazolam leads to more rapid onset of action than oral administration. None of the other agents is absorbed reliably enough intramuscularly to be used by that

Table 3-3. Characteristics of benzodiazepines

Generic name	Brand name	Approximate equivalent dosage (mg)	Oral absorption	Intramuscular absorption	Approximate half-life (hours)*
alprazolam	Xanax	0.25	Intermediate	N/A	14
chlordiazepoxide	Librium†	10–25	Intermediate	Poor	30+
clonazepam	Klonopin	1	Fast	N/A	18–50
clorazepate	Tranxene†	3.75–7.5	Fast	N/A	60
diazepam	Valium†	5	Fast	Poor	40+
flurazepam	Dalmane†	15–30	Intermediate	N/A	30+
halazepam	Paxipam	20	Slow	N/A	60
lorazepam	Ativan‡	1	Intermediate	Good	14
midazolam	Versed	5	N/A	Good	2
oxazepam	Serax†	15–30	Slow	N/A	9
prazepam	Centrax	10	Slow	N/A	60
temazepam	Restoril	30	Slow	N/A	9
triazolam	Halcion	0.5	Intermediate	N/A	3

Note. N/A = not available in this form.
*In young, healthy, normal volunteers. †Available generically. ‡Tablets available generically; injectable available only as Ativan.

route. Several agents are approved for intravenous administration, but all have some risk of respiratory depression, which is seldom, if ever, outweighed by the benefit of more rapid onset of action for psychiatric indications.

ALTERNATIVES TO BENZODIAZEPINES

Nonpharmacologic Approaches

As discussed in Chapters 17 and 20, anxiety and insomnia are usually better treated by nonpharmacologic approaches whenever possible.

Hydroxyzine and Antihistamines

Hydroxyzine (Vistaril, Atarax) and diphenhydramine hydrochloride (Benadryl) have very little abuse potential but do not have much antianxiety potential either. They may be useful more or less as placebos for some patients who just have to have pills but who may be at risk for benzodiazepine abuse. They may also be useful for patients with anxiety associated with dermatologic conditions in that they have some anti-pruritic effect. Hydroxyzine is quite painful when given intramuscularly and, of course, should not be used punitively. Always remember, too, that these drugs are much more medically serious overdoses than benzodiazepines.

Buspirone Hydrochloride

Buspirone is a promising drug that has been shown to decrease anxiety apparently without risk of habituation. Its onset of action, however, is generally over a period of days to weeks rather than minutes to hours, making it less useful under emergency circumstances. It is not cross-tolerant with benzodiazepines and, hence, does not treat the anxiety associated with benzodiazepine withdrawal (Schweizer and Rickels 1986). Some anxious patients even report an increase in "jitteriness" when beginning buspirone (Liegghio et al. 1988).

Barbiturates, Meprobamate, and Other Nonbarbiturate Sedative-Hypnotics

Abuse potential, rapid habituation, and medical dangerousness if taken in overdose make all of these drugs poor alternatives to benzodiazepines for ongoing treatment. Amobarbital sodium may be used in a dose of 250 mg as an alternative to antipsychotics or benzodiazepines for acute agitation, although respiratory, renal, or hepatic disease, porphyria, or hypotension are contraindications. An "amobarbital (Amytal) interview" may also be used diagnostically as discussed in Chapter 18. In addition, a pentobarbital challenge test to quantify degree of barbiturate dependence may, at times, be useful, as outlined in Chapter 15.

CONSIDERATIONS IN THE EMERGENCY USE OF OTHER MEDICATIONS

Antidepressants

Issues involved in starting antidepressants from an emergency service are discussed in Chapter 10. In spite of the long delay before onset of action and the risk of overdose, I believe that there are some circumstances under which cyclic antidepressants may be appropriately started from an emergency service, either for treatment of depression or for treatment of panic disorder. We cannot think of any indications for starting monoamine oxidase inhibitors on an emergency basis. Table 3-4 lists characteristics of available antidepressant drugs.

Lithium

We have had very little success in starting patients on lithium from our emergency service (see Chapter 10). The acutely manic patients that we would like to start on it generally find its effect initially dysphoric, and we have had a difficult time getting compliance. If lithium is being started, the following studies should be ordered at the time it is started: complete blood count, thyroid panel (T4, T3 uptake, and possibly thyrotropin [TSH]), and possibly an electrocardiogram. Lithium should not be started from an emergency service for patients who are dehydrated or physically ill, especially if they are suffering from cardiac or renal disorders (Jefferson et al. 1987).

Lithium intoxication sometimes leads to emergency psychiatric visits. Symptoms of mild intoxication include slight feelings of apathy, sluggishness, drowsiness, lethargy, reduced concentration power, muscular weakness, heaviness of the limbs, unsteady gait, coarse hand tremor, and slight muscle twitching. These symptoms can occur in some patients whose levels are less than 1.5 mEq/L. More severe intoxication may result from intentional overdose or dehydration or from drug interac-

Table 3-4. Characteristics of antidepressant drugs

Generic name	Brand name	Usual dosage* (mg/day)	Anticholinergic side effects	Sedative side effects
Tricyclics				
amitriptyline	Elavil, Endep†	150–300	+ + +	+ + +
desipramine	Norpramin, Pertofrane	150–300	+	+
doxepin	Adapin, Sinequan	150–300	+ +	+ + +
imipramine	Tofranil†	150–300	+ +	+ +
nortriptyline	Aventyl, Pamelor	50–100	+	+
protriptyline	Vivactil	15–60	+ + +	+
trimipramine	Surmontil	150–300	+ +	+ + +
Tetracyclics				
amoxapine	Asendin	150–450	+	+ +
maprotiline	Ludiomil	150–200	+	+ +
MAOIs				
isocarboxazid	Marplan	20–50	+	+
phenelzine	Nardil	30–60	+ +	+
tranylcypromine	Parnate	20–50	+	+
Other				
fluoxetine	Prozac	40–80	+	+
trazodone	Desyrel	150–300	+	+ + +

Note. MAOI = monoamine oxidase inhibitor. + = least severe. + + + = most severe.
*In young healthy adults. †Available in generic form.

tions (particularly diuretics) listed in Table 3-6. More severe intoxication is characterized by manifest apathy and sluggishness, drowsiness, lethargy, sleepiness, speech difficulty, irregular tremor, manifest muscular weakness, manifest myoclonic twitching, and ataxia.

Patients with symptoms of mild to moderate toxicity need a serum lithium level determination and an appropriate dosage adjustment. If the patient's level of consciousness is decreased or if levels approach 2.5 mEq/L, the intoxication should be regarded as severe and toxicology consultation should be obtained.

Anticholinergics

As noted above, prophylactic anticholinergics are often indicated when starting an outpatient on antipsychotics. Subtle extrapyramidal symptoms are one of the main reasons that patients stop taking their antipsychotics, and, hence, raising anticholinergic doses to eliminate or reduce extrapyramidal symptoms is usually a good idea as long as the patient does not have marked anticholinergic symptomatology. Amantadine hydrochloride (Symmetrel), which has an antiparkinsonian effect with less anticholinergic effect, is a reasonable alternative for some patients. Table 3-5 lists characteristics of available antiparkinsonian drugs for use with drug-induced parkinsonism.

Table 3-5. Characteristics of antiparkinsonian drugs

Generic name	Brand name	Dosage range (mg/day)	Mechanism
amantadine	Symmetrel	100–300	Dopaminergic
benztropine mesylate	Cogentin	2–6	Anticholinergic
biperiden	Akineton	2–8	Anticholinergic
diphenhydramine	Benadryl	50–300	Anticholinergic
ethopropazine	Parsidol	100–400	Anticholinergic
procyclidine	Kemadrin	10–20	Anticholinergic
trihexyphenidyl hydrochloride	Artane	4–15	Anticholinergic

Some patients abuse anticholinergic medications (Dilsaver 1988). Such abuse is probably rare, except in correctional settings, but repeated requests for more anticholinergics should be a cause for concern.

Beta-blockers

Beta-blockers are often useful in prophylactic treatment of stage fright or public-speaking anxiety. They may be useful for prophylaxis of aggressive outbursts in some patients, including some mentally retarded patients and some patients with organic brain syndromes (Ratey et al. 1986; Chapters 11 and 22). Propranolol (20–60 mg/day) may also be useful in the treatment of akathisia in patients who have not responded to anticholinergics (Adler et al. 1986). For patients with no medical problems, a test dose of 10 mg of propranolol can safely be given in an emergency room and continued if it appears to have been useful.

Anticonvulsants

Anticonvulsants, particularly carbamazepine and clonazepam, are being used increasingly in psychiatry for various indications (Gardiner and Cowdry 1986), particularly in the treatment of mood disorders (Post and Uhde 1985). These are, however, second-line drugs for psychiatric indications and should generally not be started from an emergency service.

DRUG INTERACTIONS

Patients seen on an emergency basis are frequently taking a variety of medications. It is always important to be sensitive to the possibility of adverse drug interactions, particularly those listed in Table 3-6.

Table 3-6. Clinically significant interactions between psychotropics and other drugs used in outpatient practice

	Effect of interaction
Drug interactions with antipsychotics	
Anticholinergics	Increased anticholinergic effect
Lithium	May increase CNS toxicity
Narcotics	Increased sedation, analgesia augmented, hypotension augmented, respiratory depression augmented, anticholinergic effects augmented by meperidine
Cyclic antidepressants	Increased sedation, increased hypotension, increased anticholinergic effect
L-Dopa	May exacerbate psychosis, decreased antiparkinsonian effect of L-Dopa
Amphetamines	May exacerbate psychosis by counteracting effects of neuroleptics
Barbiturates, nonbarbiturate hypnotics	Increased sedation, decreased clinical effect of neuroleptic
Isoniazid	Hepatic toxicity and encephalopathy, decreased neuroleptic effect
Reserpine, clonidine, guanethidine, bethanidine, debrisoquin	Decreased antihypertensive effect
Epinephrine	Hypotension augmented
Drug interactions with cyclic antidepressants	
Cimetidine, methylphenidate, acetaminophen, oral contraceptives, chloramphenicol, iproniazid, MAOIs	Inhibit metabolism, increasing blood levels and toxicity of antidepressants
Guanethidine, debrisoquin, bethanidine	Decreased antihypertensive effect
Quinidine, procainamide hydrochloride	Cardiac conduction prolonged

Table 3-6. Clinically significant interactions between psychotropics and other
drugs used in outpatient practice (*continued*)

	Effect of interaction
Coumarin anticoagulants	Increased bleeding
Phenytoin, barbiturates, nonbarbiturate hypnotics, dichloralphenazone, rifampin, doxycycline, griseofulvin, carbamazepine, phenylbutazone	Induces hepatic metabolism, decreasing clinical effect of antidepressant
Epinephrine	Hypotension augmented, increased bleeding in nasal surgery
Benzodiazepines	Increased CNS sedation, increased confusion, decreased motor functions

Drug interactions with MAOIs

Sympathomimetics, L-dopa, novocain (dissolved in epinephrine)	Increased blood pressure
Cyclic antidepressants	Conflicting reports on toxicity, hyperpyrexia, excitability, muscle rigidity, convulsions, coma; use with caution
Meperidine	Excitation, sweating, hypotension

Drug interactions with lithium

Indomethacin, piroxicam, sulindac, ibuprofen, phenylbutazone, naproxen, zomepirac	Increased lithium toxicity due to decreased renal lithium clearance
Thiazide diuretics, amiloride, spironolactone, triamterene, furosemide	Increased lithium toxicity due to decreased renal lithium clearance
Theophylline, acetazolamide, aminophylline	Increased renal excretion of lithium, decreasing its effect
Sodium bicarbonate, sodium chloride, urea, mannitol	Increased renal excretion, decreasing effect
Tetracycline, spectinomycin	Increased lithium toxicity due to decreased renal lithium clearance

Drug interactions with benzodiazepines

Alcohol, neuroleptics, narcotics, antihistamines, sedative-hypnotics	Increased CNS sedation

Drug interactions with carbamazepines

Lithium	Neurotoxicity with normal levels of both; combination may increase ataxia, dizziness, and feelings of unreality

Table 3-6. Clinically significant interactions between psychotropics and other drugs used in outpatient practice (*continued*)

	Effect of interaction
Cimetidine, erythromycin, isoniazid	May produce somnolence, lethargy, nystagmus, dizziness, nausea and vomiting in combination
Propoxyphene	Increased carbamazepine levels

Note. CNS = central nervous system. MAOI = monoamine oxidase inhibitor.
Source. Adapted from Glassman and Salzman (1987).

USE OF APPROVED DRUGS FOR UNLABELED INDICATIONS

All of the drugs mentioned in this chapter have been approved by the Food and Drug Administration (FDA). In a number of cases, however, I have mentioned uses for them that are not FDA "labeled indications." Some drugs mentioned that are not labeled for psychiatric indications are droperidol, pimozide, midazolam, clonazepam, propranolol, carbamazepine, and phenytoin. In addition, haloperidol is not labeled for intravenous administration.

Many physicians are concerned about the appropriateness of using approved drugs for unapproved indications; however, the FDA (1982) states:

> The FD&C Act does not, however, limit the manner in which a physician may use an approved drug. Once a product has been approved for marketing, a physician may prescribe it for uses or in treatment regimens or patient populations that are not included in approved labeling. Such "unapproved" or, more precisely, "unlabeled" uses may be appropriate and rational in certain circumstances, and may, in fact, reflect approaches to drug therapy that have been extensively reported in medical literature.

REFERENCES

Adams F: Neuropsychiatric evaluation and treatment of delirium in the critically ill cancer patient. Cancer Bulletin 36:156–160, 1984

Addonizio G, Susman LL, Roth SD: Symptoms of neuroleptic malignant syndrome in 82 consecutive inpatients. Am J Psychiatry 143:1587–1590, 1986

Adler L, Augrist B, Peselow E, et al: A controlled assessment of propranolol in the treatment of neuroleptic-induced akathisia. Br J Psychiatry 149:42–45, 1986

Baldessarini RJ, Cohen BM, Teicher MH: Significance of neuroleptic dose and plasma level in the pharmacologic treatment of psychoses. Arch Gen Psychiatry 45:79–91, 1988

Busto U, Sellers EM, Navanjo CA, et al: Withdrawal reaction after long-term therapeutic use of benzodiazepines. N Engl J Med 315:854–859, 1986

Clinton JE, Sterner S, Stelmachers Z, et al: Haloperidol for sedation of disruptive emergency patients. Ann Emerg Med 16:319–322, 1987

Dietch JT, Jennings RK: Aggressive dyscontrol in patients treated with benzodiazepines. J Clin Psychiatry 49:184–188, 1988

Dilsaver SC: Antimuscarinic agents as substances of abuse: a review. J Clin Psychopharmacol 8:14–22, 1988

Dubin WR, Waxman HM, Weiss KJ, et al: Rapid tranquilization: the efficacy of oral concentrate. J Clin Psychiatry 46:475–478, 1985

Dupuis B, Cattena J, Dumon JP, et al: Comparison of propranolol, sotalol and betaxolol in treatment of neuroleptic-induced akathisia. Am J Psychiatry 144:802–805, 1987

Food and Drug Administration: FDA Drug Bulletin 12(1):4–5, 1982

Frommer DA, Kulig KW, Marx JA, et al: Tricyclic antidepressant overdose. JAMA 257:521–526, 1987

Gardiner DL, Cowdry RW: Alprazolam-induced dyscontrol in borderline personality disorder. Am J Psychiatry 142:98–100, 1985

Gardiner DL, Cowdry RW: Positive effects of carbamazepine on behavioral dyscontrol in borderline personality disorder. Am J Psychiatry 143:519–522, 1986

Gelenberg AJ, Bellinghausen B, Wojcik JD, et al: A prospective study of neuroleptic malignant syndrome in a short term psychiatric hospital. Am J Psychiatry 145:517–518, 1988

Glassman R, Salzman C: Interactions between psychotropic and other drugs: an update. Hosp Community Psychiatry 38:236–242, 1987

Greenfeld D, Conrad C, Kincare P, et al: Treatment of catatonia with low dose lorazepam. Am J Psychiatry 144:1224–1225, 1987

Gunderson JG: Pharmacotherapy for patients with borderline personality disorder. Arch Gen Psychiatry 43:698–700, 1986

Jefferson JW, Greist JH, Ackerman DL, et al: Lithium Encyclopedia for Clinical Practice, 2nd Edition. Washington, DC, American Psychiatric Press, 1987

Laegrid L, Olegard R, Walstrom J, et al: Abnormalities in children exposed to benzodiazepines in utero (letter). Lancet 1:108–109, 1987

Lenox RH, Modell JG, Weiner S: Acute treatment of manic agitation with lorazepam. Psychosomatics 27 (suppl 1):28–31, 1986

Lerner Y, Lwow E, Levitin A, et al: Acute high dose haloperidol treatment of psychosis. Am J Psychiatry 136:1061–1064, 1979

Levinson DF, Simpson GM: Neuroleptic-induced extrapyramidal symptoms with fever. Arch Gen Psychiatry 43:839–848, 1986

Liegghio NE, Yeragani VK, Moore NC: Buspirone-induced jitteriness in three patients with panic disorder and one patient with generalized anxiety disorder. J Clin Psychiatry 49:165–166, 1988

Mac DS, Kumar R, Goodwin DW: Anterograde amnesia with oral lorazepam. J Clin Psychiatry 46:137–138, 1985

Menza MA, Murray GB, Holmes VF, et al: Decreased extrapyramidal symptoms with intravenous haloperidol. J Clin Psychiatry 48:278–280, 1987

Moleman P, Janzen G, VonBargen BA, et al: Relationship between age and incidence of Parkinsonism in psychiatric patients treated with haloperidol. Am J Psychiatry 143:232–234, 1986

Nurnberg HG, Prudic J: Guidelines for treatment of psychosis during pregnancy. Hosp Community Psychiatry 35:67–71, 1984

Owen RT, Tyrer P: Benzodiazepine dependence: a review of the evidence. Drugs 25:385–398, 1983

Plasky P, Marcus L, Salzman C: Effects of psychotropic drugs on memory: Part 2. Hosp Community Psychiatry 39:501–502, 1988

Post RM, Uhde TW: Carbamazepine in bipolar illness. Psychopharmacol Bull 21:10–17, 1985

Ratey JJ, Mikkelsen EJ, Smith GB, et al: Beta-blockers in the severely and profoundly mentally retarded. J Clin Psychopharmacol 6:103–107, 1986

Resnick M, Burton BT: Droperidol vs. haloperidol in the initial management of acutely agitated patients. J Clin Psychiatry 45:298–299, 1984

Rosebush P, Stewart T: A prospective analysis of 24 episodes of neuroleptic malignant syndrome. Am J Psychiatry 146:717–725, 1989

Schatzberg AF, Cole JO: Manual of Clinical Psychopharmacology. Washington, DC, American Psychiatric Press, 1986, pp 252–255

Schweizer E, Rickels K: Failure of buspirone to manage benzodiazepine withdrawal. Am J Psychiatry 143:1590–1592, 1986

Task Force on Late Neurological Effects of Antipsychotic Drugs: Tardive dyskinesia: summary of a task force report of the American Psychiatric Association. Am J Psychiatry 137:1163–1172, 1980

Tyrer P, Murphy S: The place of benzodiazepines in psychiatric practice. Br J Psychiatry 151:719–723, 1987

Warner MD, Peabody CA, Whiteford HA, et al: Alprazolam as an antidepressant. J Clin Psychiatry 49:148–150, 1988

Weiden PJ, Mann JJ, Haas G, et al: Clinical non-recognition of neuroleptic-induced movement disorders: a cautionary study. Am J Psychiatry 144:1148–1153, 1987

Winslow RS, Stillner V, Coons DJ, et al: Prevention of acute dystonic reactions in patients beginning high-potency neuroleptics. Am J Psychiatry 143:706–710, 1986

Chapter 4

Psychological Treatment Principles

D. Puryear, M.D.

Traditionally, emergency psychiatry has focused more on triage than on treatment, using a medical model interview for data gathering, diagnosis, and disposition. The crisis intervention approach described herein, combined with diagnostic procedures and medications, provides emergency *treatment*.

PRINCIPLES OF CRISIS INTERVENTION

Most psychiatric emergency visits occur at a time of crisis—a time when external stresses have overwhelmed the coping mechanisms that a patient ordinarily uses to deal with stress. During a crisis, an individual is anxious, is not functioning efficiently, and is trying to find relief. Crises tend to be time limited because they are so unbearable. If therapists keep in mind the following principles of crisis intervention (Puryear 1979), they will probably make good clinical decisions.

- *Immediate intervention*. A crisis is a time of danger, and a time-limited opportunity for intervention.
- *Action*. In crisis intervention, the worker very actively participates in and directs the process of assessing the situation and, together with the client, of formulating a plan of action for the client to pursue.
- *Limited goal*. The minimal goal of crisis intervention is to avert

catastrophe. The basic overall goal is to restore the client to an equilibrium state, hopefully with some growth also occurring.

- *Hope and expectations.* The worker must initially instill hope into the situation. This is done through the whole approach, including the worker's attitude and expectations of the client and about the situation.
- *Support.* The worker must provide a great deal of support to the client, primarily by being "with him or her," available to go through the process with the client. The support must be carefully given so that it is sufficient without being excessive.
- *Focused problem solving.* This is the backbone of crisis intervention; it provides the structure that shapes and supports the whole process. Basically, we try to determine "The Problem"—the basic unresolved problem that led to the crisis—and then assist the client in planning and putting into action steps aimed at resolving it. We keep our own and the client's attention focused on that problem and on the problem-solving process, and we avoid being distracted and sidetracked.
- *Self-image.* Efforts must be made to assess and understand the client's self-image, to consider carefully the effect that any of the intervention maneuvers might have on it, and to protect and enhance it. These efforts will pay off in many ways, including increased rapport, decreased defensiveness, and mobilization of the client's energies.
- *Self-reliance.* From the very onset, attention must be paid to fostering self-reliance and combating dependency. This need must be carefully balanced with the need for support.

THE INTERVIEW

Interviews are structured and are directed toward specific goals. Dynamics, transference, and catharsis are all appreciated and utilized, but the primary focus is on identifying a specific here-and-now problem to work on. Such problems are usually concrete, but they touch directly on psychological issues. To a large extent, the interview is the treatment.

Most psychiatric emergency interviews go through the same steps covered over a number of sessions in the course of a more extended crisis intervention: 1) establishing communication and rapport, 2) assessing the problem, 3) assessing resources and strengths, 4) formulating a plan, 5) mobilizing the client, and 6) closing.

The Family Interview

We begin by thinking of family, even if the patient comes in alone. It is often appropriate for the interview to include the entire family along with the patient and any others who come in with them. You, as the interviewer, see that everyone participates in a relatively equal fashion. Everyone's ideas are solicited and everyone is listened to. In this way, more information is gathered, more rapidly and more accurately. You can form an alliance with family members, develop resources, and work out a treatment plan in agreement with everyone. This saves time and avoids the family's rejecting a treatment plan negotiated with the patient alone. When this format is not working well, you can always shift gears and see people individually or in various combinations.

Being in touch with family is important to every person's sense of identity, self-worth, and feelings of connectedness and stability. Even when unaccompanied patients profess to have no family, pursuing the matter frequently leads to a long-distance telephone call. This may result in reporting to the patient that their presumptions were accurate: no one in their family wants to have anything to do with them. It may result in partially reuniting with the family, at least by telephone. The family may or may not wish to help, but the patient, at least, may obtain news of the family, and this can be supportive.

Beginning the Interview

The first step includes establishing rapport with everyone, taking charge of the interview, and beginning to establish the type of situation desired. First meet everyone, and find out who they are, what they do, and who lives together. Usually something interesting and admirable about each person is found. Establish that everyone will talk, but that you are in charge of the interview. Thus, you decide who talks when and about what. Ask questions in such a way that people talk to you rather than to each other. Do not allow people to interrupt each other, and function as a host. Your rapport and skill at being in charge will be tested and must be attended to throughout the interview. Build up this authority and rapport at the beginning, so that later in the interview, should the family members begin fighting, for example, they will stop when you tell them to. Developing this relationship increases the chances that the family will work with you in developing and following through with a plan. Establish that everyone is important and is treated with respect, and that the situation involves outlining problems and moving toward solutions rather than ventilating, blaming, assaulting, or arguing. At times, ventilation and emotionality can be useful, but, in general, they are an interference and should be limited by the psychiatrist. You can manage this, after establishing control and rapport, by focusing on factual matters, changing the topic, etc. ("I can see why you were so mad at Billy, Mr. Jones; it must have really worried you when you saw him smashing the furniture, worried you about the furniture and, of course, you're worried about what kind of problems he might have and what his future is going to be. Was that on Wednesday or on Thursday?") The psychiatrist sets up and maintains clarity of responsibility and roles. You are a consultant who assists people in resolving their problems and an expert in approaches to problem solving. You are not an expert in their problems; they are. You are not going to solve their problems for them, but will assist as they solve them. Thus, the responsibility for the problems remains with the patient and the family.

While establishing rapport, gaining control, and establishing the situation, observe the patient and family and form tentative hypotheses about what is going on. Who is going to be helpful? Who is going to be difficult and in what way? What do the patient and the family want? What are reasonable goals for the intervention? What intervention might be most helpful? This is a time of observation and tentative planning.

Checking Issues

At this point, the psychiatrist leans back and asks, "So, what's going on?" Relinquish control and shift to a more traditional open-ended interview, with people speaking spontaneously and freely. Observe how the people interact, their ideas, who speaks first, etc. Be alert to prevent emotional escalation, blaming, and other undesirable processes. During this brief phase of the interview, decide which issues to address. Begin asking more specific questions to check out the issues. Is this woman psychotic? Dangerous? Will she take medication? Could this be an organic condition? Will the boyfriend ever come back? Under what conditions? Mental status or diagnostic criteria might be assessed during this phase, or specific past history obtained.

Focused Problem Solving, Tasks, and Limited Goals

Begin to focus on a specific problem and to break it down into small steps. Motivate the patient and family to work on this particular problem. The outcome is a set of small tasks, with each person having a part in working on the problem. This may be the major problem that caused the crisis, but does not have to be. A plan that will solve the problem is not necessary. The purpose is simply to get the family and patient reorganized, reintegrated, remoralized, remobilized, and functioning once again, assuming that they will then be able to work themselves out of the crisis. The tasks should be designed so that you are sure the family will do them and will be successful. Throughout, there needs to be an emphasis on strength and assets in addition to problems. People in crisis are seen at their worst, and they are capable of much better functioning. Do not attempt to cure all of the family's problems, but to help them resolve a crisis without any catastrophe occurring. Further treatment or growth may or may not follow.

Perception, Network, and Coping Methods

Through questions, discussion, and word choice, people can be helped toward a more useful, workable perception of their problem. The network—the available people or organizations from which patients get support—can be enhanced. It is not necessary that the network provide the solution. A long-distance call to Grandmother rarely produces a magical solution, but any expression of interest and concern is supportive. It is best to help the family adjust their usual coping mechanisms or apply them in slightly different ways for this particular problem, rather than trying to use unfamiliar approaches.

Although specifically applicable to people who are in a crisis, these principles can be followed to some degree in almost every case seen in the emergency room. For example, if the patient is acutely psychotic, or if there is an organic condition, it is still useful to involve the family, formulate a plan of action, leave as much responsibility as possible with them, and assist them in dealing with their problem, whether that involves the patient taking medication, being hospitalized, or needing a neurological workup.

In the emergency interview, the psychiatrist proceeds on four tracks at once: 1) interview maintenance—managing rapport, control, and responsibility; 2) data gathering; 3) checking on issues; and 4) motion toward a goal. Continually try to help the patient and family move in a desirable direction, whether it is getting the patient to accept a fluphenazine decanoate shot, or getting the family to agree to see that the patient keeps a clinic appointment. Build a foundation for movement and gradually help the family move in that direction in the interview. This will succeed more often than simply recommending or trying to coerce or persuade them to do something.

INTERVENTIONS: CASE EXAMPLES

Crisis Intervention Approach—A Borderline Patient

A student asked me to see a patient, describing her as sullen, borderline, suicidal, and possibly needing hospitalization. I met the patient and asked a few questions without broaching the suicide issue at all. I learned that her therapist was away for a month. She said she had recently been seeing the therapist less often anyway, due to money problems. She minimized this, but I pushed, "This is really hard," trying to be empathic. We clarified that she must be careful not to say anything negative about her therapist. (Accepting her premises, such as, "You can't say anything negative about your therapist," increases rapport and leads to increased disclosure. Trying to get people to change, or to do things they can't or won't do, builds resistance and lessens rapport.) I asked if the therapist had ever been gone that long before. Acceptance is shown in the following exchange: "How did you get through this before?"—"Sleeping." "Did that help?"—"A little." "What else did you do to help get through it?"—"I'd hurt myself." "Did that help?"

She mentioned that she was thinking of suicide. I accepted that and tried to "make it real" (developing nebulous fantasies into concrete details). When questioned further, she said, "They would find me dead." I asked, "Who would find you dead?"—"My mother. She'd find me living in that pigsty." "Would your mother complain about the pigsty?" We discussed her relationship with her mother.

"You know, at first, your living in a pigsty sounded pretty negative, but now I see the positive side. You really are strong enough not to live up to all of your mother's expectations." From time to time, I then began to gently question the mother's ideas, hoping to slightly diminish their power and to lighten the emotional atmosphere. This was done tentatively and gently because negative comments about the mother (or the therapist, or the religion) would increase her defensiveness and her guilt. Because she responded positively, this was used further.

She said that she had to go home for Christmas and that this would be difficult. She "has to" go home because her family expects her to. This was accepted. No effort was made to bring about a major change in her behaviors or beliefs. The focus shifted from, "How do you survive with your therapist gone for a month?" to "Since you 'have to' go home and that's a problem, what is the best way to manage it?" Interventions included clarification of her difficulty in expressing anger, and her extreme guilt and feeling compelled to do what others wish. I indirectly interpreted that her suicidal feelings were related to her therapist's absence and to her anger about that, to "having to" go home and her anger about that, to her guilt about her anger, and to her sense of powerlessness. Support was offered for any progress—her ability to live in a pigsty, to have a little humor about the guilt, and to acknowledge that she can't acknowledge her resentment at her therapist (thereby acknowledging it). Focusing on the real problem of the Christmas trip moved away from the borderline reactions of global dysphoria and perceiving herself as totally bad.

She offered, "I refuse to go the evening before." This was endorsed. "So you're able to say 'no,' you won't go the evening before, and stick to it? What time do you have to go?" (speaking in her own idiom). Then, "What do you have to do when you get there?" (to get more specifics to work with). She described having to sit in the living room listening to them talk, feeling isolated and not really part of the family. I abruptly asked, "Do you have a Walkman, a little Walkman radio with earphones?" She did. "Are you able to lie?" She didn't think so. "Oh, that's too bad. I was thinking maybe you could tell them you got this fascinating new Walkman for Christmas and you could sit there plugged into your Walkman, not have to listen to them." She said that would be rude. I easily accepted that. "So that's really something you just couldn't do."

I asked if she would be able to take a walk. (It is better if ideas and suggestions come from her, but I do make suggestions, in a negative, tentative way, e.g., "I wonder if this might work, it probably won't," within her own framework.) She said the men could leave; I wondered if she could also. First she was negative, "I can't walk; they're right on the highway," but then, "Maybe I could walk in the pasture. There's some cattle in the pasture." I immediately asked, "Aren't you afraid?" She said she wasn't. I looked skeptical, "So you're a real country girl?" She smilingly agreed. (I was building her up, implying that I would be scared to death to walk in the pasture with the cattle, developing a somewhat different image of her than the one we started with.)

She said her therapist was seeing her at a reduced fee. I mused, "Does that make you more guilty? Does it make it harder to be mad at him for anything? Do you think it's more that you're afraid of feeling guilty or more that you're afraid he will dump you if you get mad?" (This is a veiled interpretation and implies that the concerns are unrealistic.)

We returned to discussing Christmas at home. She said she would leave early. I replied, "Since your medicine affects your vision, obviously you shouldn't drive after dark. Are you sure you'll be strong enough not to go the day before and to leave before dark?" She said, "Probably." I said, "That doesn't sound very strong." We clarified that she was 75% sure she could do it. I asked, "Can we figure out any way to raise that to 85%?" (This models that you don't always have to aim for 100%.) She said, "I always do what's ordered." I replied, "You've got lots of rebellion inside, but you don't express much of it yet." She agreed. "Well, if you're really sure about doing what's ordered, we'll use it." She nodded. "Okay, I order you not to go the evening before and to leave before dark; I guess in a pinch you could say it's doctor's orders." (Instead of just accepting her first agreement, I push the point and question her ability. This increases the probability she will do it.) "Will it be rude when you get up to go for a walk?" (It's good to bring up obstacles and objections during the session rather than letting them arise after the person has gone.) "No, they will just say I'm crazy." "So, that's one of the benefits of being crazy?" She smilingly agreed. (One uses any tools at hand, and sometimes problems turn out to be assets.) She left the emergency room with a plan of action for the holidays, including calling the student who had asked me to see her the day after she returned from her visit. (It is clear then that she does not intend to kill herself. This planned call provides continuous support and increases the chances she will follow through.)

Borderline patients tend to come to the emergency room when a relationship is breaking up, when their therapist is on vacation, when therapy is moving too fast, or when using drugs or alcohol. Some time may need to pass before the borderline patient settles down enough to work with. The borderline patient who comes in chaotically upset and intensely suicidal in the morning may be wanting to leave for a hair-dresser's appointment by the afternoon. The borderline patient will need to have contact with supportive others. Although hospitalization is sometimes necessary for safety, growth occurs through helping such patients cope with their difficulties.

Psychodynamic Intervention—A Potentially Violent Patient

A 24-year-old black man presented fearing that he was going to hurt someone. He appeared very anxious and tense, but not depressed or psychotic. He worked in a fast-food restaurant and also took one college course at night. He was very upset on the job. The other employees were lackadaisical. Being conscientious, he made up for their shortcomings. He had become furious when a fellow employee dropped some food on the floor and simply returned it to the customer's plate and served it. I said that he had certain standards that he tried to live up to, and he agreed. He eventually also revealed difficulty with his girlfriend, who was unhappy that he did not have more money, did not support his attending college, and was pressuring him to steal from his employer as other employees did.

Asked about his future, he replied, "I'm determined to make something of myself." Yet he felt very frustrated at the slowness of it, at the lack of support, and at the derogatory attitudes of others. Tension was building to where he felt he might explode at anyone. He had come close to hitting a fellow employee that day and, at times, felt like hitting his girlfriend. His only previous incidence of violence was several years earlier. He had hit a neighborhood bully with a pipe after the bully persisted in making comments about his mother. He had been raised by his grandmother and had not seen his father since he was 7 years old. I asked where he had gotten his courage and his determination to make something of himself; he assumed it was from his grandmother. I mentioned that it was hard being a boy growing up without a man around and he said, "Probably so." I said that people had very different ideas of what it meant to be a man, and that a boy needed a man he could look up to as a model. He seemed to understand. I mentioned that children and teenagers idolize rock stars and athletes, and only as boys mature do they appreciate the quiet courage and steadiness of a real man, who can set goals and strive toward them in an honest hardworking way, with consideration for others as well as for his own needs. The patient seemed to understand what I meant. I said that sometimes movies helped, and that there were a few films illustrating the difference between adolescents who felt they had to take a dare, and the man who was wise enough and strong enough to walk away from one. The patient said, "John Wayne," and I smiled and said, "Yeah."

I asked how much he loved his girlfriend; he was not sure. I asked if he met any girls at college and he said only a few, because he was not there much. I commented that it must be difficult living in a poor area with his family and friends, working in a fast-food restaurant, and yet having his eyes on another kind of life and being involved with another type of people. He nodded thoughtfully. We eventually made some tentative plans; he would continue working at the fast-food restaurant and keep his nose clean, but would spend some time each week looking for a better job, realizing that he might not find one soon. No more was said about the girlfriend. He was not interested in counseling or therapy, but said he would come back to the emergency room if he felt things were getting out of hand again. He seemed to feel much relieved and shook my hand warmly and firmly when he left.

This was a psychodynamic intervention within a crisis intervention framework. I indirectly made the interpretation, "You feel enraged because your values and sense of manhood are being challenged by your coworkers and your girlfriend. Growing up without a male figure left your sense of masculinity shaky. Yet, you are aware of your standards and values and of the benefits they will yield for you. As you continue on your course, you may change your self-image and identity a bit; you may even find a new girlfriend. It is frustrating now, and tempting to act out to 'prove' your manhood, but your reason knows better than this." I also offered him understanding, support, and John Wayne as a role model.

Special Problems: A Family Problem

Merri, an immature-looking 19-year-old, was brought to the emergency room by her mother for "immediate hospitalization" at the urging of their counselor who had just learned of Merri's suicide threat. To my dismay, this statement burst out immediately, but I diverted it and proceeded to step one, inquiring about their situation. The mother was divorced, very frightened of her violent ex-husband, and working two jobs to support herself, her 16-year-old daughter Helen, and Merri. I empathized with the fear of all three of them, the burdens on mother, and the two girls being both fearful for their mother and lacking her attention. In fact, the fear of the ex-husband was so great that the family had just moved again, and the unpacked boxes were still stacked in the living room of their apartment. Mother had been arguing with Merri, who refused to help her unpack, and this led to the suicide threat. Merri's threat was to starve herself to death, and she had eaten little for 2 days. Based on my dynamic hypothesis, I began to inquire if Merri might unpack two boxes a day if her mother worked alongside her and unpacked two others. Merri, who had been somewhat sullen and withdrawn, burst in, "I didn't refuse to unpack; it's just I won't unpack Helen's boxes." Mother said that Helen is young and upset, and Mother expects Merri, the older daughter, to be more mature. In the new apartment, the girls now share a bedroom, and Helen has her things all over the room, leaving Merri only a bed. Mother wants Merri to accept that also. I bargained that Mother would unpack Helen's boxes, and Merri would unpack everything else, and Merri would get one wall of the bedroom to do with as she pleased. (Try only for small changes.)

I inquired about the counseling. The counseling was Mother's, but she had increasingly been using her sessions to only talk about Merri, and the counselor had begun to see Merri during Mother's appointment. I suggested to the counselor by telephone that Mother have 15 minutes of every appointment alone, that every third appointment be only for Mother, and further, that she not talk about Merri on those appointments. The counselor agreed that this was a reasonable approach and told Mother by phone, "It's not fair to the girls if you don't take care of yourself." After some further work on issues, Merri and her mother left in good spirits, planning to do four boxes that afternoon, and carrying a note I had written to the counselor.

EXPECTATIONS AND IMAGES

It is important to see the patient and family as capable, functioning people, and to convey that expectation. Patients should sit in a chair rather than lying down, in their clothes rather than a hospital gown. We ask patients to do things that they can do themselves: to clean up the coffee they spill, to help other patients look up telephone numbers, to call and make their own appointments. Throughout the visit, the staff attempt to enhance positive self-images. For example:

"What do you do, Mr. Brown?"—"Nothing."
"How do you do nothing? You stay in bed all day? Watch TV, walk around the neighborhood? What?" (It is obviously impossible to do nothing.)—"Oh, I mostly watch TV."
"What kind of work have you done?"—"Oh, nothing much."
"What was your last job?"—"Carpenter."
"Oh, carpenter! What do you work on, houses or what?"—"Some houses. I built some cabinets."
"Oh! Houses and cabinets. Like with shelves, doors, and stuff?"— "Yeah."
"So, you're kind of a carpenter; you're a guy that does work with your hands then?" ("was" becomes "is")—"Yeah."
"Yeah, and who do you live with, Mr. Brown?"

Thus, we do not leave the original question with an image of a man who does "nothing." We have changed the image from an emergency psychiatric patient who does nothing to a carpenter who works with his hands and can build houses and cabinets, with shelves and doors and stuff (even though temporarily unemployed). The patient may not immediately feel better or see himself more positively, nor may his family, but this is beginning to move in the right direction. We have also begun to establish the principle that we expect specific information and not vague brush-off answers to our questions. Labels can be changed to develop images. In a previous example, an "angry man" was relabeled as a "worried father": "I can see why you were so mad at Billy, Mr. Jones; it must have really worried you when you saw him smashing the furniture, worried you about the furniture, and, of course, you're worried about what kind of problems he might have and what his future is going to be."

RESPONSIBILITIES

The areas of responsibility of the psychiatrist and the patient and the family should be kept clear. People under stress tend to regress. They may manifest extreme dependency and magical wishes for rescue by an omnipotent mother figure. You as the psychiatrist should divert these tendencies, providing support as necessary, doing for the patient and family only what they are unable to do for themselves and not accepting responsibility for solving their problems for them. Be cautious about giving advice; you may do well to give it indirectly or negatively, or to attribute it to the family: "From your last comment, it sounds like you were starting to think about all your relatives, and wondering if there's any you might call?" "I just had a crazy idea; it doesn't make any sense. I wondered for a moment if you could call your girlfriend to clarify whether she has any intention of ever coming back, but really you're too upset for that right now." If you offer advice, you are liable to find that the patient or family gives three good reasons why that advice won't work and then sits and looks at you expectantly. By offering advice, you signed a contract to come up with the solution for them. Because your effort was a failure, the second effort is now awaited. That is very likely to be a failure, too. If the family hasn't done something fairly obvious they will have good reasons for not having done it. You frequently have to repeatedly hand the responsibility back: "Well, where am I supposed to stay tonight?"—"That really is an issue, isn't it? What ideas have you come up with so far?"

The psychiatrist functions as a consultant, an expert in helping people work on their problems, rather than as a magical rescuer, expert at solving other people's problems for them.

TIME

In emergency psychiatry, the issue of time arises at many different points and in many different forms. Do not fall into the trap of mentally taking a "Polaroid snapshot" of the patient. The patient may appear ragingly psychotic and highly dangerous or may be professing intense suicidal determination. If you had only 5 minutes available, there would be no alternative but prompt hospitalization. However, the fact that a patient is psychotic and dangerous right now does not mean that this will be the case in 3 hours, after healthy doses of neuroleptics, contact with supportive staff members and perhaps family members, and beginning discussion of stresses. Someone who is psychotic and dangerous may need to be hospitalized, but someone who *was* psychotic and dangerous does not necessarily require hospitalization.

People in a crisis, or under stress, or with borderline problems have a narrowed focus on immediacy. The statement, "My girlfriend left me; I have nothing to live for," has suicidal implications that must be attended to, but it can also be translated as, "I want my girlfriend back, and right now!" Inquire into the girlfriend's complaints before she left and then help the patient develop a strategy to maximize the possibility of her eventual return. This introduces the concept of striving toward a goal over time as opposed to requiring that goal immediately and with certainty. "Well, I understand you told me you don't have a drinking problem at all, but still, that was your girlfriend's complaint. So, do you think if you attended Alcoholics Anonymous twice a day for the next 3 weeks and could stop drinking, and could prove it to her, that she might be willing to talk to you about possibly getting back together?" The suicide risk is asked about *after* helping the patient develop other options.

Help expand the time perspective of patients: "Mr. and Mrs. Smith, I certainly don't envy you, or Tony. Being a teenager is hard, and trying to raise one nowadays is even harder. I don't know how you all have managed putting up with this for the last 2 years, and I don't know how you're going to make it through the next 2. Of course, once he's 18, he's at least legally an adult and in some ways your burden won't be so heavy." This shifts some attention from the immediate crisis, for which the parents desperately want an immediate magical solution, to the idea of an ongoing process, one that has been going on for 2 years and will very likely continue for at least 2 more, from the urgency of the moment to the slowly unfolding future, bleak though it may be. Without empty words of encouragement (which never work), the possibility is indirectly raised that things may get better and that this won't last forever. Some empathy is expressed, both for the parents and Tony, without making anyone feel attacked. The crisis is defused by redefining it, and the parents can be induced to enter a program to learn how to best deal with these severe problems. Some treatment resources will also be offhandedly offered to Tony; however, it is doubtful that he will be interested. "It takes a great deal of courage to begin to face problems and work on them. Many of the teenagers we see just aren't mature enough to do that or aren't in bad enough trouble yet."

Yet is a useful word. It can chip a hole in a wall of negativism, introduce a ray of hope into darkness, and slightly alter perceptions. It also makes suggestions indirectly: "So you really haven't gotten around to doing much crying about your mother's death yet?" "So you've been so upset you really haven't had a chance to make a list of people you might be able to spend the night with yet?"

Time issues arise in the tense of the language used ("I used to be a carpenter."—"So you're a man who builds things with his hands, right?") in assessing and enhancing a suicidal person's investment in the future ("Here you are at 20 and things are really a mess. What are you hoping you can have arranged for yourself by the time you're, say, 25?"), in delaying assessment of suicide risk until other options are developed, and in waiting for a borderline patient to settle down.

REFERRALS

Making referrals effectively requires knowing what the resources have to offer and clarifying with the patient the specific purpose of the referral. Appointments are more likely kept if the patient leaves with a specific time and place in hand rather than just a telephone number. Before referring a patient for psychotherapy, I ask, "Have you ever had therapy or counseling before? How did it go for you?" I may need to select an alternative type of therapy, or help the patient understand why it wasn't useful and how they could make it different this time. "Who do you have you can talk to? Do you find that helpful?" "You talked to Mr. Adams here (the trainee) about some of your problems. What was that like for you? How do you feel now? Do you think having someone to talk to regularly might be of help?" The patient's responses help the psychiatrist to induce the patient into therapy, to deal with resistance, or to decide not to recommend therapy at all. I anticipate with the patient the difficulties that might arise and what might make it hard to keep the appointment. I try to diminish magical expectations and tell the patient that therapy will not be easy or quick. If the referral is for therapy, part of the interview can help the patient get an idea of what therapy might be like: "Well, obviously you've got a good-enough mind to be able to think about yourself some. You've begun to wonder if losing Jack, as painful as that is, is just another episode in some kind of problem with men. You were able to think of some examples and some possibilities, and had the guts to wonder if you may be doing something wrong. You might be the kind of person who's strong enough to use therapy. Do you think it might be helpful to have someone to talk with and to help do this kind of figuring things out?"

I may challenge the patient, "I'm not sure you'll be able to do it. I don't think you're ready yet, but later you may become interested." This may motivate them to go now or may plant a seed for the future. I follow up, "Your appointment is Wednesday; I want to call you Thursday and see how it went." This markedly increases the chance that they will keep the appointment, and provides a safety net if something goes wrong.

SUMMARY

Psychological emergency treatment is an approach and an attitude. We are having psychological impact on our patients whether we are aware of it or not. We work to help patients and families shift out of a disorganized, demoralized, and immobilized state of crisis. With a specific plan for dealing with a concrete problem, they can safely work themselves out of the emergency or crisis situation.

Emergency psychiatry is one of the most challenging and most rewarding aspects of psychiatry. The psychiatrist deals within medical issues and is able to combine medication and psychological interventions to produce quick and visible results and to create possibilities for long-term benefit.

REFERENCE

Puryear DA: Helping People in Crisis. San Francisco, CA, Jossey-Bass, 1979

SUGGESTED READINGS

Adler G: Borderline Psychopathology and Its Treatment. Northvale, NJ, Jason Aronson, 1985

Caplan G: The Principles of Preventive Psychiatry. New York, Basic Books, 1964

Guggenheim F, Weiner M (eds): Manual of Psychiatric Consultation and Emergency Care. New York, Jason Aronson, 1984

Haley J: Problem Solving Therapy. San Francisco, CA, Jossey-Bass, 1976

Hoffman L: Foundations of Family Therapy. New York, Basic Books, 1981

Kroll J: The Challenge of the Borderline Patient. New York, WW Norton, 1988

Langley DG, Kaplan DM: The Treatment of Families in Crisis. New York, Grune & Stratton, 1968

Chapter 5

Social Treatment Principles

J.R. Hillard, M.D.

A person seeks emergency psychiatric evaluation and treatment when the level of symptomatology or distress reaches the point that it can no longer be handled by his or her ordinary social network. Emergency psychiatric care is meaningful only in the context of a patient's overall social environment. Furthermore, a psychiatric emergency service is meaningful only in the context of the overall mental health system in the community. Every biological and psychological intervention is also a social intervention. Often social interventions are the most important response to underlying biological or psychological problems.

PSYCHIATRIC EMERGENCY CARE IN THE SOCIAL ENVIRONMENT

Appropriate psychiatric emergency care can be given only when the clinician understands a patient's social needs and resources as well as biological and psychological needs and resources. In this context, "social" is used to subsume economic, interpersonal, and cultural components (see also Chapter 28). Every emergency visit must be understood within the context of a patient's hierarchy of needs:

- Self-actualization needs
- Esteem needs (e.g., self-respect, success)

71

- Belonging and love needs
- Safety needs (e.g., security and order)
- Physiological needs (e.g., hunger, thirst)

As described by Maslow (1943), a "lower need" must be fulfilled before a higher one can emerge. If a patient is anxious and homeless, a psychotherapy referral to help with self-actualization is unlikely to be helpful unless it is accompanied by referrals that will help the patient meet more basic needs.

Every visit must also be understood in the context of a patient's social network, that is, the whole set of people with whom the patient interacts. Questions to answer include 1) What is the meaning of this visit in the context of the patient's family, in the context of the patient's livelihood (e.g., job or welfare payments), and in the context of the patient's community? 2) Who decided that this situation was an emergency? 3) Who decided that it was psychiatric? 4) What sources of care have been tried first? 5) What are the expectations of everyone involved (Gaines 1979; Wood et al. 1984)?

Hospitalization as a Social Intervention

Hospitalization, which is thought of as a biomedical intervention, is clearly also a social intervention with distinct social costs and benefits. Costs may include financial burdens from hospital charges or from lost wages, negative labeling of the patient by family and the community, and disruption of the patient's ongoing support system in the community. Benefits of hospitalization may include providing respite for family or other care givers and providing evaluation and treatment impossible on an outpatient basis within the realistic constraints of transportation and supervision.

Other Social Interventions

In addition to hospitalization, social interventions routinely performed by psychiatric emergency services include

- Sanctioning of the sick role by providing temporary excuses from obligations such as work
- Mobilizing family members to provide a more positive environment
- Finding temporary housing
- Mobilizing other community resources (e.g., case management, welfare entitlements, and support groups)

A psychiatric emergency service, of course, cannot be a comprehensive social service agency, but it must be able to provide appropriate referral and, in some cases, transportation to the appropriate specialized agency.

PSYCHIATRIC EMERGENCY CARE IN THE MENTAL HEALTH SYSTEM

Psychiatric emergency care is offered in numerous settings. All psychiatric facilities need to be equipped to deal with some emergencies. Emergency care was one of the original five essential services (along with inpatient, outpatient, partial hospitalization, and consultation/education services) that were originally mandated for federally funded comprehensive community mental health centers. In practice, most urban areas have gone to some degree of centralization of emergency services for efficiency reasons. In any given community, a patient will end up in a hospital emergency room or in specialized psychiatric emergency facilities whenever the nonemergency system is unable to provide needed help. In any given community, the resources not provided by the nonemergency system define what is "an emergency."

The degree of deinstitutionalization in a given community will have a major bearing on the population of patients in the community who are at risk for psychiatric emergency hospitalization (Bassuk 1980). If there is a case management system in place, many problems that would otherwise be dealt with by emergency services can and should be dealt with instead by the case management team (Witheridge 1989).

FUNCTIONS OF A SPECIALIZED EMERGENCY FACILITY

All specialized emergency facilities have an evaluation and referral function available around the clock, or at least during certain hours. In addition, psychiatric emergency services may include any of the following:

- Brief treatment service allowing patients to return to the emergency room for a limited number of sessions of crisis intervention treatment
- A holding area that allows prolonged evaluation and treatment in the emergency room for a period of hours to days (Gold Award 1987; Ianzito et al. 1978; Walker et al. 1973)
- Telephone counseling services (Hornblow 1986)
- Mobile crisis service to respond to psychiatric emergency patients

unable to come in to the hospital (Bengelsdorf and Alden 1987)

When a number of these services are located in the same facility, there can be a positive synergism between them (e.g., a patient may call the telephone service, be visited by the mobile crisis service, and later be able to come in to the emergency room for follow-up). The following support services are important to a centralized emergency facility.

• Police are needed to help with restraints and for transporting patients when necessary.
• Legal consultation (as discussed in Chapter 6).
• Telecommunications that may be hooked into the 911 system. At times it is also useful to be able to trace telephone calls (see Chapter 8).

Figure 5-1 shows the flow of patients into and out of a centralized psychiatric emergency facility. A frequent problem arises when an outpatient therapist or family member or police officer brings a patient to the emergency service wanting hospital admission, and the available hospitals do not believe that the patient fits their admission criteria. It is easy for emergency personnel to end up fighting with both the inpatient and outpatient system. In general, it is best to try to avoid fighting with anyone and to let them fight with each other instead. It is worthwhile to put a lot of effort into relationships with both inpatient and outpatient personnel. Emergency service workers are in a position to do favors for both and frequently need favors in return because they are on the border between systems. Emergency service workers are at risk for having negative feelings projected onto them by other systems. If they are known to people in the other systems in a personal way, this projection is less likely.

An emergency service cannot function as "a facility of last resort" (Bassuk 1985, p. 11) and needs to have some resources available to hospitalize patients when clinically necessary. A system that patients frequently need but cannot obtain hospitalization in is a system to get out of.

In addition to the mental health system, psychiatric emergency service workers need to have working relationships with and working definitions of services involved with the criminal justice system, which in many areas are trying to deinstitutionalize many clients; i.e., the adult and child protective service system; the medical/surgical care system (e.g., what degree of alcohol withdrawal should lead to a medical as

Figure 5-1. Psychiatric emergency service in the context of the mental health system. HMO = health maintenance organization.

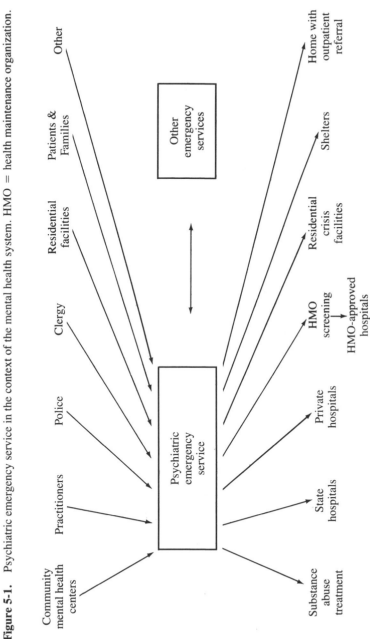

opposed to a psychiatric admission); the mental retardation and substance abuse systems, which in many areas are separate from the mental health system, functionally and administratively; and the voluntary shelter system, which in many cases will provide the only available referrals for patients.

GENERAL GUIDELINES FOR MAKING APPROPRIATE SOCIAL INTERVENTIONS

- Conceptualize your task as that of finding the most appropriate available resources for the patient.
- If minimally adequate resources are sometimes not available, bring this to the attention of appropriate agencies. Planners will often be interested in input from emergency services.
- If minimally adequate resources are frequently not available, consider working someplace else.
- Know the available mental health and social service resources in the community. Know the constraints that different hospital programs and health maintenance organizations put on patient admission (Olfson 1989). These constraints are ever increasing (Greenberg et al. 1989; Swift 1986), and appropriate patient care must take them into account. Referring a patient to someplace that rejects him or her is, at best, nontherapeutic and may be countertherapeutic, in terms of decreasing the likelihood that the patient will seek help in the future.
- Always communicate with the ongoing care givers about each case. Make sure that your emergency care is consistent with the patient's ongoing treatment plan.
- Remember that in the climate of deinstitutionalization, family members are likely to be the most consistent ongoing care givers and need to be treated as both cotherapists and "secondary consumers" (Perlmutter 1983).
- Try to preserve an open-door policy in the service as much as possible.
- Try to have as clear an understanding as possible with other agencies, i.e., about which one has primary responsibility for a given patient.

REFERENCES

Bassuk EL: The impact of deinstitutionalization on the general hospital psychiatric emergency ward. Hosp Community Psychiatry 31:623–627, 1980

Bassuk EL: Psychiatric emergency services: can they cope as last resort facilities? in Emergency Psychiatry at the Crossroads (New Directions for Mental Health Services, No 28). Edited by Lipton FR, Goldfinger SM. San Francisco, CA, Jossey-Bass, 1985

Bengelsdorf H, Alden DC: A mobile crisis unit in the psychiatric emergency room. Hosp Community Psychiatry 38:662–665, 1987

Gaines AD: Definitions and diagnoses: cultural implications of psychiatric help-seeking and psychiatrists' definitions of the situation in psychiatric emergencies. Cult Med Psychiatry 3:381–418, 1979

Gold Award: Brief psychiatric inpatient care for acutely disturbed patients. Hosp Community Psychiatry 38:1203–1206, 1987

Greenberg WM, Seide M, Scimeca MM: The hospitalizable patient as a commodity: selling in a bear market. Hosp Community Psychiatry 40:184–185, 1989

Hornblow AR: The evolution and effectiveness of telephone counseling services. Hosp Community Psychiatry 37:731–733, 1986

Ianzito BM, Fine J, Sprague B, et al: Overnight admissions for psychiatric emergencies. Hosp Community Psychiatry 29:728–730, 1978

Maslow AH: A theory of motivation. Psychol Rev 50:370–396, 1943

Olfson M: Psychiatric emergency room dispositions of HMO enrollers. Hosp Community Psychiatry 40:639–641, 1989

Perlmutter RA: Family involvement in psychiatric emergencies. Hosp Community Psychiatry 34:255–257, 1983

Swift RM: Negotiating psychiatric hospitalization within restrictive admissions criteria. Hosp Community Psychiatry 37:619–623, 1986

Walker WR, Parsons LB, Skelton WD: Brief hospitalization on a crisis service: a study of patient and treatment variables. Am J Psychiatry 130:896–900, 1973

Witheridge TF: The assertive community treatment worker: an emerging role and its implications for professional training. Hosp Community Psychiatry 40:620–624, 1989

Wood KA, Rosenthal TL, Khuri R: The need for hospitalization as perceived by emergency room patients and clinicians. Hosp Community Psychiatry 35:830–832, 1984

Chapter 6

Legal Issues

J.R. Hillard, M.D.

If you don't get sued twice a year, you are not doing enough cases.
—Anonymous neurosurgeon

Professional liability claims against psychiatrists and other mental health professionals have increased markedly in recent years (Slawson and Guggenheim 1984). Clinicians in emergency settings are particularly at risk for such actions because of high patient volume, high level of patient dangerousness, and brief clinician-patient contacts. On the positive side, the average malpractice premium for self-employed psychiatrists remains only about one-quarter that of the average physician ("MD's Liability Rates" 1986). Furthermore, courts have generally been willing to consider the realistic limitations that an emergency setting imposes on a clinician's ability to perform definitive assessments (Tancredi 1982). Clinicians can gain additional protection by building clinical activities into their routines, a strategy for managing the risk of litigation.

This chapter will 1) outline general principles of malpractice, informed consent, and confidentiality in an emergency setting; 2) outline legal issues related to specific clinical problems; and 3) suggest specific institutional and individual actions that can minimize risk. This chapter focuses on general concepts rather than details of specific cases. Case citations are available in the references cited and in the Suggested Readings noted at the end of this chapter.

79

MALPRACTICE

Liability for malpractice results when the following four elements of negligence are met in a professional (medical) setting:

- The clinician has a legal *duty* to a patient or client or third party. (A doctor-patient relationship exists.)
- The clinician has *breached* that legal duty.
- The patient or client has legally recoverable *suffered damages*.
- The breach of legal duty has *directly caused* the damages.

The plaintiff in a malpractice action against a clinician must prove, by a preponderance of the evidence, that all four of these conditions existed in order to prove the case.

Duty

In a psychiatric emergency setting, the clinician has a legal duty to evaluate within some reasonable period of time anyone who requests evaluation (Julavits 1983) or who is legally brought in for evaluation. The clinician also has the legal duty to provide whatever emergency (see below) treatment is indicated and to refer the patient appropriately, given available resources, for treatment that cannot be provided in the emergency setting. As will be discussed later in this chapter, a clinician, under some circumstances, also has a legal duty to protect third parties who may be injured by a patient.

Breach of Legal Duty

A clinician is negligent if he or she fails to provide the standard of care that a reasonably prudent practitioner in the same specialty would provide under like or similar circumstances. In the past, the reference group for the "standard of care" has generally been the practitioners in the same locality. However, most jurisdictions currently favor a reference group consisting of practitioners nationwide who provide similar professional services (Tancredi 1986). A practitioner need not do what a majority of colleagues would have done under similar circumstances, but the actions taken need to be endorsed by at least a "respectable minority" of practitioners to be considered to have met an acceptable standard of care. The "controversy" sections of this manual highlight some of the areas in the practice of emergency psychiatry where there exists a respectable minority opinion. A crucial point to keep in mind is that making a wrong judgment is not the same as being negligent. If a patient commits suicide soon after leaving the emergency room, negligence is not assessed on the basis of what is known about the case after the fact, but on the basis of what was known or should have been known at the time the patient was seen. If an appropriate evaluation was conducted, and if reasonable conclusions were drawn from it and reasonable treatment was carried out, care is not likely to be found to have been negligent.

Damages

Damages may be physical, financial, or emotional (e.g., "pain and suffering") but can generally be compensated only financially. It is the charge of the judge and jury to reduce all damages to specific dollar amounts. Lawyers now have access to data on the dollar amount of recent judgments in a particular locality and are able to state with some degree of accuracy what a given type of injury is "worth" in that locality (e.g., death by suicide of a father with a wife and a child under 5 years of age).

Direct Causation

Perhaps nowhere is the difference between "medical thinking" and "legal thinking" more pronounced than in relation to the question of direct causation. Physicians, particularly psychiatrists, tend to conceptualize outcomes as "overdetermined." For example, a psychiatrist might conceptualize a patient's suicide as the result of an unfortunate childhood, plus a physical illness, plus an unsupportive family, plus financial problems, plus unavailability of public transportation to the community mental health center. A lawyer might view the proximate cause for the suicide as having been the physician's failure to foresee that the patient was incapable of complying with an outpatient referral. In general, the best test for whether a given act of negligence was the direct cause of damages is whether the damages were reasonably foreseeable on the basis of what the clinician knew or should have known.

Common Types of Malpractice

Common forms of malpractice alleged in psychiatric emergency settings are

- Failure to diagnose suicide risk, risk of violence, or medical illness
- Inappropriate somatic treatment
- Inappropriate seclusion and/or restraint
- Failure to protect third parties from injury by dangerous patients

If the standard of care outlined in this book is followed and documented, it is unlikely that a malpractice suit will be lost, even given an unfortunate outcome.

INFORMED CONSENT

Medical treatment for a patient can generally be undertaken only with the patient's informed consent. Informed consent exists when the following three conditions hold:

- The patient is *competent* to give informed consent.
- The patient has been given *adequate information* to make informed consent possible.
- The consent is given *voluntarily*.

Competence

Each state has a statute that defines general competence to handle affairs. Individuals who are incompetent according to that statute can have a guardian appointed by the court, and the guardian's judgment will substitute for that of the patient in clinical as well as in other situations. The guardian is charged by the court to act in the "best interests" of the incompetent individual.

Each state also has a statutory definition of when an adolescent has reached "the age of consent." Ordinarily, parents will be guardians for minors unless guardianship has been transferred, or unless the adolescent has been "emancipated" according to the laws of that state. When dealing with minors, it is a good idea to clarify who their guardians are, almost as quickly as determining their pulse, temperature, and blood pressure. Efforts should be made to gain "assent" (a standard less than consent) from the minor in addition to consent from the guardian (Appelbaum 1989).

Patients who have not been adjudged as in need of a guardian may still be incompetent to make a specific decision. To be competent to make a specific clinical decision, a patient should 1) be aware of the clinical situation, 2) have some factual understanding of the issues involved in the decision, and 3) be able to manipulate the information rationally (Appelbaum and Roth 1981). These issues will be discussed later in this chapter under "Specific Clinical Problems."

Adequate Information

Adequate information is that information that a "rational person" would need to make an informed decision on a given issue. In a decision about medical treatment, this should include information about exactly

- What the recommended treatment is
- What the risks as well as benefits of the recommended treatment are
- What alternative treatments are available
- What positive and negative consequences of alternative treatments and of *no* treatment may be

Voluntary Decisions

Treatment decisions that are in any way coerced are not voluntary. For example, a patient who was told, "You can't leave the emergency room until you have had your medication," is not a patient who can give informed consent for the medication.

The major exception to the necessity of obtaining informed consent for treatment occurs when the treatment is required as an emergency. The law creates an "implied" consent in the true emergency situation and, thus, protects the clinician.

CONFIDENTIALITY AND PRIVILEGE

Confidentiality is the legal duty that prevents the disclosure of information about a patient obtained in the doctor-patient relationship to a third party without the patient's permission. *Privilege* is the duty that specifically prevents disclosing confidential information in court without a patient's permission. In general, even the fact that a patient is seeking emergency evaluation and treatment is confidential information.

Specific exceptions to disclosure that can arise in the psychiatric emergency setting include

- Communication within the team that is caring for the patient at a given agency. However, communication with clinicians caring for the patient through other agencies is not acceptable unless the patient consents or unless another exception to confidentiality applies.

- When the patient is incompetent—in which case, the guardian's consent must be obtained. In the case of incompetent patients without guardians or family, the clinician must go ahead and attempt to act in the best interests of the patient.
- When reporting is required by law. Many states, for example, require the reporting to government agencies of child abuse or neglect, even when only suspected by the clinician. Many states also require a relative to be informed when a patient is involuntarily hospitalized.
- When the clinician is ordered to testify by a judge—either in open court or by a court order—the clinician must comply. A subpoena simply requires that the physician appear in court, but it is not equivalent to an order to testify.
- When it is necessary to contact third parties to adequately evaluate a patient. This exception is particularly clear when a patient is brought in to be evaluated for involuntary hospitalization and it is impossible to make a reasonable decision about hospitalization without obtaining information from third parties.
- When there is a risk of physical harm to an identifiable third party (see below).

WHAT IS AN EMERGENCY?

A situation in which a patient, due to mental disorder, poses an immediate risk to life and limb of self or others is certainly an emergency (e.g., an acutely assaultive, paranoid patient). Some jurisdictions have accepted broader definitions that include danger to the treatment environment (e.g., a loud and intrusive but nonviolent psychotic patient) or situations in which the potential for rapid decompensation exists (Wexler 1984). It is useful to understand the definition as established in your particular state, if one has been established at all.

WHO IS LIABLE: THE CLINICIAN OR THE INSTITUTION?

If an employed clinician is guilty of malpractice, the doctrine of "respondeat superior" has made the employer (hospital, agency, etc.) liable. Recent case law has found hospitals and agencies liable in cases where there is no employment relationship, but there is a contract for services or simply that the involved physician has privileges at the institution. The liability arises out of what courts are calling "apparent authority." In effect, a patient relies on a particular hospital or agency for medical services and does not realize that the clinician is not an employee. The courts treat the clinician as an employee. Hospitals and agencies have also been found liable for hiring clinicians with less than competent track records as far as malpractice actions. Recently, there has been an increasing tendency toward individual liability for nonphysician clinicians, such as nurses, social workers, and even chaplains.

WHO CAN BE FOUND GUILTY OF VIOLATING A PATIENT'S CIVIL RIGHTS?

Section 1983 of the Civil Rights Act states that "every person who under color of any statute, ordinance or regulation . . . of any state . . . subjects . . . any citizen . . . to the deprivation of any rights, principles or immunities secured by the constitution and the laws shall be liable to the party injured in the action" (quoted in Knapp and VandeCreek 1987, p. 651). This act has been used by members of the activist mental health bar to bring about changes in the mental health system. A side effect has been that individual clinicians have, at times, been sued for actions that are actually in compliance with state law. This act provides just one more reason for not working in a system that does not adequately protect the rights of patients, including the right to treatment.

SPECIFIC CLINICAL PROBLEMS

Emergency psychiatry presents many situations in which legal duties are in conflict with one another. This section will discuss some of these situations and suggest some general approaches to them.

Duty of Confidentiality Versus Duty to Protect Third Parties

The famous *Tarasoff* decision of 1974 first focused professional attention on a legal duty to protect third parties who may be injured by a patient, a legal duty that may include a duty to warn the potential identifiable victims. The concept was that a clinician had a duty to warn society of impending harm and this duty, on balance, outweighed the duty of confidentiality to an individual patient. Post-*Tarasoff* decisions in various jurisdictions have been quite inconsistent, and several states have enacted statutes to limit potential scope of duty to third parties (Mills et al. 1987). As always, it is a good idea to be aware of cases and statutes that apply in your state. If there has not been a clarification of exact duties in your state, as is probably the case, a reasonable approach is to assume that a legal duty to protect identifiable third parties does, under some circumstances, outweigh duty to patients' confidentiality. If there has been a clear physical threat toward an identifiable third party, or if physical violence toward an identifiable third party is reasonably foreseeable, there is probably a duty to protect that third party. Ordinarily, that duty should be discharged by using the state commitment laws to involuntarily hospitalize the patient. In cases where the patient is not an appropriate subject for involuntary treatment (as might be the case if a patient has an antisocial personality disorder but no other mental disorder), notifying the potential victim and the police is probably appropriate. If the cause for concern about potential violence is adequately documented, there will be little risk of liability for breach of confidentiality. Some recent cases have extended this "duty to protect" to a disturbing degree (e.g., to liability for damage to property that was not really foreseeable [Stone 1986]). At this point, however, such cases are still very much the exception.

Duty of Confidentiality Versus Duty to Report Past Crimes Admitted by Patients

Clinicians are generally under no obligation to report past crimes a patient may have committed. There is nothing to warn society about, because the crimes have already occurred. On balance, the confidentiality outweighs the duty to report a past crime (Applebaum and Meisel 1986). If identifiable third parties are at risk from future crimes, the duty to protect, as noted above, may apply. In many jurisdictions, as noted earlier, suspected child abuse or neglect may be an offense that a physician is specifically required to report.

Duty to Exercise State Commitment Laws Versus Duty to Avoid False Imprisonment

If a physician fails to use the state commitment laws to involuntarily hospitalize a patient who clearly falls under those laws, the physician may have breached a legal duty. If a physician uses the state commitment laws to involuntarily hospitalize a patient who clearly does not fall under those laws, the physician may be guilty of having falsely imprisoned the patient. If force was necessary, the physician is probably exposed to battery charges also. In real clinical situations, it is often unclear whether a given patient meets the commitment laws. The only way to cope with this situation is to thoroughly understand the relevant laws and to try to apply them in good faith. Liability for false imprisonment or battery is unlikely unless the physician acted maliciously or with reckless disregard for the truth or if false information was used to commit the patient (e.g., if a physician claims to have examined a patient whom he or she had never set eyes on). It is critical that the clinician fully document in the chart the rationale for whatever action was taken.

Duty to Avoid Unnecessary Restraint Versus Duty to Protect Patients in the Treatment Area

If the necessity of restraints is documented and if patients in restraints are monitored frequently and treated with respect, the physician is unlikely to lose a suit for unnecessary restraint.

Right to Treatment Versus Right to Refuse Treatment

This conflict in regard to psychotropic medication is less problematic in the emergency setting than in the inpatient setting. If a patient truly poses an immediate risk to self or others if not medicated, he or she falls under the emergency exception to informed consent and can be medicated involuntarily. If the patient meets state commitment laws, he or she can be admitted and the inpatient service can deal with these issues. If the situation is not an emergency and the patient cannot be hospitalized, discharge is appropriate.

In terms of right to refuse treatment, the issue is competency. Requests, often from surgeons, to "declare this guy incompetent so we can get on with the case" are often related to underlying communication problems between doctor and patient and often involve competent patients. It is reasonable to have a higher index of suspicion that a patient may be incompetent if the patient is making what seems to be a very irrational medical decision. Under such circumstances, it is particularly important to look for subtle forms of incompetence (Gutheil and Bursztajan 1986), such as that involving a patient who can describe the condition and the recommended treatment but who seems unable to manipulate the information rationally (e.g., a severely depressed patient who says, "Yes, I know that if I don't have the procedure I might die, but what's to live for anyway?").

RISK MANAGEMENT STRATEGIES

For the Clinician

- Do what is clinically appropriate. A good-faith attempt to care for the patient in a clinically appropriate way is generally the best defense to fall back on.
- Know the state statutes and any hallmark common-law court verdicts relevant to mental health.
- Remember that imminent risk to life and limb usually overrides other considerations such as confidentiality, informed consent, or false imprisonment.
- Try, as much as possible, to get informed consent from the patient and the family, even if a patient is to be hospitalized involuntarily.
- Talk with the patient and family enough that they do not leave angry. Effective communication can prevent lawsuits in certain situations.
- Document evaluation and treatment and clinical decision making in the medical record. Specifically,
  - Make sure that the assessment and plans are supported by the subjective and objective data recorded.
  - Include pertinent negatives (e.g., patient has no previous suicide attempts).
  - Document contact with third parties.
  - Explain rationale for controversial decisions (e.g., "Although this patient poses some long-term risk of suicide, hospitalization is not indicated since his long-term treatment plan calls for maximum effort at outpatient problem resolution and since the acute risk of suicide is past, as evidenced by . . .").
  - Make sure that any negative feelings you may have about the patient are not reflected in the chart.
- Seek consultation or independent assessment of difficult patients.
- Routinely request and examine old records and get, with the patient's consent, information from other clinicians treating the patient.
- Accept the probability of eventually being sued. Make sure that you have legal consultation available and adequate professional liability insurance.

For the Institution

- Provide adequate staffing.
- Provide as safe an environment as reasonably possible.

- Provide risk management and legal backup.
- Provide patient relations and ombudsman service.
- Provide adequate medical and surgical backup.
- Have written, and easily followed, policies and procedures and documentation protocols.
- Have periodic quality-assurance audits.
- Screen patients quickly after they arrive to determine which need immediate attention and which can wait.
- Make consultation available, at least by phone.
- Have explicit understandings with referral agencies, disposition sites, and managed care systems.
- Have orientation meetings with appropriate institutional resources to clarify any potential problems, conflicts, etc.
- Have sound credentialing policies to make sure you have a competent clinical staff.

REFERENCES

Appelbaum PS: Admitting children to psychiatric hospitals: a controversy revived. Hosp Community Psychiatry 40:334–335, 1989

Appelbaum PS, Meisel A: Psychiatrists not obligated to report patients' past crimes. Psychiatric News, March 1986

Appelbaum PS, Roth LH: Clinical issues in the assessment of competency. Am J Psychiatry 138:1462–1467, 1981

Gutheil TG, Bursztajan H: Clinicians' guidelines for assessing and presenting subtle forms of patient incompetence in legal settings. Am J Psychiatry 143:1020–1023, 1986

Julavits WF: Legal issues in emergency psychiatry. Psychiatr Clin North Am 6:335–345, 1983

Knapp S, VandeCreek L: A review of tort liability in involuntary civil commitment. Hosp Community Psychiatry 38:648–651, 1987

MD's liability rates rose an average of 20% in 1985. American Medical News, October 24–31, 1986, p 2

Mills MJ, Sullivan G, Eth S: Protecting third parties a decade after *Tarasoff*. Am J Psychiatry 144:68–74, 1987

Slawson PF, Guggenheim FG: Psychiatric malpractice: a review of the national loss experience. Am J Psychiatry 141:979–981, 1984

Stone AA: Vermont adopts *Tarasoff*: a real barnburner. Am J Psychiatry 143:352–355, 1986

Tancredi LR: Emergency psychiatry and crisis intervention: some legal and ethical issues. Psychiatric Annals 12:799–806, 1982

Tancredi LR: Psychiatric malpractice, in Textbook of Psychiatry. Edited by Michels R. Philadelphia, PA, JB Lippincott, 1986

Tarasoff v Regents of the University of California, 188 Cal Rptr 129, 529 P2d 553 (1974)

Wexler DB: Legal aspects of seclusion and restraint, in Psychiatric Aspects of Seclusion and Restraint. Edited by Tardiff K. Washington, DC, American Psychiatric Press, 1984

SUGGESTED READINGS

Beck JC: The Potentially Violent Patient and the *Tarasoff* Decision in Psychiatric Practice. Washington, DC, American Psychiatric Press, 1985

Gutheil TG, Appelbam PS: Clinical Handbook of Psychiatry and the Law. New York, McGraw-Hill, 1982

Simon RI: Clinical Psychiatry and the Law. Washington, DC, American Psychiatric Press, 1986

Simon RI: Concise Guide to Clinical Psychiatry and the Law. Washington, DC, American Psychiatric Press, 1988

Tardiff K: Psychiatric Uses of Seclusion and Restraint. Washington, DC, American Psychiatric Press, 1984

Chapter 7

Ethical Issues

T. Perlin, Ph.D.

When a trained member of a treatment team in the psychiatric emergency service (PES) approaches a potential patient for the first time, two questions emerge: 1) "What is happening with this person?" 2) "What is the right thing to do for this person?" The answer to the second question can never be purely medical, for doing the "right thing" always entails judgments about moral, legal, and sociological matters. Ethics is embedded in decisions made in the setting of emergency psychiatry. A few examples will suffice: 1) Determining the *competence* of a patient may influence a claim the police have regarding the criminal responsibility of the person. 2) Assessing the *dangerousness* of the patient may determine the short- and long-term liberty of the person. 3) Evaluating the *degree of rationality* of the patient may control the future treatment choices for this person. Finally, doing the "right thing," often conditional on the availability of scarce resources ("Do we have a bed upstairs?"), may be decisive for the patient's future as a client in the mental health and medical care system. No judgment in the PES is simply psychiatric.

The following case is provided to allow examination of some specific ethical dilemmas.

> J.R., a 44-year-old man, enters the PES and tells the resident that he has recently lost his job and his life is "no fun." He seems clearly upset but reports no prior history of mental illness or treatment. His wife has been

threatening to leave him and to take their two teenage children with her. His appetite is down. He has no close relatives nearby. He has been thinking about suicide. When asked for a reason, he states, "It's either that or kill *her*." The doctor recommends a temporary hospitalization to "check things out." J.R. refuses.

The dilemmas for the resident are several. Professionals who deal with suicidal patients are potentially liable for "inappropriate release of a patient, inappropriate hospitalization of a patient, or for the inappropriate care of a patient in the emergency facility itself" (Hillard 1983). Decisions about assessment, confinement or release, and the involvement of third parties are inherently ethical. They center around issues of justice, fairness, compassion, and honesty.

Myths About Emergency Ethics

Dealing with J.R. suggests many difficulties. Responsible answers to the questions his case poses require *advance* discussion of ethics in the PES. As a first step, certain myths about emergency ethics need to be addressed. Keep these in mind throughout the chapter discussion.

Myth #1. Potential psychiatric patients cannot know their own best interests.

Myth #2. Quick decisions do not allow time for reasoned choices; we have to go by the "seat of our pants."

Myth #3. In ethics, there can be no right or wrong answer; it's all a matter of opinion.

Myth #4. When uncertain, always err on the side of intervention.

Myth #5. PES staff always do "what's best for the patient."

This chapter attempts to deal with the real-life difficulties encountered in making ethical decisions in the PES. After a brief description of ethics per se, I will deal with the most frequently encountered problems in emergency psychiatry from the perspective of ethics.

What Is Ethics

Knowing what is right through the rational process of choosing the most morally desirable course of action is, in the most general sense, the substance of ethical decision making. But choosing the right over the wrong begs the question, How do we know what is right? How do we think controversial issues through? How do we make ethical judgments at all?

Ethical reasoning is an inherently problematic, yet useful, mode of thought. Like much of medical diagnosis, it is filled with uncertainty. But it is far superior, in process and consequence, to mere opinion giving with data or to forceful assertion without analysis. Some basic definitions in clinical medical ethics may serve to clarify this process.

- **Ethics**: the study of values, rights, duties, and obligations
- **Principles**: fundamental doctrines claiming that acts have validity without specific regard to their consequences
- **Rights**: an acknowledged interest within a moral or a legal system that (usually) imposes an obligation on others

The challenge for staff in the PES is in devising a method of examining difficult ethical decisions in a systematic and sustained manner. To respect principles or to consider rights will not be sufficient. Principles are often hard to discover; rights are sometimes in conflict. What is needed is a clear framework for ethical decision making that takes into account these basic definitions.

Clinical medical ethicists make use of two essential frameworks in the analysis of difficult cases. The first is the *utilitarian* approach, which attempts to balance benefits and burdens for affected parties, with a view to achieving the best possible consequences. The second is the *deontological*, or duty-based, approach, which urges acting in accordance with principles per se, without specific regard for results, but with concern for the goodness of the act itself.

- **Utilitarianism**: The promotion of the best long-term interest of everyone concerned should be the moral standard. Utilitarians look to *consequences* of acts for moral justification. They attempt to maximize good (or pleasure, or right) over harm (or evil, or wrong). Utilitarianism claims that rights and duties have no independent standing, that they derive from the goal of maximizing the overall good.
- **Deontology** (from Greek *deon*, meaning duty): An action's or rule's consequences are not the only criteria for determining the morality of an action. Deontologists look to the *features* of the act itself, without regard for the consequences. They emphasize maxims, rules, and principles (e.g., that promises must be kept). Morals, insist the deontologists, are based on fundamental principles and not on mere results.

Making use of these perspectives demands a cogent and manageable process of ethical decision making. The ethical workup serves as a complement to the diagnostic workup in PES or other emergency settings. It attempts to widen the data base to include ethical issues, to make explicit criteria for decision making, to examine the rationale used in making judgments, and to spell out the differences between using a utilitarian versus a deontological perspective in specific cases. The ethical workup is merely a tool; it does not dictate action. Rather it provides a model for the critical analysis of ethical problems. Steps in the ethical workup follow.

1. Describe all the relevant medical, psychiatric, and psychosocial facts in the case.
2. Describe the ethical (and legal) perspectives and responsibilities of the physicians, house staff, and other hospital personnel (including the institution itself) and of the patient and his or her relatives and friends.
3. Note the principal value conflicts in the case. For example, is the physician attempting to treat the patient against the patient's wishes?
4. Determine possible courses of action. Attempt, in proposing such courses of action, to respect stated values.
5. Choose and defend a course of action. State why one value (or set of values) was chosen over another in the case. Discuss the result of such a choice for both participants in the case and for society in general. Ask, In the present situation, whose "agent" are we?

The Special Situation of PES Ethics

Time constraints ("We need a decision *now*") are clearly significant in the PES. But there are other impediments to the process of clear reasoning and careful planning that temper ethical decision making. Acknowledging these problems is a first step toward anticipating, and then resolving, them. Some distinctions between emergency psychiatry and others types of interventions follow (Iserson et al. 1986).

- The patient is often brought into the PES situation involuntarily, or at least with mixed motives.
- The patient has virtually no choice in accepting the physician.
- Sources of data about the patient are often self-reports, at least until confirming data are available.
- Anxiety, pain, alcohol or substance use, and altered mental status may impede the accessibility of information.

- The capacity of the patient to make an informed decision may be compromised.
- The PES staff usually represent the policies and interests of the hospital administration; this may conflict with the needs of patients and staff members.

Going back to the case study, as J.R. heads for the emergency room door, an ethical decision complements a medical dilemma: What is to be done? The resident in this treatment-refusal situation—an all too common one—might be taken back at first. An effort might be made to get J.R. to wait. Additional staff would be called. The patient would be told that his depression was impairing his judgment, and he would be held, involuntarily, for observation. J.R. might yell about a lawsuit.

At a conference the next day, the case would be discussed. After a factual recapitulation, a series of questions would emerge about actions taken. Had the resident let the patient go, some remarks like, "Well, we'll probably see him again over the weekend," or "I hope he has a therapist out there," might well follow.

Had the resident arranged for J.R. to be held, things would go quite differently. Had the patient admitted, several hours later, that he had a gun at home, the hospitalization would be validated. Had J.R., after some beneficial medication, expressed his gratitude for being held, the involuntary hospitalization would have been justified (Stone 1984).

But this follow-up clearly has a missing dimension: ethical analysis and evaluation. We should not skip over the underlying ethical questions: Why should patients give consent? Who determines "best interest"? How are projected consequences of hospitalization or release assessed? What justifications can be given for the limitation of autonomy?

Paternalism Versus Autonomy

PES staff treat patients, especially those who seem suicidal or homicidal, with care and caution and always in the belief that a decision should be made for the good of that patient. To benefit a patient, especially one temporarily incapacitated, seems right in itself. It may well be. But this approach must be called by its proper name: *paternalism*. In the ambiguous setting of treatment refusal, paternalism may result in resistance to the patient's expressed desires; limitations on patient liberty, if only temporarily; compromise of a potential therapeutic alliance; and potential legal complications. Yet, rather than allow a depressed person to commit suicide, PES staff necessarily act paternalistically.

The empirical evaluation of dangerousness—itself a subject of methodological conflict professionally—presumes predictive value. But holding a patient is more than a statistical activity. It symbolizes a moral claim: that patients in the mental health system differ from many other medical clients because their autonomy is either in doubt or is (at the moment) nonexistent. To be autonomous is to be self-legislating, to be able at minimum to look at evidence, to weigh it, and to make a judgment. But is autonomy possible for persons with compromised mental statuses? Can a nonrational person act freely?

In the conflict between paternalism and autonomy, we see questions about the notion of mental disease and the ethical ambiguities that arise from it. If psychiatrists and other professionals could make "regular and reliable distinctions between peculiar and psychotic people" (Chodoff 1984, p. 388), there would be little worry. But the difficulties of differentiating potential mental patients from the idiosyncratic "normal" are substantial—predictions are inexact. And the liberty of coerced parties is at stake (Morse 1982).

What guidance from ethics can there be about removing decision making from a patient who may or may not be capable of exercising reasonable choice? Three factors may be considered in seeking assistance in this situation:

- Are there moral or value considerations at stake for the patient? For example, is the conflict rooted in religious doctrine (conventionally understood)? Does the desire to make the controversial decision originate in the patient's "values history," i.e., beliefs and perspectives developed over time (McCullough 1984)?
- Whose needs are at stake in this controversy? Do the desires of the professional staff, or the hospital administration, supersede the desires of the individual patient? Are institutional concerns paramount? Should they be tempered by fidelity to the rights of the patient and his or her claim to liberty?
- What are the differences between short- and long-term autonomy? Is it responsible to detain, deter, or coerce a patient in the expressed interest of autonomy? How can such paternalism be justified?

Clearly, the mental status of the PES patient will weigh heavily in the ethical dimensions of treatment choice. But the assessment of competence—beyond legal requirements that eventuate in court orders—is a vexing issue. In the PES, diminished capacity to reason should not be prima facie evidence of incompetence to exercise treatment choices. The mental status of a patient based on age, history, diagnosis, or physical and/or mental condition does not tell us what we need to know about the patient's competence to make autonomous choices. We would ask these additional questions:

- Can the patient make a voluntary, deliberate choice?
- Does the decision reflect the patient's past or present values?
- Does the patient understand the consequences of either accepting or refusing recommended interventions?

Examining these questions distributes the burden and balances the natural temptation to impose treatments on PES patients.

COMMONLY ENCOUNTERED ISSUES

PES decisions will, inevitably, be "judgment calls." How dangerous must a patient be to be involuntarily institutionalized? What kinds of justifications can be found for the limitation of liberty? What degree of certainty is required to validate a recommendation by a PES staff member?

Suicidal Threats or Behavior

Medical values ("preserve life," "do no harm") and psychiatric practice (suicide hot lines, taking suicidal ideation seriously) suggest that suicide presents one of the rare instances of value coherence. Suicide is wrong; it must be prevented; it is the ultimately destructive act. Religious and secular commentators—from the Talmud and the Roman Catholic Church to the writings of the deontological thinker Immanuel Kant—sustain this impression. To be "for life" is to abhor self-destruction. But such virtual unanimity does not deny the utility of an ethical analysis of suicide.

First, the ethical basis of intervention is quite logical: All medical personnel have a moral obligation to help those in pain. Suicide is closely linked to major psychiatric disorders, such as depression. Successful suicides are irreversible. Thus, responsible medical personnel must prevent suicide (Heyd and Bloch 1984).

Second, even for those who do not state that all suicidal behavior is psychopathological per se, good reasons remain for intervening. If suicide is not evidence of mental illness, it is either a "cry for help" or a demonstration of patient ambivalence. In either case, it calls for responsible intervention. Whatever the hidden agenda, we must not allow the patient to die.

Still, agreement on the rudiments of an ethical response to threatened suicide does not close the discussion. Rather, it opens us to other, equally grave, concerns. Suicidal ideation or behavior makes us ponder

- What sorts of promises should be made to suicidal patients?
- What are the limits of protection that should be offered to suicidal patients?
- Is paternalistic intervention always therapeutic, or does it support the manipulative patient in unpredictable ways?
- Can suicide ever be "rational" (Battin 1982)?
- Can intervention with suicidal patients be justified on the basis of the needs and interests of an "affirming therapeutic profession" (Ciccione and Clements 1984)?

If we involuntarily institutionalize suicidal patients—in their best interests—we claim to help them regain the freedom lost temporarily to psychiatric disorder, overwhelming stress, or difficult interpersonal relationships. In other words, we limit autonomy to guarantee autonomy? Can psychiatry fulfill the promise made in this latter phrase?

Privacy and Confidentiality: The Violent Patient

Confidentiality is one of the oldest and most consistently held doctrines in medical ethics. Based on the safeguarding of privacy, confidentiality is the foundation on which persons establish and maintain relationships of intimacy. Psychiatrists have access to deep personal and secret information about individuals and families; confidentiality is the basis of trust in the therapeutic relationship.

Patients expect privacy in health care, and institutions have policies designed to protect such information. Disclosure of clinical information requires the informing of patients and their consent. Third parties are given confidential information only after patients have permitted such disclosure.

In PES settings, complications over issues of confidentiality arise when multiple claims are placed on staff. Such questions as, Whose agent is the psychiatrist? What rights do family members have? Are potentially incompetent patients capable of understanding waivers of confidentiality? What exceptions should there be to the doctrine of confidentiality? Patients who are severely disturbed are, at times, likely to divulge information unawares.

The exception to the general rule of confidentiality centers around the possibility of "dangerousness" to others. However, the unpredictability of such dangerousness makes the premature revelation of private information a touchy ethical problem. The recently enunciated maxim in psychiatric circles is that "protective privilege ends where public peril begins" (Karasu 1984). Certainly the well-publicized aftermath of the *Tarasoff* case has instigated the radical rethinking of patient confidentiality as a moral absolute in psychiatry. Without remarking on the legalities of the case, it is sufficient to state that PES staff now must concern themselves with threats to designated third parties and that they must, on occasion, breach promises of secret keeping to patients (Beck 1985). The grounds for such a breach are both deontological and utilitarian. PES staff clearly have moral obligations to nonpatients. Preserving life as a moral maxim may require a *Tarasoff* warning.

On the consequentialist side, public policy seems to demand that the privacy of a single patient be sacrificed if a solid "hunch" makes it evident that some other designated person(s) may be in substantial danger. In this balancing act, it is the individual who is sacrificed to the good of society.

Emergencies frequently entail behavior that appears, at the very moment, to be dangerous and disruptive. Such violent actions may in fact be criminal. The language of rights—to privacy, to autonomy, and to freedom—is never absolute. No one believes that another person can act violently with impunity. But for patients in the PES, management of violent behavior in the short run—with seclusion or restraints or via forced medication or through the filing of criminal charges against assaultive patients—opens up several ethical issues. For example:

- Courts, and conventional practice, advocate the "least restrictive means" of control for patients deemed in need of restraint or treatment. What are the implications of making such a judgment?
- Patients have a right to treatment, and to refuse treatment in given settings. Do staff members have any established rights in violent situations, save the opportunity to leave a job after the fact?
- To what extent is voluntariness on the part of a violent patient compromised by threatening to restrain the patient? What are the consequences of forcing treatment by compelling compliance through seclusion, restraint, or criminal charges?
- Should violent patients without major mental disorders be discharged

to "the street"? Where do the obligations of PES staff to society as a whole begin, and end?

Every interaction with the criminal justice system—whether through warning police in a *Tarasoff* situation or "punishing" a violent PES patient through prosecution—carries with it the dilemma of moving the conceptual understanding of behavior from medical to moral or legal. "Acting out," no longer a product of psychopathology, becomes simply "bad" and is thus punishable by criminal sanction.

Informed Consent and Involuntary Commitment

Treating patients whose mental status is unclear presents a bundle of ethical problems. As one source has pithily put it: "The damaged organ is the consenting organ." The impediments to gaining consent from authentically psychotic patients are considerable; those who can neither understand or speak must have surrogates make their decisions. At the other end of the spectrum are patients with "problems in living," whose disorders are surely impediments to their granting of informed consent.

By law and practice, all patients being offered treatment, medication, or specific procedures must be told the nature of their condition, disease, disorder, or problem. The nature and purpose of the proposed treatment must be given in specific language that can be commonly understood. The risks and consequences of the proposed treatment, and any feasible alternatives to the treatment, must be stated. The patient's prognosis if the proposed treatment is not given must be described.

Can potential psychiatric patients in the PES freely grant a truly informed consent? Problems abound for those patients whose competence (see above) may be in doubt. For patients demonstrably psychotic —deemed dangerous to self or others, for example—the "emergency exception" to the requirement of informed consent will apply (Macklin 1982). But what of patients presently taking medication that may impede the understanding of the medical situation? What level of informed consent is appropriate for the patient—at the moment acting out in anger due to the failure to take psychotropic medication—who resists treatment?

In the PES, where decisions must be made swiftly, there will be less time to establish the relationship necessary to discuss, with time allowed for questions and responses, the content of proposed treatments in the detail that might be possible in outpatient settings. Still, data about the efficacy of the treatment, the incidence and prevalence of side effects of drugs, and the short- and long-range prospects with and without treatment should be stated clearly, efficiently, and in a noncoercive manner. The goal, which is not always met, in seeking informed consent is to establish the fact that the PES patient is indeed making a choice based on a secure understanding of the factual issues and does indeed appreciate the nature of the situation in medical and psychological perspective. Patients with debilitating delusions will obviously not meet such a minimalist test. Others should be offered an opportunity to exercise autonomous choice. For those who cannot make such a choice, a useful rule of thumb for the practitioner is: *Attempt to restore competence to consent in the most noncoercive manner possible.*

Involuntary civil commitment, procedures for which will vary from jurisdiction to jurisdiction, is a last alternative. Its rationale, medically and ethically, is overtly paternalistic: to protect the patient who cannot exercise decision-making power. Grounds for such commitment also vary, but include demonstrable dangerousness to self or others, the inability to care for oneself (though "care" is specified in meaning less often than is desirable), dangerousness to property, and the controversial notion of "in need of treatment." There is considerable doubt about the consistency with which civil commitment standards are applied in psychiatric emergency rooms (Segal et al. 1986). Because an emergency situation prevents the fullest development of data and perspective, the likelihood of erring on the side of incarceration is considerable.

Some questions of ethics involved when considering involuntary care follow.

- Is the refusal of offered treatment seen as a *major* reason for attempting to commit the patient?
- What weight should be put on temporary factors (e.g., alcohol use, drug abuse) in the assessment that might lead to alternative discussions about the patient's capacity to be left at liberty?
- What other interests (family, societal) are at stake in the commitment decision?
- What are the likely effects of involuntary commitment (in the long and short run) on presenting problems (e.g., psychotic decompensation)?
- Will the treatment available—if successful—justify the abridgment of liberty made necessary by commitment?

The struggle over involuntary commitment may be seen as pitting a "benevolent paternalism" against a "civil liberties" emphasis on physical freedom (Chodoff 1984). It will not be easily solved. But it is undeniably more than a medical issue: it is a difficult, perhaps intractable, moral problem.

RATIONING HEALTH CARE

The proliferation of PES sites (from fewer than 160 in 1963 to more than 2000 at present) has demonstrably changed the face of psychiatric diagnosis and treatment outside the state hospital setting (Wellin et al. 1987). But though the original assumption about the PES was that it would treat *acute* problems, the parallel deinstitutionalization movement has thrust *chronic* patients into the emergency room in vast numbers. This contextual aspect must not be neglected in assessing the policy dimensions of emergency psychiatry. The PES serves as a "gatekeeper," with all that difficult phrase entails.

Thus, the legal and ethical battles fought during the past 25 years have created a situation that must, necessarily, permeate the decision making of PES staff who must determine who is or who is not served, and in what way(s). Stone (1984) has captured that setting most vividly: "Yet madness has not gone out of the world as was hoped, in fact madness is more visible than ever before . . . One can see chronic mental patients in the streets of every major city in the United States."

All expensive medical treatments are rationed today. The medical care budget in this nation, although rising out of proportion to population growth and inflation, is insufficient to meet demand. Remarkable new technologies, the aging of American society, and raised expectations about the quality of life all combine to impinge on a limited medical care system. Society seems clearly unable to provide treatments to all who might benefit.

Given the necessity of distributing scarce resources, what framework or set of principles should be utilized? Two such approaches are predominant: the utilitarian and the egalitarian (a deontological perspective; see above). Put simply, we should decide who gets what either on the basis of results or on the basis of fairness.

The scarcity of psychiatric resources will remain a policymaker's nightmare. But its impact on actual decisions at the micro level is considerable. If there are only three remaining beds tonight at the only hospital that will accept indigent patients, a decision is forced on the PES staff. Only a certain amount of bending, coaxing, cajoling, or "fudging" will help; and only in the short run. The ethics of working within the current system is an ethics of compromise.

A second policy issue surrounds the issue of justice. For PES patients and staff, what rights should be guaranteed as a matter of policy? How should such rights or claims be judged and enforced? The recent effort by the National Center for State Courts, in their *Guidelines for Involuntary Civil Commitment* (1986), is a noble start in the right direction (Keilitz 1988). But this attempt to blend the medical and legal dimensions of the problem suggests that PES dilemmas are rarely simple and rarely "solved." Balancing the interests of individual and society will always be a difficult task. But the discussion must proceed.

Finally, we must recognize that the medical, legal, and ethical decisions made about the fate of persons seen in the PES are economic and financial. The availability of a bed; the presence (or absence) of an insurance card; the willingness of a family member to transport the patient to a community mental health center; the resources of city, county, and state agencies for mental health support; the slice of the national budget available for such services—these all influence PES decisions every day, and in ways that force hard choices on an often stressed staff who must make allocation decisions immediately with insufficient resources.

THE MYTHS ADDRESSED

The topic of ethics in emergency psychiatry is, quite patently, difficult and complex. Problems abound; counterexamples multiply. Yet some measures can be taken to address such dilemmas. Let us briefly address the five common myths noted earlier from the context of our discussion.

Myth #1. Potential psychiatric patients cannot know their own best interests.

Response. Even when patients cannot absolutely know their best interests, the assumption must be—in law and in common morality—that they retain their autonomy until the contrary is demonstrated. Working from this value base, all efforts will be expended to try to attain and support patient competence in a supportive atmosphere.

Myth #2. Quick decisions do not allow time for reasoned choices; we have to go by the "seat of our pants."

Response. There is no PES ethical issue that will not profit from sustained discussion and the development of useful, general policies in advance. Reasoned choices need not be abandoned during the rush to decide. They should be the product of anticipated crises and previously resolved difficulties. Use of the ethical workup described earlier may aid this process.

Myth #3. In ethics, there can be no right or wrong answer; it's all a matter of opinion.

Response. Though there is, in a secular age, no absolutely certain right answer to many serious ethical dilemmas, there are clear, cogent processes and overt perspectives that can be used and applied consistently to ethical issues. Table 7-1 lists three tests to use in determining what's right. The utilitarian and deontological viewpoints should be addressed systematically. At the very least, the value bases for decisions will be made explicit.

Table 7-1. What's right? Three informal tests

- *Impartiality Test.* Would you be willing to have this action performed if you were in the other person's (the patient's) place?
- *Universalizability Test.* Are you willing to have this action performed in all relevantly similar circumstances?
- *Interpersonal Justifiability Test.* Are you able to provide good reasons to justify your action to others?

Source. Adapted from Iserson et al. 1986, pp 40–41.

Myth #4. When uncertain, always err on the side of intervention.

Response. Erring on the side of intervention, especially in life-threatening emergency circumstances, is surely a wise policy. But it should not become a clichéd rationale for coercion or minimization of the rights of patients or staff. Erring on the side of engagement would be morally preferable.

Myth #5. PES staff always do "what's best for the patient."

Response. The notion of "agency," i.e., just who are PES staff working for, deserves special scrutiny. Competing interests do exist in emergency psychiatry, and the "balancing act" needed to reach an ethical decision is a remaining problem.

REFERENCES

Battin MP: Ethical Issues in Suicide. Englewood Cliffs, NJ, Prentice-Hall, 1982

Beck JC: The Potentially Violent Patient and the *Tarasoff* Decision in Psychiatric Practice. Washington, DC, American Psychiatric Press, 1985

Chodoff P: Involuntary hospitalization of the mentally ill as a moral issue. Am J Psychiatry 141:384–389, 1984

Ciccione JR, Clements C: Forensic psychiatry and applied clinical ethics: theory and practice. Am J Psychiatry 141:395–399, 1984

Heyd D, Bloch S: The ethics of suicide, in Psychiatric Ethics. Edited by Bloch S, Chodoff P. Oxford, Oxford University Press, 1984

Hillard JR: Emergency management of the suicidal patient, in Psychiatric Emergencies: Intervention and Resolution. Edited by Walker JI. Philadelphia, PA, JB Lippincott, 1983, p 120

Iserson K, Sanders A, Mathieu D, et al: Ethics in Emergency Medicine. Baltimore, MD, Williams & Wilkins, 1986

Karasu T: Ethical aspects of psychotherapy, in Psychiatric Ethics. Edited by Bloch S, Chodoff P. Oxford, Oxford University Press, 1984

Keilitz I: An introduction to the National Center for State Courts' Guidelines for Involuntary Civil Commitment. Hosp Community Psychiatry 39:397, 1988

McCullough LB: Medical care for elderly patients with diminished capacity: an ethical analysis. J Am Geriatr Soc 32:150–153, 1984

Macklin R: Some problems in gaining informed consent from psychiatric patients. Emory Law Journal 31:345–374, 1982

Morse SJ: A preference for liberty: the case against involuntary commitment of the mentally disordered. California Law Review 70:54–103, 1982

National Center for State Courts: Guidelines for involuntary commitment. Mental and Physical Disability Law Reporter 10:409–514, 1986

Segal SP, Watson MA, Nelson S: Consistency in the application of civil commitment standards in psychiatric emergency rooms. Journal of Psychiatry and Law 14:125–148, 1986

Stone AA: Law, Psychiatry, and Morality: Essays and Analysis. Washington, DC, American Psychiatric Press, 1984

Tarasoff v Regents of the University of California, 188 Cal Rptr 129, 529 P2d 553 (1974)

Wellin E, Slesinger DR, Hollister CD: Psychiatric emergency services: evolution, adaptation and proliferation. Soc Sci Med 24:475–482, 1987

PART II

SPECIFIC PROBLEMS

Chapter 8

Suicide

J.R. Hillard, M.D.

Patient suicide is the outcome we worry about the most. It is what we most commonly admit patients to the hospital for fear of. It is one of the main things that psychiatric emergency services were set up to prevent, and it is one of the main things we get sued for failing to prevent.

In a statistical sense, we know what the risk factors are for suicide. In a large population of patients, we can predict fairly accurately how many will kill themselves in a given year. It is very difficult, however, to predict exactly which individuals will kill themselves or which of the limited number of resources at our disposal will make a difference in a particular case (Clark et al. 1987; Pokorney 1983).

RISK FACTORS

Everything ever written about suicide has mentioned risk factors, and this chapter will too. Be forewarned, though, that generic risk factors are, at best, only a little bit helpful in assessing an individual case and are, at worst, misleading.

Shaded sections indicate areas of legitimate diversity of professional opinion in the literature. See Preface for further discussion.

Demographic Factors

The relationship of demographic factors to completed suicide has been quite consistent across a very large number of studies. Males, both in the general population and across a wide range of clinical populations, have a higher rate of suicide than females, usually two to four times higher ("Advance Report" 1986). Whites and American Indians have a consistently higher rate than blacks and Latin Americans ("Advance Report" 1986). Divorced, widowed, or separated individuals have rates higher than single individuals, who have rates higher than married individuals (Roy 1982).

Children still have very low rates of suicide. Adolescent rates have risen markedly in recent years, but are still lower than rates in older age groups (Maris 1985). Older adults tend to have slightly higher rates than younger adults ("Advance Report" 1986).

Attempted suicides, as opposed to completed suicides, are more common among females, among younger individuals, and possibly among blacks (Weissman 1974). This is generally attributed to the use of less lethal means of attempt in these groups and to the use of attempts as a means of communication. Although overall rates of completed suicide have been fairly constant for decades in the United States, rates of attempted suicide appear to have increased markedly in the last 20 years.

Diagnosis

Risk of suicide is strongly concentrated in just a few diagnostic groups: mood disorders, schizophrenia, and psychoactive substance abuse (Hillard et al. 1983; Martin et al. 1985; Roy 1982). Other disorders that may be associated with suicide are delusional disorder, brief reactive psychosis, schizoaffective disorder, anxiety disorders (Coryell et al. 1986), and borderline and antisocial personality disorders.

Social Factors

Connections with other people protect against suicide. Isolation, or rupture of connections, is associated with suicide. Living alone is strongly associated with suicide (Roy 1982). Being unemployed, particularly recently unemployed, is also associated (Roy 1982). A significant involvement with any religious group tends to protect against suicide, but nominal involvement does not.

Plan
Mean
Intent

PMI

Past History and Family History

Past attempts at suicide are associated with future attempts and with future completed suicide. This is the case across the whole range of patient diagnoses (Roy 1983). Risk of suicide is associated with a history of suicide by relatives and is most closely associated with suicide by closest relatives.

ASSESSMENT OF RISK BY TYPE OF PRESENTATION

Patients Without Recent Suicidal Ideation or Attempt

Every individual needing emergency psychiatric evaluation or treatment must be regarded as potentially at risk for suicide. The information in Table 8-1 should be elicited and documented for every emergency psychiatric patient.

In general, it is a good idea to ask about suicidal ideation, as outlined below, even if the patient does not mention it spontaneously. However, it is generally better if suicidal ideation is not the first topic discussed. Often, suicide is easier for patients to talk about than feelings of

Table 8-1. Information to be gathered and documented for every potentially suicidal patient

- Is the patient in a relatively high-risk (i.e., male, white or American Indian, older or unmarried) or low-risk demographic group for suicide?
- Is the patient in a relatively high-risk (i.e., major affective disorder, substance abuse, or psychosis) or low-risk diagnostic group for suicide?
- What degree of acute stress and emotional turmoil is the patient currently experiencing?
- To what extent is the patient socially isolated?
- Does the patient have a past history of suicide attempts?
- Does the patient have a family history of suicide?
- Has the patient communicated suicidal ideation or intent to clinicians or to family or acquaintances
    Directly? (see Table 8-2)
    Indirectly? (e.g., giving away valued possessions, talking about no longer "being around" by some date in the near future)
- Is the patient able to speak about the future with any degree of hope?

aloneness or shame or guilt. Focusing too much on suicide too early in the interview may make it difficult to learn much else.

Patients With Suicidal Ideation

Talking about suicidal ideation is socially unacceptable under most circumstances. The clinician needs to make it as easy as possible for patients to talk about their suicidal thoughts (see Chapter 1). If a patient with depression or with acute emotional turmoil does not spontaneously mention suicide, it is reasonable to say something like, "It sounds as though you are in a lot of pain. Have thoughts of suicide crossed your mind? Have you had any of that?" If the patient can admit any ideation at all, then the issues in Table 8-2 should be addressed. (For a more quantitative approach to this assessment, see Beck's Scale for Suicide Ideation [Beck et al. 1979].) If the patient has a suicide plan and the means of carrying it out, there is cause for grave concern, even if the patient does not feel able to carry out the plan. Intense ideation or suicidal impulse that patients are worried they cannot control is also a

Table 8-2. Information to be gathered and documented for patients with suicidal ideation

---

- Does the patient have a plan for how he or she would kill himself or herself?
  - Does the patient have access to the means for carrying out the plan?
  - Does the patient feel able to carry out the plan?
  - Has the patient already taken steps to carry out the plan (e.g., written a note, saved up pills, made a will)?

- What is the ideation like?
  - Frequency—occasional, frequent, or continuous
  - Intensity—fairly easy versus almost impossible to put out of mind
  - Sense of control over ideation or impulse—"I'm in control of it" versus "It's stronger than I am"
  - Recency of onset—just today versus present for years

- What is the motivation for the thoughts of suicide?
  - Degree of wish to die
  - Degree of wish to communicate pain or anger to the living
  - Voices or forces telling the patient to commit suicide

- Are there deterrents to the attempt (e.g., religion, family, fear)?

- Does the patient actually expect to make an attempt?

- Is the patient less agitated and preoccupied with suicide at the end of the interview than at the beginning?

---

source for grave concern. The patient who speaks of "hearing voices saying to kill himself" is the psychiatric equivalent of the cardiac patient who complains of "crushing chest pain radiating to the left arm and left jaw." Such a patient must be regarded as at imminent risk of death, and in need of further evaluation.

Unfortunately, just as there are some patients who have learned what they need to say to gain medical admission, there are patients who have learned what they need to say to gain psychiatric admission. Some clinical findings that suggest hospital-seeking, as opposed to death-seeking, suicidal ideation include lack of depressed affect or agitation, a history of multiple nonproductive hospitalizations, and evidence of attempts to conceal past history.

Patients With Recent Suicide Attempts

Possible attempts.   Any injury or near injury that comes to the physician's attention should be evaluated to assess what, if any, suicidal component may have been present in it. "Accidental" overdoses in adults and adolescents would definitely fall into this category, as would many single-vehicle automobile accidents. Such an evaluation should usually include 1) how the patient has been feeling since the accident, 2) how the patient was feeling before the accident, 3) whether the patient thought of suicide, and, finally, 4) inquiry as to whether the accident might have been a sort of suicide attempt.

Definite attempts.   Every suicide attempt, no matter how medically insignificant, should be evaluated in terms of how much "wish to die" is embodied in it. Every suicide attempt, no matter how medically serious, should be evaluated in terms of how much of an attempt to communicate is embodied in it. The degree of ongoing wish to die has important implications for immediate treatment and must be assessed in a variety of ways. Asking the patient, "Did you expect to die from this attempt?" can yield useful information, but there is useful information that it cannot yield. For various reasons, a patient may be afraid to be honest, or the underlying motivation may not be entirely conscious. Even if an attempt represented a conscious wish to die when made, that wish may have been denied or repressed by the time the patient is evaluated. It is important to assess intent to die as it can be inferred from action, in addition to assessing it as stated by the patient. For these reasons, a medically serious attempt should be regarded with concern even if the patient states it was "just to get them to listen." Conversely, an attempt that is recognized as quite unlikely to have been fatal (e.g., ingestion of 20 5-mg diazepam tablets) may have been believed by the patient to have been dangerous. The information in Table 8-3 should be elicited from patients after suicide attempts, in addition to the information in Tables 8-1 and 8-2. (For a more quantitative approach to this assessment, see Beck's Suicidal Intent Scale [Beck et al. 1974].) Those patients at greatest immediate risk for subsequent completed suicide are those who had a significant wish to die and who, after the attempt, are in no better frame of mind than they were before it. About 1% of all patients who attempt suicide will go on to completed suicide within the next year (Roy 1983); however, 99% will not. This rate of 1% per year, however, is about 100 times as great as the rate in the general population.

TELEPHONE CALLS

Any telephone number for psychiatric services, especially psychiatric emergency services, will get telephone calls from people talking about suicide. Most of these are from lonely people who do not feel they deserve to be listened to unless they are about to die. Some, however, represent an immediate threat of death. The first determination that needs to be made rapidly is whether the patient has already ingested an overdose. If yes, it is necessary to locate the patient and notify police or life squad to bring the patient to the medical emergency room. It is a good idea to make arrangements with the telephone service ahead of time for tracing calls. Under these circumstances, if a patient is unwilling or unable to reveal his or her whereabouts, a call can be traced, in most areas, if the party stays on the line for at least 60 minutes. In many areas, a call can be traced much more rapidly than this.

The other common situation requiring special care is the patient who claims to be holding a gun, because an instantaneous lapse can lead to a fatal outcome. Negotiations should center on getting the patient to relinquish the weapon.

Most other situations are best dealt with by "talk and time." Unfortunately, except in a specialized telephone counseling facility, time is seldom available. It is best to have an arrangement for transferring calls to the telephone counseling line, but this is often not possible. Under these circumstances, it is necessary early in the conversation, after determining that the patient has not already overdosed and does not have a gun, to let the caller know that is is not possible to talk at length. Some patients will be angry that "you do not care about me." Usually, the best

Table 8-3. Information to be gathered and documented for patients examined after a suicide attempt

- Medical seriousness of the attempt
- Stated intent of the attempt
  - Does the patient say it was an attempt
    To die?
    To get away or to end the pain?
    To communicate degree of pain to others?
    To get high, or to calm down, or to fall asleep?
    Some combination of the above?
  - Does the patient say he or she believed
    Death was an unlikely result?
    Death was possible, but unlikely?
    Death was probable or certain?
- Inferred intent of attempt
  - Did the patient make preparations for death (e.g., making a will)?
  - Did the patient communicate an intent to die before the attempt (e.g., leaving a note)?
  - Was there evidence of premeditation (e.g., hoarding of pills)?
  - Did the patient take precautions for or against discovery?
    Was discovery likely given the location and timing of the attempt?
    Did the patient drop hints to others?
    What was the delay between the attempt and the patient being found?
  - To what degree was the attempt impulsive and what is the patient's degree of impulse control?
  - Was the patient under the influence of drugs or alcohol at the time of the attempt? Is the patient at continuing risk for drug and alcohol abuse?
- Reaction to the attempt
  - Does the patient feel that important people in his or her life have responded appropriately to the attempt?
  - Does the patient regret the attempt, or only the failure of the attempt?
- Patient's state of mind at interview
  - Is the patient still confused and disoriented due to intoxication or emotional turmoil?
  - Is the patient able to form a relationship, or is the patient hostile and uncommunicative?
- Plans for the future
  - Does the patient feel he or she can control suicidal impulses in the near future?
  - Can the patient visualize and talk about the future with some degree of hope?
  - Is the patient able to collaborate with planning for his or her future treatment?

stance to take is to provide the following information: 1) You would be glad to see them, if they could come in to see you in person. 2) Telephone counseling services, which you feel good about, are available. 3) Here is how to get in to see you, and here is the number for the telephone counseling.

USE OF HOSPITALIZATION

Hospitalization is never without costs but it is often without benefit. Some of the social costs are discussed in Chapter 5. On the other hand, hospitalization is sometimes the only mechanism available to make reasonably certain that suicidal patients will not kill themselves in the immediate future. In addition to protection, the hospital offers more rapid initiation of diagnosis and treatment than would ordinarily be possible on an outpatient basis. Furthermore, some forms of treatment are ordinarily available only on an inpatient basis, most notably electroconvulsive therapy. Table 8-4 summarizes situations in which hospitalization of suicidal individuals must be considered. Patients in these categories do not necessarily require hospitalization, but their medical record requires an indication that hospitalization was considered and an explanation of why it was rejected.

Table 8-4. Situations in which hospitalization must be considered

---

- The patient expresses the intention to commit suicide and has a definite plan and the means to carry it out.

- The patient has strong suicidal impulses and presents evidence of being unable to control those impulses.

- The patient is acutely psychotic and has acute suicidal ideation of any degree.

- The patient has made a medically very serious attempt with some suggestion of intent to die.

- The patient evidences less serious suicidal ideation or a less serious suicide attempt, both medically and in terms of intent, plus one or more of the following:
  - Major depression
  - Lack of, or exhaustion of, the support system in the community
  - Need for intensive diagnostic or treatment resources not available on an outpatient basis
  - Failure of outpatient treatment
  - An escalating pattern of suicide
  - Substance abuse plus mental illness

Degree of suicide risk is always balanced against degree of support available in the community. Patients at high risk of suicide can sometimes be managed on an outpatient basis if a very supportive family and appropriate outpatient resources are available, whereas patients who are only moderately suicidal may need to be hospitalized if no social supports can be found.

All 50 states have laws allowing for involuntary hospitalization of mentally ill persons who are imminently suicidal. Exact wording varies by state in terms of 1) what constitutes mental illness, with some states specifically including, or excluding, substance abuse or mental retardation; and 2) what constitutes imminent risk, with some jurisdictions being much more liberal than others in terms of what is included as imminent. All states now have a system of checks and balances with judicial review at various points in the process. It is, of course, important to know the applicable state laws to use them effectively. Very little is gained by having patients released from the hospital by a judge just a few days after having been put there against their will.

Threshold for Involuntary Hospitalization

All state commitment statutes leave a lot up to professional judgment. In dealing with the large group of patients who show moderate risk of suicide, different professionals operate with different thresholds for involuntary hospitalization. Some professionals contend that releasing a patient after a suicide attempt may be colluding with denial of illness. They would further take the position that completed suicide is such a catastrophic outcome that it is acceptable to involuntarily hospitalize some individuals for whom hospitalization is perhaps not entirely necessary in order to avoid releasing any for whom it is necessary.

Those advocating a high threshold would argue that unless there is very substantial evidence that the patient is likely to commit suicide in the next few days, hospitalization should be avoided. These professionals are concerned about the negative effects of hospitalization and about the negative effects of being forced into treatment. Can treatment be forced? Does use of force destroy the therapeutic alliance? If the therapist attempts to hospitalize involuntarily, will the patient be less likely to seek professional help at the next crisis? We would advocate a moderately high threshold for involuntary hospitalization.

ALTERNATIVES TO HOSPITALIZATION

If a patient can be promptly and safely evaluated and treated on an outpatient basis, that is usually preferable to inpatient treatment. Different communities have different outpatient resources available, and different programs referred to by the same name (e.g., crisis stabilization center) may have very different treatment capabilities from each other. It is important to understand what is available in a given community.

In some cases, it is possible for an emergency service or private practitioner to set up an informal alternative to hospitalization by seeing patients and, if possible, their families on a daily basis using the treatment principles outlined below.

Emergency Psychotherapy of the Suicidal Patient

Making the assessment therapeutic. Suicidal patients usually have characteristic cognitive distortions (Rush and Beck 1978). They have often suffered a recent loss and feel alone and unlovable. They tend to have a hard time trusting or taking comfort from anyone. They tend to exhibit the "cognitive triad" of depression: negative view of their present, negative view of their past, and negative view of the future. They tend to believe and take heart in whatever is consistent with these negative views and to discount or externalize whatever is inconsistent with them. Suicidal people are acutely aware of their pain and are unable to see any way out of it. Life, with its infinite choices, is boiled down for them to only one choice—"Do I go on living with unbearable, unending pain or do I kill myself?" Their sense of time is often distorted, leaving them with a very limited ability to imagine the future and with a limited ability to experience the past prior to their present circumstances. It is seldom useful to try to convince patients how much they have to live for. They can seldom hear it. What they do hear is the therapist arguing with them and criticizing them. It is more helpful if patients can feel that the therapist can appreciate and share their pain. It also can be useful to point out, rather than dispute, the patients' cognitive distortions, and to help patients label them as abnormal and as temporary.

The process of the interview itself can be therapeutic in that it starts with the present illness and moves on to explore the past. It starts with the patient and moves on to explore relationships with others. The process can help widen the patient's constricted cognitive world.

It is also useful to help patients become aware of their ambivalence about suicide. At times, it is appropriate to identify specifically to patients after an overdose that there must have been a part of them that wanted to die (e.g., the part that led them to take the pills), or else they wouldn't be talking to you, but that there also must have been a part that wanted to live (e.g., the part of them that warned a relative to look for them) or else they wouldn't be talking to you. It may at times be useful to tell patients explicitly that "I want to work with the part of you that wants to live. I'm glad that part of you will have another chance."

It is often tempting to point out the angry component of a patient's suicide attempt. That component is often so blatant (e.g., the patient who takes an overdose in his car in his ex-wife's driveway), but so unrecognized by the patient. To work with a patient on a long-term basis requires that the anger be dealt with at some point, but that point is almost never during the first interview. The patient who attempts suicide has, in a sense, been willing to die rather than admit the anger. The therapist probably cannot get the patient to admit it either and may come across as accusatory and rejecting when trying to.

No-Suicide Contracts

The no-suicide contract has been advocated as a therapeutic technique. In one version, the suicidal patient is asked to make a decision and state out loud that "No matter what happens, I will not kill myself, accidentally or on purpose" for a specific period of time or without coming back to the emergency room (Drye et al. 1973). At times, I have seen notes in emergency room charts stating, "Patient released after making a no-suicide contract." I am always skeptical of such contracts because they are only valid for people capable of making contracts, which, I think, excludes most people with much risk of suicide. Every completed suicide represents many broken promises to many significant people. One more promise to someone the patient barely knows is unlikely to be the deciding factor. Contracts of this sort, however, may be more useful in dealing with nonlethal self-destructive behavior, which can be interpreted as asking for help. At times it is very therapeutic to work out with such a patient other ways of asking for help that do not necessitate real or potential tissue damage.

SPECIFIC CONSIDERATIONS BY DIAGNOSIS

Depression

Depressed patients are probably the most obviously suicidal people the clinician sees. It is easy to imagine how their hopelessness and inability to experience pleasure or regeneration will ultimately, and predictably, lead to suicide, if unchecked. Prospective studies of suicide among depressed individuals have, however, contained some surprises. Fawcett et al. (1987) found that the characteristics of depressed patients that were most closely correlated with suicide within 1 year were not those related to the overall severity of depression, but those related to intensity of depressive turmoil (agitation), hopelessness, loss of pleasure, psychotic thinking, and rapid mood cycling. They found risk of suicide greater for those with *fewer* previous episodes of depression and in those abusing drugs or alcohol.

The prospective study of suicide in psychiatric patients by Martin et al. (1985) showed a much higher rate of suicide among patients with secondary depression (i.e., those with depression that developed on top of a preexisting psychiatric disorder) than among those with primary depression. Studies like these are, of course, difficult to apply to clinical situations. Fawcett et al., for example, found predictors of suicide within 1 year to be different from those that predicted suicide within 1–5 years. It may be that still another set of factors best predict suicide among depressed persons during the period that really concerns us most—the first few days or weeks after the patient comes to our attention. It is probably wise, however, to pay particular attention to anxiety and to preexisting disorders as being factors that may make a particular depressed patient at particularly high risk for death by suicide.

Schizophrenia

Schizophrenic patients, particularly those who are young, are at high risk for suicide (Breier and Astrachan 1984; Drake et al. 1985). One study of psychiatric emergency service patients showed young schizophrenic patients to have the highest rate of any psychiatric emergency patients (Hillard et al. 1983). Their suicides are often difficult to predict or, even in retrospect, to understand (Breier and Astrachan 1984). Patients with acute hallucinations commanding them to kill themselves are at high risk, but patients with other sorts of command hallucinations are apparently not at higher risk (Hellerstein et al. 1987). Some patients, however, state that they have had hallucinations urging suicide more or less continuously for many years. As is usually the case for chronically psychotic patients, how patients compare with their baseline levels of thought disorder and affect are most important to assessing short-term outcome. A particular situation to be dealt with cautiously is the chronically schizophrenic patient who seems perhaps less thought disordered but more depressed than at baseline. This period of "postpsychotic depression" may be a time of particularly increased risk for suicide (Drake et al. 1985).

Borderline Personality

Repetitive suicide attempts or gestures form one of the diagnostic criteria for borderline personality disorder. Characteristic countertransference reactions have been proposed as another (Kernberg 1975). A frequent pattern is for a particular borderline patient to come for emergency treatment repetitively after suicide attempts that arise after interpersonal rejection, real or imagined, either in everyday life or in therapy situations. These patients frequently demand hospitalization and frequently elicit negative reactions from care givers, who do not like being threatened or manipulated any more than does anyone else (Maltsberger and Buie 1974). (See Chapter 19 for suggestions regarding the assessment and treatment of borderline patients with suicidal ideation or attempts.) Keep in mind that concomitant substance abuse or affective disorder greatly increases the risk of serious suicide attempts in borderline patients (Fyer et al. 1988).

Deliberate Self-harm Syndrome

This is a proposed syndrome that often occurs among patients with borderline personality, but that can occur among patients with other personality disorders. According to Pattison and Kahan (1983), it is characterized by

- Onset in late adolescence
- Multiple episodes of self-harm behavior
- Multiple types of self-harm behavior
- Low lethality of self-harm behavior
- Behavior continuing over many years
- Predominant psychological symptoms of despair, anxiety, anger, and cognitive constriction

- Predisposing factors of lack of social support, homosexuality, substance abuse, and suicidal ideation
- Associated depression and psychosis

The same principles outlined above for dealing with borderline patients should generally be followed in dealing with these individuals.

Substance Abuse

Substance abusers probably pose the most difficult management problems of any suicidal patients. Prospective studies of psychiatric emergency patients consistently show substance abusers to have rates of suicide as high as do depressive patients (Hillard et al. 1983). Among completed suicides in patients younger than age 30, one major study has found that the majority had a principal psychiatric diagnosis of substance abuse (Fowler et al. 1986). A common presentation is the acutely intoxicated person who has taken an overdose, or who has self-inflicted lacerations, and who after sleeping in the emergency room overnight, says he did not really intend to kill himself. If such a patient has a mental illness in addition to substance abuse, hospitalization is usually appropriate because of the difficulty in diagnosis and treatment of such dual-diagnosis patients on an outpatient basis. If there is no evidence of mental illness other than substance abuse, involuntary substance abuse treatment may be appropriate in states that permit it. In states that do not permit involuntary treatment of substance abuse with self-destructive behavior, patients with isolated episodes of suicidal behavior while intoxicated may need to be released. Repetitive self-destructive behavior while under the influence of alcohol, however, may be regarded as evidence of mental illness in addition to substance abuse.

Recent clinical research has confirmed the importance of interpersonal loss in precipitation of suicide among substance abusers (Rich et al. 1988). Substance abusers with recent losses and suicidal ideation or attempts must be regarded as at special risk of completed suicide.

LEGAL ISSUES

Courts have generally appreciated the difficulty of predicting suicide under emergency circumstances. If all the points listed in Tables 8-1 through 8-3 are discussed in the patient's chart, and the disposition is consistent with them, the clinician is unlikely to lose a judgment, even in the face of a completed suicide. Even with less extensive documentation, clinicians will probably not lose these suits as long as it is clear that they have examined the patient, made a reasonable attempt to assess risk of suicide, and formulated a consistent treatment plan. Particularly dangerous situations occur, however, if 1) there is evidence of negative feeling about the patient in the chart (e.g., "probably trying to get into the hospital to avoid going to jail"); 2) the patient requests hospitalization, and the clinician has not documented clearly why it was refused; 3) the patient had a psychiatric disorder indicating high risk for suicide, and there is no indication at all that suicide risk was assessed; and 4) important sources of collateral information were neglected (e.g., no attempt was made to contact the patient's therapist or family). Chapter 6 discusses how to deal with conflict between duty to exercise commitment laws and duty to avoid false imprisonment.

WHEN WE FAIL

In spite of our best efforts, some emergency patients will successfully kill themselves. One study has estimated that over half of all psychiatrists have had the experience of working with a patient who subsequently committed suicide (Chemtob et al. 1988). Very natural, but very maladaptive, responses to such an event include excessive self-doubt, blaming the victim, and scapegoating other staff or other agencies. Expect these reactions from your staff and from yourself. Try to objectively review the medical record and notify your legal backup, but do not allow focus on the legal issues to prevent focus on emotional responses. Facilitate open discussion of cases. Try not to withdraw from caring for severely ill patients.

REFERENCES

Advance report of final mortality statistics, 1984. Monthly Vital Statistics Report 35 (6, suppl 2), September 26, 1986

Beck AT, Schuyler D, Herman I: Development of Suicidal Intent Scale, in The Prediction of Suicide. Edited by Beck AT, Resuik HP. Bowie, MD, Charlo Press, 1974, pp 76–78

Beck AT, Kovacs M, Weisman A: Assessment of suicidal intention: the Scale for Suicide Ideation. J Consult Clin Psychol 47:343–352, 1979

Breier A, Astrachan BM: Characterization of schizophrenic patients who commit suicide. Am J Psychiatry 141:206–209, 1984

Chemtob CM, Hamada RS, Bauer G, et al: Patients' suicides: frequency and impact on psychiatrists. Am J Psychiatry 145:224–228, 1988

Clark DC, Young MA, Scheffner WA, et al: A field test of Motto's risk estimator for suicide. Am J Psychiatry 144:923–926, 1987

Coryell W, Noyes R, House JD: Mortality among outpatients with anxiety disorders. Am J Psychiatry 143:508–510, 1986

Drake RE, Gates C, Whitacker A, et al: Suicide among schizophrenics: a review. Compr Psychiatry 26:90–100, 1985

Drye RC, Goulding RL, Goulding ME: No-suicide decisions: patient monitoring of suicidal risk. Am J Psychiatry 130:171–174, 1973

Fawcett J, Scheftnor W, Clark D, et al: Clinical predictors of suicide in patients with major affective disorders: a controlled prospective study. Am J Psychiatry 144:35–40, 1987

Fowler RC, Rich CL, Young D: San Diego suicide study, II: substance abuse in young cases. Arch Gen Psychiatry 43:962–965, 1986

Fyer MR, Frances AJ, Sullivan T, et al: Suicide attempts in patients with borderline personality disorder. Am J Psychiatry 145:737–739, 1988

Hellerstein D, Frosch W, Koenigsborg HW: The clinical significance of command hallucinations. Am J Psychiatry 144:219–221, 1987

Hillard JR, Ramm D, Zung WWK, et al: Suicide in a psychiatric emergency room population. Am J Psychiatry 140:459–462, 1983

Kernberg O: Borderline Conditions and Pathological Narcissism. New York, Jason Aronson, 1975

Maltsberger JT, Buie DH: Countertransference hate in the treatment of suicidal patients. Arch Gen Psychiatry 30:625–633, 1974

Maris R: The adolescent suicide problem. Suicide Life Threat Behav 15:91–109, 1985

Martin RL, Cloninger R, Guze SB, et al: Mortality in a follow-up of 500 psychiatric out patients, II: cause-specific mortality. Arch Gen Psychiatry 42:58–66, 1985

Pattison EM, Kahan J: The deliberate self-harm syndrome. Am J Psychiatry 140:867–872, 1983

Pokorney AD: Prediction of suicide in psychiatric patients: report of a prospective study. Arch Gen Psychiatry 40:249–257, 1983

Rich CL, Fowler RC, Fogarty LA, et al: San Diego suicide study: relationship between diagnoses and stressors. Arch Gen Psychiatry 45:589–592, 1988

Roy A: Risk factors for suicide in psychiatric patients. Arch Gen Psychiatry 39:1089–1095, 1982

Roy A: Family history of suicide. Arch Gen Psychiatry 40:971–974, 1983

Rush AJ, Beck AT: Cognitive therapy of depression and suicide. Am J Psychother 32:201–219, 1978

Weissman MM: The epidemiology of suicide attempts 1960–1971. Arch Gen Psychiatry 30:737–746, 1974

Chapter 9

Medical Treatment of Overdoses

K. Merigian, M.D.

Overdose or suspected drug ingestion is a leading cause for both medical and psychiatric emergency room visits. Anyone working in emergency medicine needs to understand the basics of suicide assessment, and anyone working in emergency psychiatry needs to understand the basics of toxicology assessment.

Medical management of acute self-poisoning has become controversial over the past decade (Foulke et al. 1988; Kulig et al. 1985; Merigian et al. 1988; Wason 1987). Traditional gastric emptying procedures, use of cathartic, treatment with activated charcoal, and the therapeutic use of toxic screens have come under close scrutiny. Currently, investigators remain undecided as to universally accepted protocols for evaluation and treatment of acute self-poisoning.

The incidence of intentional overdoses seems to be on the rise. In 1984, the number of self-poisonings as reported by the American Association of Poison Control Centers (AAPCC) was 35,931 (Litovitz and Veltri 1985). The number for 1986 was 61,788 (Litovitz et al. 1987).

This brief chapter will give an overview of self-poisoning with

---

Shaded sections indicate areas of legitimate diversity of professional opinion in the literature. See Preface for further discussion.

specific focus on a general medical approach to intoxications. Detailed information concerning individual pharmaceutical agents will not generally be discussed, with the exception of those agents responsible for delayed toxicities.

AGENTS MOST COMMONLY INGESTED

Several authors have identified the most commonly ingested agents in suicidal poisoning (Brett 1988; McCoy and Trestrail 1988). Geographical location seems to alter the frequency; however, ethanol, benzodiazepines, antidepressants, anticonvulsants, nonsteroidal inflammatory agents, aspirin, acetaminophen, and nonbenzodiazepine nonbarbiturate sedative-hypnotics are most commonly ingested (Kulig et al. 1985).

Self-poisonings are almost always multiple ingestions, with ethanol being the most frequent common constituent. The central depressant effects of ethanol or sedatives and hypnotics alone are usually well tolerated; however, combination of the two can be deadly.

The 1986 AAPCC report (Litovitz et al. 1987) identified antidepressants as the major cause of mortality in poisonings, followed in order by analgesics, sedative-hypnotics, stimulants and street drugs, cardiovascular drugs, alcohols and glycols, gases and fumes, chemicals, asthma therapies, cleaning substances, insecticides, and hydrocarbons. No association was made between suicide attempt, drug ingestion, and fatality in the report. Frommer et al. (1987) reported that "cyclic antidepressants are responsible for a disproportionate share of both intensive care unit admissions and mortality when compared with other drug ingestions, and probably represent the most common life-threatening drug ingestion worldwide" (p. 521).

CLINICAL ASSESSMENT OF POISONINGS

Patients present to an emergency unit at various times in their postingestion course (Kulig et al. 1985). Most commonly, patients are initially evaluated 2–4 hours postingestion. Theoretically, patients become symptomatic at that time and seek medical attention to reverse the untoward effects of their ingestion.

Before the development of the toxic screen, clinicians depended on the clinical signs of poisoning to diagnose patients. Complete clinical assessment is essential in evaluating and treating poisonings, because treatments for most acute poisonings must be delivered before toxic screen results are available. In addition, poisons requiring antidotes (i.e., cyanide, atropine, organophosphates) are not routinely identified in most "stat" toxic screens.

The total assessment of the patient includes a precise medical history and focused clinical examination. The history should include

- Type of agents ingested
- Time of ingestion
- Amount ingested
- Symptoms pre- and postingestion
- Time since symptoms began
- Allergies
- Past medical and family history

Patients may not remember every ingested agent, or the specific time that the ingestion took place. These unknowns may not be important if the patient is asymptomatic, alert, awake, and without remarkable physical signs.

The focused clinical assessment of self-poisoning begins with the recording of vital signs and temperature. In addition, a short screening test for cognitive impairment is helpful in objectifying a decreased mental status.

Signs and Symptoms

Most commonly, poisonings are manifested in a constellation of signs and symptoms. For example, a patient who ingested an organophosphorous insecticide 1 hour before evaluation should manifest "cholinergic poisoning," i.e., salivation, lacrimation, defecation, vomiting, pinpoint pupils, bradycardia, and bronchorrhea. Physical examination should be directed to these areas. Table 9-1 shows several toxidromes (i.e., syndromes associated with poisoning) associated with intoxications. Rarely, patients may present with one sign or symptom of a toxidrome. However, these atypical presentations are difficult to diagnose and should be properly evaluated by trained medical toxicologists.

Clinical signs of poisoning are reliable indicators of ingestion and should correlate with the patient's history. Patients who remain asymptomatic and clinically stable despite massive-ingestion histories (Table 9-2) are not at risk for delayed compromise, except in the case of drugs that "slow release" or have late toxicities, discussed later in this chapter.

Table 9-1. Common poisons and their associated toxidromes

Poison	Symptoms and signs
Analgesics	
Acetaminophen	Abdominal pains, nausea, vomiting, anorexia (acute signs)
Aspirin	Hyperventilation, flushing, elevated temperature, tinnitus, nausea, vomiting
Narcotics	
Heroin, morphine, codeine, meperidine (Demerol)	Pinpoint pupils, decreased respirations, hypotension, coma
Antidepressants	
Cyclic antidepressants	Decreased mental status, tachycardia, hyperreflexia, cardiac conduction delay, seizures
Monoamine oxidase inhibitors	Delayed toxicity, hypertension, tachycardia, muscular rigidity, hyperthermia
Lithium	Decreased mental status, hyperreflexia, nausea, vomiting, polyuria, tremor, coma, seizures
Sedatives and hypnotics	
Benzodiazepines	Coma, normal blood pressure, normal pulse, decreased reflexes
Barbiturates	Decreased mental status, coma, hypotension, decreased aspirations, blisters, hypothermia
Nonbarbiturates	Fluctuating coma, decreased reflexes, decreased respirations, hypothermia

Cholinergic agents
Organophosphates, carbamates

Bradycardia, constricted pupils, salivation, lacrimation, bronchorrea, defecation

Anticholinergic agents
Atropine, scopolamine

Tachycardia, dilated pupils, fever, agitation, delirium, dry skin, dry mucous membranes

Table 9-2. Definition of asymptomatic overdose

	Yes	No
Vital signs		
Is systolic blood pressure between 160 and 110 mmHg?	___	___
Is diastolic blood pressure between 100 and 60 mmHg?	___	___
Are respirations between 8 and 20?	___	___
Is pulse between 60 and 110?	___	___
Is temperature between 99.5°F and 97.5°F?	___	___
Cognitive examination		
Is the patient's cognitive examination intact grossly?	___	___

If all questions are answered Yes, the patient is an asymptomatic overdose.

Source. Adapted from Merigian et al. 1988.

TREATMENT OF ACUTE OVERDOSE

Traditional management of acute overdoses has included gastric-emptying procedures, use of cathartics, and activated charcoal and antidote delivery ("General Consideration" 1986; Boehnert et al. 1985). Most patients tolerate self-poisonings well, and mortality from poisonings is less than 1% if the patient reaches the hospital; of patients who die, most die before reaching a health-care facility (Callaham and Kassel 1985). With the advent of supportive care equipment (ventilators, pharmaceutical agents for blood pressure control, dialysis, hemoperfusion, cardiac monitors, and portable electroencephalographs and X-ray machines), we rarely witness severe physiologic compromise that cannot be normalized.

Gastric emptying was first noted as a recognized therapy for overdoses and self-poisoning before the twentieth century. In 1895, German physicians used a rubber tube with a bulb pump to empty gastric contents in overdoses. Since that time, routine gastric emptying has been practiced without hesitation if patients present to physicians with even the slightest history of drug ingestion. Standard gastric-emptying procedures including induced emesis from syrup of ipecac or large-bore nasogastric tube lavage have been utilized to help decontaminate the stomach. Both of these procedures have associated risks, and neither can be used in every patient. After gastric emptying, further stomach decontamination is achieved with administration of oral activated charcoal. Many physicians use cathartics to "purge" the poison and poison-charcoal complex from the intestine.

Routine gastric emptying has come under close investigation by several investigators (Foulke et al. 1988; Kulig et al. 1985; Merigian et al. 1988; Wason 1987). In a prospective randomized study of 738 overdoses, gastric emptying did not shorten symptomatic patients' course of illness in the emergency room or hospital when compared with charcoal therapy alone (Merigian et al. 1988). It appears that gastric emptying is not needed in every overdose. More data are needed to characterize patients who will benefit from it.

Ipecac use or gastric lavage should be used in an emergency room setting with direct physician supervision. Because the efficacy of gastric emptying is questionable, psychiatrists should not use these procedures routinely in their evaluation and treatment of overdose. The only instances when gastric emptying may be helpful are those when patients have ingested drugs not absorbed by charcoal (i.e., lithium or iron) or the poisons themselves cause delayed gastric emptying (i.e., jimsonweed).

We believe that 50–100 g of oral activated charcoal is sufficient therapy in most reported overdoses. In cases of decreased mental status or coma, naloxone and dextrose should be given as well as oral activated charcoal. "Medical clearance" should translate to a patient with normal vital signs and normal cognitive function. Patients with abnormal vital signs such as tachycardia, hypo- or hypertension, fever, or decreased mental status should be admitted for medical observation and supportive therapy.

Antidotes

There are few agents that have been approved for use as antidotes in acute poisonings (Table 9-3). Oral activated charcoal has been mislabeled as an antidote, as it does not "reverse" the acute effects of poisoning. Heightened clinical suspicion and history are the only diagnostic aids in poisonings requiring antidote delivery.

With the exception of short-acting narcotic overdose, most patients requiring antidotal therapy should be admitted to a medical observation area for a 24-hour evaluation period. In addition, patients who overdose on hypoglycemic agents (insulin injections or oral hypoglycemic agents) should also be admitted.

Physostigmine is a reversible cholinesterase inhibitor that reverses central and peripheral signs of anticholinergic poisoning (Taylor 1985). In skilled hands, the use of this agent in suspected overdose is safe and effective (Walker et al. 1976). However, cardiac monitoring, blood pressure measurement, and close physiologic observation should be undertaken while the drug is administered. We believe physostigmine should be used by toxicologists and trained emergency physicians if the diagnosis of anticholinergic poisoning is entertained.

DELAYED TOXICITY

Medical clearance of most reported or alleged overdoses usually requires observation, supportive care, and antidote delivery when appro-

Table 9-3. Commonly ingested drugs and their antidotes with dosages

Intoxicant	Antidote	Dosage
Organophosphates	Atropine	1–2 mg iv, repeat until eyes dilate
Carbamates	Pralidoxime	1–2 g iv over 5 minutes
Iron	Deferoxamine mesylate	15 mg/kg body wt per hour iv
Digoxin	Fab fragment	65 mg/1 mg digoxin
Methanol	Ethanol	Maintain 100 mg/dl iv
Beta-blockers	Glucagon	1–5 mg iv
Opiates, narcotics	Naloxone	2 mg iv
Atropine, scopolamine	Physostigmine	1–2 mg iv
Carbon monoxide	Oxygen	100% mask or hyperbaric chamber
Benzodiazepines	Flumazenil	Dosage still being studied

priate. An unfounded fear of the clinician is the return of toxic signs or symptoms despite adequate treatment and evaluation.

There are few agents that will allow presentation of an asymptomatic patient 6 hours postingestion. *Amanita* (mushroom) poisoning, diphenoxylate (Lomotil) ingestion, monoamine oxidase inhibitor intoxication, acetaminophen poisoning, iron ingestion, cyclic antidepressant overdose, and nonbarbiturate sedative and hypnotic intoxication have all been implicated in "delayed" toxicities. Few authors have been able to adequately characterize any of these agents as causing delayed signs or symptoms from an asymptomatic state.

Cyclic antidepressants have been implicated in sudden-death episodes as few as 24 hours postingestion to 7 days postingestion (Nicotta et al. 1981; Serafimovski et al. 1975). Many authors have investigated these anecdotal reports. Recent work by Pentel and Sioris (1977) and Callaham and Kassel (1985) has shown no sudden-death syndrome as a manifestation of delayed cyclic antidepressant poisoning. In fact, if after 6 hours of observation the patient is asymptomatic from an overdose of cyclic antidepressants, no problems related to the ingestion will be later identified.

Reports of patients having asymptomatic presentations followed by "crashing" are usually misrepresented. These reports usually downplay the sleepy or minimally symptomatic presentation and focus on the "shock state." If one scrutinizes these case reports, patients had early signs of poisoning, and poisoning progressed in an unusually slow fashion. In fact, the only true reports of delayed toxicities have been identified in *Amanita* poisonings and monoamine oxidase inhibitor intoxications (Linden et al. 1984; Olson et al. 1982).

Physicians should be aware of delayed toxicities as manifested in sustained-release tablet ingestion, or "enteric-coated" ingestions. However, asymptomatic subclinical or subacute poisoning requires observation and charcoal administration.

REFERENCES

Boehnert MT, Lewander WJ, Gaudreau HP, et al: Advances in clinical toxicology. Pediatr Clin North Am 32:193–211, 1985

Brett A: Implications of discordance between clinical impression and toxicology analysis in drug overdose. Arch Intern Med 148:437–441, 1988

Callaham M, Kassel D: Epidemiology of fatal tricyclic antidepressant ingestion: implications for management. Ann Emerg Med 14:1–9, 1985

Foulke GE, Albertson TE, Derlet RW: Use of ipecac increases emergency department stays and patient complication rates (abstract). Ann Emerg Med 17:165, 1988

Frommer PA, Kulig KW, Marx JA, et al: Tricyclic antidepressant overdose: a review, JAMA 257:521–526, 1987

General consideration of poisoning, in Poisoning Toxicology, Symptoms, Treatment. Edited by Arena JM, Drew RH. Springfield, IL, Charles C Thomas, 1986, pp 3–173

Kulig K, Bar-or D, Cantrill SV, et al: Management of acutely poisoned patients without gastric emptying. Ann Emerg Med 14:562–567, 1985

Linden CH, Rumack BH, Strehlke C: Monoamine oxidase inhibitor overdose. Ann Emerg Med 13:1137–1144, 1984

Litovitz T, Veltri JC: 1984 annual report of the American Association of Poison Control Centers national data collection system. Am J Emerg Med 3:423–450, 1985

Litovitz T, Martin T, Schmitz B: 1986 annual report of the American Association of Poison Control Centers national data collection system. Am J Emerg Med 5:405–445, 1987

McCoy D, Trestrail J: Finding of ten years of clinical drug screening. Vet Hum Toxicol 30:34–38, 1988

Merigian KS, Hedges JR, Pesce A, et al: Prospective evaluation of gastric emptying in self poisoned patient (abstract). Ann Emerg Med 17:165, 1988

Nicotta MB, Rivera M, Pool JL, et al: TCA overdose: clinical and pharmacologic observations. Clinical Toxicology 18:599–613, 1981

Olson KR, Pond SM, Seward J, et al: *Amanita phalloides*, type mushroom poisoning. West J Med 137:282–289, 1982

Pentel P, Sioris L: Incidence of late arrhythmias following TCA overdose. Clinical Toxicology 10:149–158, 1977

Serafimovski N, Thorball N, Asmussen I, et al: Tricyclic antidepressive poisoning with special references to cardiac complications. Acta Anaesthesiol Scand [Suppl] 57:55–63, 1975

Taylor P: Anticholinesterase agent, in The Pharmacological Basis of Therapeutics. Edited by Goodman LS, Gilman AG, Rall TW, et al. New York, Macmillan, 1985, pp 110–129

Walker WE, Levy RC, Hanenson IB: Physostigmine, its use and abuse. JACEP 5:436–439, 1976

Wason S: Gastrointestinal decontamination of the poisoned patient—a critical review. Drugs of Today 23:455–465, 1987

Chapter 10

Mood Syndromes

J.R. Hillard, M.D.

Mood (or affective) syndromes are among the most common problems leading to emergency treatment. They are among the most lethal problems treated by psychiatrists and can result from a wide variety of causes. Appropriate emergency treatment must be based on rapid and accurate assessment of the severity of a given mood syndrome and on an understanding of disorders that may underlie a specific presentation.

This chapter will use the following terms as defined in DSM-III-R (American Psychiatric Association 1987, pp. 213–214):

- "A *mood syndrome* . . . is a group of mood and associated symptoms that occur together for [at least] a minimal duration of time" (e.g., major depressive syndrome, manic or hypomanic syndrome).
- "A *mood episode* . . . is a mood syndrome that is not due to a known organic factor and is not part of a nonmood psychotic disorder."
- "A *mood disorder* is determined by the pattern of mood episodes. For example, the diagnosis of major depression is made when there have been one or more major depressive episodes without a history of manic or unequivocal hypomanic episode."

Shaded sections indicate areas of legitimate diversity of professional opinion in the literature. See Preface for further discussion.

Each mood syndrome will be delineated. The underlying disorders that can cause each syndrome will be discussed, and the emergency treatment implications for each syndrome will be outlined.

MAJOR DEPRESSIVE SYNDROME

Major depressive syndrome is characterized by a history of at least 2 weeks of either 1) depressed mood most of the day, nearly every day, or 2) markedly diminished interest or pleasure in all, or almost all, activities most of the day, nearly every day. A diagnosis of major depressive syndrome requires that at least five depressive symptoms have been present nearly every day during the same 2-week period. Depressive symptoms, in addition to those above, are 3) significant weight loss or appetite changes, 4) insomnia or hypersomnia, 5) psychomotor agitation or retardation, 6) fatigue or loss of energy, 7) feelings of worthlessness or guilt, 8) decreased concentration or indecisiveness, and 9) recurrent thoughts of death or suicide.

Assessment

In assessing depressive syndromes, as in other interviews, it is generally best to let patients describe their condition in their own words first, to ask for clarification of specific symptoms alluded to, and to probe for characteristic symptoms not mentioned spontaneously. It is most important to distinguish depressive syndromes from subclinical mood fluctuations, and to distinguish mild from severe depressive syndromes. These distinctions may be difficult to make due to the diverse ways patients with different personality styles tend to present their symptoms. Assessment may also, at times, be difficult due to a patient's intentionally misleading the clinician (e.g., to avoid or to precipitate hospitalization). Most depressive symptoms can be assessed only by history, and not by examination. Whenever possible, independent confirmation of symptom severity and duration should be sought (e.g., from family members). The patient's behavior during the interview may also help to confirm the character of the symptoms. Bright affect during the interview is usually not consistent with a protracted mood of depression. Careful tracking of the interview by the patient is not consistent with extreme inability to concentrate. Psychomotor changes are extremely difficult to simulate or to override and, therefore, serve as a good indication of a true depression.

In every patient with depressive syndrome, the following need to be assessed:

- Suicidal ideation (see Chapter 8)
- Violent or homicidal ideation, a frequently overlooked concomitant (Rosenbaum and Bennett 1986)
- Severity of syndrome, as measured by symptoms and, perhaps more important, by degree of functional impairment
- Presence of psychotic symptoms, either mood congruent (e.g., delusions of guilt, disease, or punishment) or mood incongruent (e.g., thought insertion or persecutory delusions without depressive themes)
- Presence of medical disorders

Differential Diagnosis

A major depressive syndrome is not classified as an episode of a major depressive or bipolar disorder if the syndrome is 1) due to an organic mood disorder, 2) due to uncomplicated bereavement, or 3) superimposed on a psychotic disorder (including schizoaffective disorder).

Organic mood syndrome. An enormous number of physical conditions and an enormous number of drugs have been associated with depressive syndromes (McNeil 1987). The literature on this subject, however, must be regarded with some skepticism because much of it is based on small numbers of case reports, many of them failing to distinguish between major depressive syndromes and other nonspecific depressive reactions. Depressive symptoms are a likely consequence of any number of life stresses and disappointments, including physical illnesses. Furthermore, major depression is common enough (2–8% prevalence in the general population [Helzer et al. 1985]) that it is likely, by chance, to have co-occurred with most of the more common medical problems and medications. With these caveats in mind, the following causes of organic depressive disorder should be considered, particularly in patients with atypical presentation (e.g., depression plus features of dementia) or in patients in whom there is a clear temporal relationship of medical and depressive symptoms.

- *Medications.* The medications listed in Table 10-1 are those most convincingly associated with depression. Other medications, including oral contraceptives (McNeil 1987), may be associated with individual cases. Patients taking any of the medications in Table 10-1 or other medications that seem to bear a clear temporal relationship to depressive symptoms should be started on antidepressant treatment only after careful consideration has been given to their existing

Table 10-1. Drugs most convincingly associated with major depressive syndrome

• Cardiovascular medications	• Neurologic medications
Reserpine	Barbiturates
Methyldopa	Ethosuximide
Clonidine	Baclofen
Propranolol	L-Dopa
• Anti-inflammatory medications	• Anticancer medications
Steroids	Decarbazine
Indomethacin	Hexamethylamine
Sulindac	Vincristine
• Psychotropic medications	Vinblastine
Antipsychotics	L-Asparaginase
Benzodiazepines	• Gastrointestinal medications
Disulfiram	Cimetidine

Source. Adapted from Estroff and Gold 1986.

medication regimen. This will ordinarily entail consultation with patients' other physicians and ordinarily cannot be done on an emergency basis.

• *Physical illness.* Secondary depression can develop in the context of any physical illness. Table 10-2 lists illnesses that may have a physical role in initiating and maintaining a major depressive syndrome. If a patient who is known to have one of these disorders has developed depression, the possibility of an organic mood syndrome should be considered. (The special problems of diagnosing depression in the face of dementia are discussed in Chapter 12.) When depression is an early symptom, the underlying illness usually will not present a classic picture that can be diagnosed during the emergency encounter, and the confirmatory laboratory findings will usually not be ready soon enough to help with emergency decision making either.

A reasonable approach to screening for physical illnesses in depressed patients should include 1) vital signs, 2) a survey of past medical history, and 3) a review of symptoms. If the patient has abnormal vital signs, a history of illnesses that can cause mood syndromes, or an unusual pattern of physical complaints, a physical examination and screening laboratory tests (e.g., complete blood count, electrolytes, blood glucose, blood urea nitrogen or creatinine, and possibly a urinalysis or chest X ray) should be completed. It is not as important to make a definitive diagnosis as it is to make sure that

Table 10-2. Common medical disorders most convincingly associated with depressive presentations

● Endocrine	● Infections
Diabetes mellitus	Viral hepatitis
Hyper- or hypofunction of the thyroid	Viral encephalitis
Hyper- or hypofunction of the parathyroid	Viral pneumonia
Hyper- or hypofunction of the adrenal cortex	● Neoplastic
(i.e., Cushing's or Addison's disease)	Pancreatic cancer
● Central nervous system	Other neoplasms
Parkinson's disease	● Metabolic
Multiple sclerosis	Uremia
Myasthenia gravis	Hyponatremia
Huntington's chorea	Hypo- or
Stroke	hyperkalemia
Tumors	● Other
Wilson's disease	Systemic lupus
Dementia	erythematosus
Cardiopulmonary hypoxia	Rheumatoid arthritis
	Nutritional
	deficiencies

Source. Adapted from McNeil 1987 and Hall 1980.

patients with severe medical or surgical problems are admitted to those services instead of to psychiatry, and to make sure that the inpatient or outpatient facilities to which patients are referred will complete a more detailed physical evaluation. (See Chapter 2 for more discussion of physical assessment.)

● *Psychoactive substance use disorders.* Fifty percent or more of alcoholic patients suffer from short periods of severe affective disturbances, often with suicidal ideation. Persistent alcohol abuse may lead to a full-blown depressive syndrome. Such alcohol-induced syndromes, however, generally clear rapidly on cessation of drinking, even without psychotropic medication (Schuckit 1985). Abuse of other sedative-hypnotics and opiates is also associated with organic affective syndromes which may clear with the cessation of substance abuse (Rousaville et al. 1982). Withdrawal from amphetamines (Schuckit 1984) or cocaine (Gawin and Kleber 1986) and other stimulants (including those available over-the-counter, such as phenylpropanolamine) is also commonly associated with affective symptoms that frequently meet criteria for major depressive syndrome.

   History of psychoactive substance abuse must be carefully searched for in all patients with depressive symptoms, and detoxification should generally be completed before initiation of antidepressant medication.

Uncomplicated bereavement. Death of a loved one can be associated with symptoms of great enough severity and duration to qualify as a major depressive syndrome. Ordinarily, however, uncomplicated bereavement is not associated with extreme feelings of worthlessness or guilt, and the degree of the patient's reaction is regarded as "within normal limits" by the patient and family. If symptoms of a major depressive disorder persist more than a few weeks, or if they are worsening over a period of weeks, a major depression may have arisen out of the grief reaction and will probably need to be treated. Treatment of grief reactions will be discussed later in this chapter.

Depression superimposed on psychosis. Major depressive syndromes develop frequently in patients with psychotic disorders. DSM-III-R does not allow a diagnosis of major depressive disorder in such patients. They must be diagnosed as depression not otherwise specified or as schizoaffective disorder. The period immediately after recovery from psychosis may be a time of particular risk for depression (Siris et al. 1984). Depressive symptoms are a source of considerable morbidity and, in fact, mortality among psychotic patients. As noted in Chapter 8, suicide risk can be difficult to assess in psychotic patients, and hospitalization or other intensive treatment referral must be considered.

Dysthymia. Dysthymia is characterized by depressed mood and symptoms most of the day, more days than not, for at least a 2-year period, without a major depressive episode during the first 2 years, and without a history of mania or hypomania. Dysthymic symptoms wax and wane, and it is not uncommon for a major depressive episode to develop on top of a dysthymic episode (so-called double depression [Miller et al. 1986]). When symptoms worsen, requests for emergency psychiatric treatment are common. Dysthymia is frequently associated with personality disorders and, unless complicated by development of a major depressive disorder, should be treated in a similar manner to a personality disorder, i.e., as an acute manifestation of a chronic problem. If the patient can be helped to see the chronic nature of the problem rather than be allowed to focus solely on the recent precipitants for its worsening, referral for ongoing treatment may be facilitated. Cyclothymia, i.e., 2 years of alternating dysthymic and hypomanic (see below) symptoms, is usually best approached in a similar manner.

ADJUSTMENT DISORDER WITH DEPRESSED MOOD

Adjustment disorder with depressed mood refers to a depressive reaction to identifiable psychosocial stressors that occurs within 3 months of onset of the stressors, has persisted for 6 months or less, and does not meet criteria for any other specific mental disorder. By definition, an adjustment disorder must cause impairment in occupational or social functioning or in relationships with others. At times, adjustment disorders may be associated with serious suicide risk and may necessitate hospitalization. The diagnosis should not be used for episodes that are merely one instance of a pattern of overreactions to stress.

An adjustment disorder can be conceptualized as a failure to cope with stressors in a patient's usual ways. With prompt treatment, a patient may be able to develop better coping skills than before. If treatment is delayed, a patient may develop chronic maladaptive coping strategies. Treatment of adjustment disorders should be started as soon as possible after their onset. This is an important indication for at least a few sessions of treatment in the emergency setting. Adjustment disorders present a situation in which therapy delayed is therapy denied. (See Chapter 17 for a discussion of adjustment disorder with anxious mood.)

EMERGENCY TREATMENT OF DEPRESSIVE SYNDROMES

Emergency treatment of depressive syndromes is more related to severity and to degree of suicide risk than it is to specific etiology. If there is a major risk of suicide (see Chapter 8), inpatient psychiatric treatment is necessary. Hospitalization may also be required if 1) the patient has a medical problem (e.g., severe cardiac conduction abnormality) that would complicate outpatient treatment; 2) outpatient treatment has been tried and failed; 3) the patient is unable to care for self or family; 4) substance abuse is complicating treatment; or 5) depression is severe, and outpatient resources are not realistically available.

Outpatient referrals need to be made forcefully. Depressed patients do not have enough energy for anything—not even for seeking treatment. They are not able to believe that anything can make the future better— not even treatment. It is not surprising that they frequently fail to follow through with outpatient referral. When referring depressed patients, it is important to 1) express confidence that treatment can help them; 2) express confidence in the facility or person (preferably the latter) that they are referred to; 3) involve family members in support of the patient until the appointment and in making sure that the patient keeps the appointment; and 4) follow up by phone to see if the referral has been completed.

If outpatient treatment is not immediately available, acutely depressed patients should be asked to return to the emergency room for ongoing evaluation and treatment until a referral can be completed. This is necessary because depressed patients are at continuing risk for becoming suicidal, because they are easily discouraged by obstacles such as waiting lists, and because they are often socially withdrawn and need considerable encouragement to approach another therapist.

Treatment of Uncomplicated Bereavement

Ordinarily, it is best to help the patient and family to conceptualize bereavement as normal, to encourage family support, and to encourage participation in funerals and other religious rituals related to the death of a loved one. At times, it is appropriate to prescribe benzodiazepines, particularly for sleep, for patients whose level of anxiety makes it impossible for them to deal with funerals or to do the work involved in dealing with the death. At times, it is also important to deal with maladaptive family reactions to a death, such as projection of everyone's feelings of inability to cope onto one individual who is scapegoated and designated as the patient.

Normal grief reactions can be complicated by ambivalent feelings toward the loved one, by family conflicts, by secrets involving the loved one, or by traumatic circumstances surrounding the loss (Melges and DeMaso 1980). Such problems, and others, may give rise to unresolved grief reactions that may be prolonged, delayed, or distorted (Lindamann 1944). Distorted grief reactions may give rise to major depressive disorders, generalized anxiety disorder, or posttraumatic stress disorder (see Chapter 17). It is very important to distinguish between normal grief reactions, which usually do not require specific mental health interventions, and complicated reactions that are likely to become worse without specific intervention (Barry 1981).

If the grief reaction has been delayed more than about 3 months or has persisted without signs of improvement for more than about 3 months, a complicated reaction should be strongly suspected. An outpatient referral for short-term supportive therapy should ordinarily be offered to anyone who has felt it necessary to seek emergency evaluation for symptoms related to grief.

Starting Tricyclics From the Emergency Room

There is a lot to be said against starting tricyclic antidepressants from the emergency room: 1) The drugs are a bad overdose. 2) The full therapeutic effect will not be evident in most cases for 2 or more weeks. 3) The medications have many side effects. 4) Patients often conceal substance abuse problems that may underlie a depressive syndrome, and for which tricyclics may not be indicated. 5) It is difficult to rule out physical causes of depression on an outpatient basis. 6) The clinician to whom the patient is referred for ongoing care should optimally have a chance to see the patient unmedicated and to choose the medication to be used. 7) Depression often remits spontaneously.

On the other hand: 1) It is often impossible to complete an outpatient referral for several weeks or more, particularly in the public sector. 2) It is not really humane to leave patients in a depressed state any longer than is avoidable. 3) If prescribed in small doses, tricyclics are not a life-threatening overdose. 4) Problems of side effects and differential diagnosis may not be much worse from the emergency room than they are from the outpatient clinic. 5) Diagnosis and treatment of depression is now standard enough that clinicians receiving a referral are likely to view the illness in a similar way to the referring clinicians.

We take the position that if a patient can be seen within a few days by a clinician who can follow the patient on an ongoing basis, it is better to allow that clinician to start medication. If a patient cannot be seen that rapidly, starting tricyclics from the emergency service can be appropriate if 1) the patient can be assessed for physical causes of depression as described above, 2) ongoing substance abuse can be ruled out, 3) the patient has a major depressive disorder rather than a dysthymia, 4) the patient can be followed in the emergency setting until picked up by another agency.

MANIC AND HYPOMANIC SYNDROME

Manic syndrome is characterized by abnormally and/or persistently elevated expansive or (perhaps most often) irritable mood, along with three or four, if mood is only irritable, of the following symptoms:

- Grandiosity
- Decreased need for sleep
- Pressure of speech
- Flight of ideas
- Distractibility
- Increased activity
- Irresponsible activities

If the disturbance is severe enough to cause marked impairment in occupational or social functioning, a manic syndrome is present; if not, a hypomanic syndrome is present.

Differential Diagnosis

A manic syndrome is not classified as an episode of mood disorder if the syndrome is due to organic affective syndrome, which can be caused by the same spectrum of physical illnesses as can major depressive syndrome (Krauthammer and Klerman 1978), or if it is superimposed on a psychotic disorder, including schizoaffective disorder.

Acute mania is often associated with psychotic features, either mood congruent (e.g., related to inflated sense of worth, power, knowledge, or identity or special relationship to a deity or famous person) or mood incongruent. Differentiation from other acute psychotic syndromes can be difficult, as discussed in Chapter 16, and is, at times, not possible in an emergency situation.

Medicating manic or hypomanic patients on an outpatient basis usually does not work well. The acute effects of either antipsychotic drugs or lithium are usually felt by the patient to be unpleasant, and compliance rates can be low. Inpatient treatment is usually preferable to outpatient treatment. If a manic patient refuses hospitalization and does not meet state commitment laws, antipsychotic medications are probably a better choice acutely than is lithium because they bring about symptom control more rapidly and may be experienced as producing less dysphoria than lithium.

References

American Psychiatric Association: Diagnostic and Statistical Manual of Mental Disorders, 3rd Edition, Revised. Washington, DC, American Psychiatric Association, 1987

Barry MJ: Therapeutic experience with patients referred for prolonged grief reactions. Mayo Clin Proc 56:744–748, 1981

Estroff TW, Gold MS: Medication-induced and toxin-induced psychiatric disorders, in Medical Mimics of Psychiatric Disorders. Edited by Extein I, Gold MS. Washington, DC, American Psychiatric Press, 1986, pp 163–198

Gawin FH, Kleber HD: Abstinence symptomatology and psychiatric diagnosis in cocaine abusers: clinical observations. Arch Gen Psychiatry 43:107–113, 1986

Hall RCW: Depression in Psychiatric Presentations of Medical Illness: Somatopsychic Disorders. Edited by Hall RCW. Jamaica, NY, Spectrum Press, 1980, pp 37–63

Helzer JE, Robins LN, McEvoy LT, et al: A comparison of clinical and Diagnostic Interview Schedule diagnoses: physician reexamination of lay-interviewed cases in the general population. Arch Gen Psychiatry 42:657–666, 1985

Krauthammer C, Klerman GL: Secondary mania: manic syndromes associated with antecedent physical illness or drugs. Arch Gen Psychiatry 35:1333–1339, 1978

Lindamann E: Symptomatology and management of acute grief. Am J Psychiatry 101:141–148, 1944

McNeil GN: Depression, in Handbook of Psychiatric Differential Diagnosis. Edited by Soreff SM, McNeil GN. Littleton, MA, PSG Publishing, 1987, pp 57–126

Melges FT, DeMaso DR: Grief resolution therapy: reliving, revising and revisiting. Am J Psychother 34:51–61, 1980

Miller IW, Norman WH, Dow MG: Psychosocial characteristics of double depression. Am J Psychiatry 143:1042–1044, 1986

Rosenbaum M, Bennett B: Homicide and depression. Am J Psychiatry 143:367–370, 1986

Rousaville BJ, Weissman MM, Crits-Christoph K, et al: Diagnosis and symptoms of depression in opiate addicts. Arch Gen Psychiatry 39:151–156, 1982

Schuckit MA: Drug and Alcohol Abuse: A Clinical Guide to Diagnosis and Treatment, 2nd Edition. New York, Plenum, 1984, pp 97–99

Schuckit MA: The clinical implications of primary diagnostic groups among alcoholics. Arch Gen Psychiatry 42:1043–1049, 1985

Siris SG, Rifkis A, Reardon ET, et al: Course-related depressive syndromes in schizophrenia. Am J Psychiatry 141:1254–1257, 1984

Chapter 11

Violence

J. Parks, M.D.

Violence to self or others is a common cause for psychiatric emergency service visits. Violence toward oneself—suicide—is discussed in Chapter 8. However, remember that 16–27% of violent psychiatric patients have been reported also to be suicidal (Skodol and Karasu 1978; Tardiff and Sweillam 1980).

Earlier research reported that the mentally ill are less likely to be violent than the general population. However, this was based on police reports and arrest records, and many violent acts never reach the attention of police because charges are not brought because the person is "ill." More recent findings do not support the proposition that the mentally ill are less violent, but offer no support that they are more violent. Overall, reports of assaultiveness in psychiatric emergency patients have ranged from 4 to 60% (Rossi et al. 1985; Skodol and Karasu 1978; Tardiff and Sweillam 1980); most report that around one-third of admissions are preceded by violence (Jacobs 1983).

Shaded sections indicate areas of legitimate diversity of professional opinion in the literature. See Preface for further discussion.

PREDICTION OF VIOLENCE

Since the early 1970s, the conventional wisdom has been that psychiatrists and psychologists have no expertise in predicting violence and are wrong twice as often as they are correct in their predictions (Dubin 1981). However, the studies that led to these conclusions were all based on attempts to predict violence to be committed in a community during a period of years after institutionalization. It is not surprising that such attempts were unsuccessful (Monahan 1984). The actual clinical task in emergency psychiatry is to predict violence over a period of hours or days, rather than years, and that is much less difficult. Several studies have indicated that some reasonable short-term prediction of violence is, in fact, possible (Rofman et al. 1980; Rossi et al. 1985; Yesavage et al. 1982).

Risk of violence among psychiatric patients has been associated with the following factors:

- *Demographic*—male, young (15–24 years old), poor, uneducated, unemployed, minority, no supportive social network (Skodol and Karasu 1978)
- *Diagnostic*—organic brain syndrome (including intoxications), psychosis, personality disorders (discussed at length later in this chapter)
- *Past history*—violence, early victimization
- *Psychological*—low frustration tolerance, low self-esteem, low tolerance for interpersonal closeness, low tolerance for criticism, tendency toward projection and externalization

INTERVIEW OF PATIENTS AT RISK TO BECOME VIOLENT

Predictors of Potential Violence During the Interview

Patients very seldom become acutely violent without some period of building tension and escalation of threatening behavior. The following clues suggest a serious risk of violence within the next few minutes:

- Posture—sitting on the edge of the chair, gripping armrests
- Speech—increasingly loud, strident, or profane

- Pacing—increased motor restlessness
- Affect—angry or irritable
- Increased startle reflex
- Loss of "directability," i.e., unable or unwilling to attempt to follow directions
- Agitated, intoxicated, or paranoid state
- Violent acts in the very recent past
- Motor tension—clenched fist or jaw

Physically Approaching the Patient

- Always remember that your body posture, facial expression, and voice tone are still understood even by patients so impaired by delirium, psychosis, anger, or fear that they cannot process and understand your words.
- Allow more physical space than usual. Kinzel (1970) reports that the body buffer zone, the area where if intruded on one feels the other person is too close, is four times larger in violent than in nonviolent persons and is greater to the rear than to the front, a reversal of the pattern in nonviolent people. Therefore, do not approach patients from behind; however, do not face them directly because this can be perceived as confrontational.
- Be careful about direct eye contact, which can also be experienced as confrontational or invasive.
- Keep your hands to the midline of your body where they will be more ready to ward off a blow, but do not fold them akimbo or at your waist, which is again confrontational.
- Keep your facial expression neutral, accepting, and attentive.
- To avoid being in easy striking range, stand either close side by side where you will be difficult to swing at or at least 1½ arms' length away so the patient will have to move toward you to strike.
- Never turn your back, and stay near the door or an escape route. If you must retreat rapidly, do not turn to run, making yourself easy to grab from behind; do not attempt to run backward, making yourself easy to knock over. You should turn sideways, presenting a smaller body profile of less vulnerable anatomy as a target. Keep your eyes on the assailant and your arms up in front of your face and neck without closing your fists. Then move rapidly away from the assailant by moving your foot nearest him or her across behind your other foot and then moving the front foot across in front away from your assailant and repeat the pattern. This allows you to retreat rapidly while

protecting yourself, to look quickly where you are going, and to return your attention to the assailant without turning your whole body. Practice this before attempting it during an actual assault.

- Ideally, you and the patient should be equal distance from the door so the patient will not feel "cornered." If the physical shape of the interview room makes this impossible, consider conducting the interview in an open area. If there is no choice but that either you or the patient be nearer the door, however, let it be you.
- Potentially violent patients should be placed in a quiet area of the emergency room where they can be constantly observed. They should not be near patients who are agitated or disturbing and they should not be alone and unobserved.
- Sometimes patients will behave in a more aggressive or more threatened way around staff who are the same sex as themselves or sometimes around staff of the opposite sex. If this seems to be the case, try to assign a staff member of the sex that the patient is less agitated by.

Verbally Approaching the Patient

- The interview should be pursued in a calm, direct, reassuring manner. Convey an attitude of respect and the expectation of good behavior.
- Referring to patients by surname with title, e.g., Mr./Ms./Mrs., is preferred to first names.
- Be ready to explain your own behavior and find an opportunity to do so. This will make the patient feel more in control by knowing and understanding what to expect.
- If the patient is psychotic or intoxicated or has an organic brain syndrome, keep your questions, requests, and comments very simple and brief and repeat information to the patient several times.
- Inquire about and encourage verbal expression of feelings. This will reduce the pressure to express them in action as well as expand your information base.
- Constantly clarify that talking and feeling are acceptable but that acting violently is not.
- Make it clear that the patient will be held responsible for his or her actions.
- Encourage *detailed* fantasies of the results of uncontrolled rage, especially consequences such as police, courts, and prison.
- Acknowledge the patient's ability to harm others, then establish your position that this would not be acceptable and that the staff will act to

prevent harm to the patient or to others. Do not let this sound like a threat, but state it as a matter of fact and balance it with a statement that you will do what you can to help.

"Counterprojective" Approaches

Havens (1980) has used what he terms counterprojective remarks to diminish the adversarial aspect of the interaction and to build an alliance. Clinicians must assume on the basis of stimulus generalization that they will be seen as part of the hostile and threatening world the patient is fighting against. They must verbally and psychically remove themselves from the camp of the enemy to the position of the patient's ally. This is accomplished by means of a verbal strategy with three components: 1) The remarks should point "out there" away from the clinician and the patient. 2) A perceived enemy "out there" that is not present in the emergency room should be talked about. 3) Feelings about this enemy similar to the patient's should be expressed. For example, after the police have brought the patient and departed, the clinician might say, "The police don't give anyone a chance, four of them against one of you doesn't seem fair." Such remarks should, obviously, not reinforce frank delusions that the patient has and should not appear to sanction physical violence toward outside individuals. A related approach to making yourself a smaller target for projection is commenting on similarities that you and the patient share (e.g., same sports-team preferences, being married, having children).

Other Strategies to Minimize Patient Threat

Sometimes utilizing an appeal to narcissism will redirect the patient, especially in personality-disordered patients with a lack of conscience: "That guy's trying to provoke you into attacking him so he can have the police put you in jail, why give him the satisfaction?" (Rosenbaum and Beebe 1975). Offering the patient something to eat or drink or a cigarette can attenuate tension and build an alliance (Dubin 1981). It will be harder for the patient to be enraged with someone who is feeding him or her.

Often the presence of a family member or friend will calm and reassure the patient. They almost always encourage the patient to cooperate with the interview and treatment. In the rare instance in which their influence makes the situation worse, valuable information about the social environment antecedents of the patient's violence has been gained.

Weapons. On entering the emergency department, patients should be asked if they are armed with any weapons. They should be informed that the hospital is a safe place and therefore they will not need to keep their weapon on their person while they are at the hospital. Instruct patients to leave weapons on a nearby table along with any other valuables they would like kept safe. Tell patients that another staff member will come to inventory and secure their possessions; then go with the patient to another area of the emergency room. Never take weapons directly from patients or approach or pick one up in their presence. Anyone who needs to carry a weapon feels vulnerable without it. The weapon represents power as well as safety so it is more frightening to hand it over to another than to put it down. Before hospital admission, patients should be searched for weapons. In some centers where weapon carrying is common, it may be appropriate to search patients when they first arrive to be seen. This procedure is usually well tolerated by patients (McCulloch et al. 1986). Metal detectors, either hand held or walk through, can be a useful adjunct to search procedures but cannot substitute for a more individual approach.

Security forces.   Treating aggressive and violent patients without a trained security force as part of the treatment team is not a good idea. Patients can often sense a clinician's anxiety, and this often leads to increased agitation and violence. The presence of adequate security forces increases the clinician's sense of safety and confidence, thereby facilitating more effective evaluation and treatment. If patients are at high risk for violence, they should be interviewed from the doorway, with security guards present where they can be seen by patients. It is sometimes reassuring for patients to know there are enough staff to keep them from losing control and hurting themselves or others (Dubin 1981). Security should be summoned in a manner such that the patient does not know they are coming until their arrival. A silent security call button, a discreet phone call, or an intercom code-name page are several options. The security forces should be met at the door by the clinician or another staff member and rapidly briefed as to what they can expect from this particular patient and their role in the situation. This briefing will significantly increase their effectiveness and facilitate mutual trust and confidence. If security forces are to be used, they should be numerous enough to rapidly overwhelm the patient.

Restraint.   When an aggressive, potentially assaultive patient cannot be managed by the preceding interventions and cannot be talked to, reasoned with, persuaded, contained, delayed, or denied, the humane and effective response to protect patient and staff is physical restraint

(Lion 1972; Skodol and Karasu 1978; see Chapter 3). One study of the use of restraint in a psychiatric emergency room reported that 24% of patients were put in restraint (Telintelo et al. 1983). Of those restrained, 60%, usually psychotic or intoxicated men, required restraint immediately. The other 40%, usually psychotic men, registered and waited first, then were restrained later in response to agitation, confusion, or perceived elopement risk. Half of their restrained patients were released from restraints before leaving the emergency room; 42% were not hospitalized. In most emergency services, the rate of restraint should be less than 10%. A 24% rate, as in the study above, should probably lead to a quality-assurance audit to ensure that all of the restraints were, in fact, appropriate.

The restraining team must have a designated leader and an agreed-on plan with backup options if the initial maneuver fails. When restraint is decided on, a minimum of five staff members (i.e., one for each limb, plus one to direct the process) should be available to implement the restraint. More staff may be required depending on the patient (e.g., an additional one for the head). Patients should be informed that they are being restrained for their own safety and that no harm will come to them. There should be no negotiation, but patients should be informed of each step in the procedure (i.e., "We're going to move you to the other stretcher," "We're going to turn you over"). If patients are delirious due to intoxication or head injury and vomiting is a possibility, they should be restrained on their stomach with their head to one side to avoid aspiration; otherwise, they should be restrained on their back. Either four-limb, three-limb, or two-limb contralateral leg and arm restraints are used. Two-limb ipsilateral and single-limb restraints should never be used because patients may twist their limbs and injure themselves struggling to get free. In most cases, a patient will initially be put in four-limb restraints. After the patient has regained control, first an arm and then the contralateral leg will be released. Table 11-1 outlines recommended standards for the implementation of seclusion and restraint. Each of these has been required by a specific court ruling, although all have certainly not been required in all rulings.

Once a patient has been restrained, a decision about emergency medication can be made as outlined in Chapter 3.

HISTORY AND EVALUATION

Once the safety of patient and staff has been secured, a complete history and evaluation are done. The following specifics should be inquired into:

- History of present situation
  - Has anyone been harmed?
  - Thoughts of harming someone—a particular person or people
  - Plans to harm—have preparations been made, weapons in possession, access to weapons
  - Under what conditions would the patient feel impelled to act?
  - Current alcohol or drug use, behavior when intoxicated
  - Current anxiety or depression
  - Current quarrels, jealousy, provocations
  - Driving habits—reckless or aggressive
  - Attitude toward punishment and other negative consequences
  - Degree to which violence is normal in current social circle
  - Suicidal thoughts or plans

- Past history
  - Previous violent thoughts, plans, or acts; against whom and why; why didn't the patient act at that time, if plan wasn't carried out; premeditated or impulsive; punishments or consequences
  - Arrests, prison
  - Fighting, reckless driving, vandalism
  - Sanctioned violence—military, police
  - Head trauma, psychosis, seizures, encephalitis, meningitis, menstrual history and symptoms
  - Victim of violence
  - Family history of violence

- Childhood
  - Parental brutality or seduction
  - Degree to which violence was normative in family and culture of origin
  - Fire setting, bed-wetting, cruelty to animals

Table 11-1. Recommended standards for seclusion and restraint

---

- Examination by qualified mental health professional before restraint
- Examination by psychiatrist within 2 hours of restraint
- Patient checked every 15 minutes
- Patient reevaluated within 12 hours
- Careful records be kept of seclusion and reasons for it
- Patient be allowed to use bathroom once an hour
- Patient be bathed every 12 hours

Source. Adapted from Appelbaum 1983.

Whenever possible, the history should be obtained from and corroborated by the patient's friends and family. Unless they contact you on their own initiative, you must obtain permission to contact them. Chapter 6 discusses issues related to confidentiality and the "duty to warn" potential victims of patient violence.

DIFFERENTIAL DIAGNOSIS

In psychiatry, loss of control resulting in violence is a specific criterion in 11 DSM-III-R (American Psychiatric Association 1987) Axis I diagnoses, 3 of them intoxications, and 3 Axis II diagnoses (Table 11-2). Overall, violence can be conceptualized in three broad diagnostic categories: organic, nonorganic psychotic, and nonorganic nonpsychotic.

Organic Etiology

Organic causes of violence include intoxication and other organic brain syndromes. Organic brain syndromes have been reported to be the underlying etiology in 6.4–11.0% of violent patients (Rossi et al. 1985; Skodol and Karasu 1978; Tardiff and Sweillam 1980). It is the least predictable etiology because it often involves fluctuations of consciousness. It is also the most difficult to manage because the patient often cannot be influenced by persuasion or a show of force. Violence asso-

Table 11-2. DSM-III-R diagnoses that specify violence in criteria

Axis I
- Intermittent explosive disorder
- Adjustment disorder with disturbance of conduct
- Organic personality disorder—explosive type
- Alcohol idiosyncratic intoxication
- Alcohol intoxication
- Amphetamine intoxication
- Phencyclidine intoxication
- Antisocial personality disorder
- Borderline personality disorder
- Paranoid personality disorder (implied)
- Sexual sadism

Axis II
- Antisocial personality disorder
- Borderline personality disorder
- Sadistic personality disorder

ciated with organic brain syndromes is often without focus. The most effective intervention is reduction of stimulation.

Etiologies of organic brain syndromes are many, and 59% of all of these patients have been reported to be belligerent in the emergency room (Elliott 1987). Commonly reported etiologies for organic brain syndromes associated with aggression are

- Trauma
- Alzheimer's disease or multi-infarct dementia
- Mental retardation
- Intermittent explosive disorder (discussed later in this chapter)
- Infectious meningitis and encephalitis
- Tumor, especially frontal and temporal lobe particularly in the area of the amygdala and hippocampus
- Metabolic, especially hypoglycemia
- Seizure—This is controversial at this time; however, many patients with temporal lobe epilepsy are reported to show aggressive behavior.
- Hypoxia—due to lung disease or carbon monoxide poisoning
- Intoxication—Of all violent patients, in 4–23%, loss of control is at least in part due to intoxication (Marten et al. 1972). Although intoxication with any substance can be associated with violence, amphetamines, cocaine, phencyclidine (PCP), and pathological alcohol intoxication are most likely to be associated with violent behavior.

> **Intermittent explosive disorder.** According to DSM-III-R, intermittent explosive disorder is characterized by a history of several discrete episodes of serious assaultive acts or destruction of property in which the degree of aggression is out of proportion to psychosocial stressors. Furthermore, the individual is supposed to have no signs of impulsiveness or aggressiveness between episodes and not to suffer from borderline or antisocial personality, organic personality syndrome, psychotic disorder, conduct disorder, or intoxication with a psychoactive substance.
>
> DSM-III-R notes that "many doubt the existence of a clinical syndrome . . . that is not symptomatic of one of the disorders that must be ruled out before a diagnosis of intermittent explosive disorder can be made" (p. 321). We are among that "many." Elliot (1987) provides a more extensive discussion of this issue.

Nonorganic Psychotic Etiology

Nonorganic psychosis is the most common condition predisposing patients to violence. Of all violent psychiatric patients, 32–44% are psychotic when they lose control and become violent (Rossi et al. 1985; Skodol and Karasu 1978; Tardiff and Sweillam 1980). Their management is complex because maintenance antipsychotic medication often causes akathisia, which may predispose to violence. Increasing doses of antipsychotic medication for these patients in an attempt to tranquilize them would increase their agitation in this case (Keckich 1978). Psychotic violence is usually preceded by a period of rising tension and increasing agitation. Anticholinergics, or perhaps a beta-blocker such as propranolol, may be useful (as outlined in Chapter 3) under these circumstances. Usually, even the most psychotic patients will not become violent if they are confronted by a show of force—enough police or staff to assure that they will be overwhelmed.

Nonorganic Nonpsychotic Etiology

Patients with borderline, paranoid, or antisocial personality disorders are the most prone to violence and are discussed further in Chapter 19. Violence may also occur in individuals who are not mentally ill but who are from violent subcultures and can probably occur in practically anyone in the face of enough provocation.

Nonorganic nonpsychotic violence tends to be the most predictable in that it is most reliably preceded by a period of rising tension. It is also the most responsive to a show of force as described above.

EMERGENCY PHARMACOTHERAPY FOR VIOLENT PATIENTS

Pharmacological treatment of violence is controversial (Eichelman 1988; Jacobs 1983). A wide variety of substances may have a beneficial effect on violence over a period of time, but for short-term control of violent behavior, antipsychotics or benzodiazepines continue to be the mainstays of treatment. As discussed in Chapter 3, benzodiazepines may disinhibit violent behavior in some patients, although that reaction is apparently rare. Either 5–10 mg haloperidol po or im or 1–2 mg lorazepam po or im is a reasonable choice for patients needing "rapid tranquilization." Haloperidol is probably to be preferred in patients who are obviously psychotic, who are elderly, who are currently intoxicated on sedative-hypnotics, or who have had adverse reactions to benzodiazepines in the past.

PROSECUTION OF VIOLENT PATIENTS

Few assaults by patients identified as mentally ill are prosecuted. Police and courts view this as a psychiatric problem, and mental health care givers either do not hold the patient responsible in their own minds or else fear that prosecution would exacerbate the patient's mental illness. Hoge and Gutheil (1987) reported on nine patients who were charged with assault. In two cases, the patients improved after charges were filed; but in three cases, the courts refused to cooperate, and the staff was demoralized as a result. In none of the cases did the patient's mental illness become worse. The advantages of pressing charges include

- Making a public record and fulfilling the mental health professional's duty to protect society from potentially dangerous patients
- Helping maintain clinical objectivity toward the patient by removing moral considerations to the proper agency—the court
- Possibly deterring future violence by behavior training
- Possibly engendering a more responsible self-image in the patient by avoiding the infantilizing effect of not being held responsible for one's own behavior

Disadvantages include

- Possible alienation of the patient from the mental health care system.
- If the patient is incarcerated, the prison or jail may have less effective mental health care than is available in the community. This can be mitigated by the use of "pocket probation" in which the patient is brought before the clerk of the court and told that the file will be kept open for a year and that if the patient appears again the charges will be fully prosecuted.
- Demoralization of staff when the court is uncooperative.

When managing patients with a previous history of violence, they should, in most cases, be informed that prosecution is an option if they are violent again. After all cases of violence, a clinical report should immediately be written. The patient should be evaluated as soon as possible by an independent consultant to determine mental state at the time of the assault. Then a team meeting should be held to weigh advantages and disadvantages of prosecution. This process should be formally stated in an administrative protocol.

INJURY TO STAFF

When a member of the care team is injured by a patient, the team's effectiveness and morale are damaged. Health-care providers usually react to assault by a patient with denial and self-blame, the usual response of any victim (Phelan et al. 1985). Many assaults are not recorded, anger is unexpressed, and the patient is not blamed, especially if psychotic. The victim usually minimizes or denies any sequelae to the assault. Engel and Marsh (1986) have stressed the necessity of an administrative protocol mandating the following:

- Immediate medical and emotional care
- Legal and practical advice
- Follow-up treatment including psychosocial counseling
- Well-timed investigation of the incident
- Documentation of incident and injury

We also recommend a team meeting to review the incident and debrief staff. A mixed reaction from staff regarding this policy should be anticipated because it implies admitting feelings of vulnerability at work and with patients and, therefore, threatens the staff's self-image of being strong and in control; however, over the long term, morale and objectivity toward violent patients will improve and staff burnout will decrease.

REFERENCES

American Psychiatric Association: Diagnostic and Statistical Manual of Mental Disorders, 3rd Edition, Revised. Washington, DC, American Psychiatric Association, 1987

Appelbaum PS: Legal considerations in the prevention and treatment of assault, in Assaults Within Psychiatric Facilities. Edited by Lion JR, Reid WH. New York, Grune & Stratton, 1983, pp 173–190

Dubin W: Evaluating and managing the violent patient. Ann Emerg Med 10:481–484, 1981

Eichelman B: Toward a rational pharmacotherapy for aggressive and violent behavior. Hosp Community Psychiatry 39:31–39, 1988

Elliot FA: Neuroanatomy and neurology of aggression. Psychiatric Annals 17:385–396, 1987

Engel F, Marsh S: Helping the employee victim of violence in hospitals. Hosp Community Psychiatry 37:159–162, 1986

Havens L: Explorations in the uses of language in psychotherapy: counterprojective statements. Contemporary Psychoanalysis 16:53–57, 1980

Hoge SK, Gutheil TG: The prosecution of psychiatric patients for assaults on staff: a preliminary empirical study. Hosp Community Psychiatry 38:44–49, 1987

Jacobs D: Evaluation and management of the violent patient in emergency settings. Psychiatr Clin North Am 6:259–269, 1983

Keckich WA: Neuroleptics—violence as a manifestation of akathisia. JAMA 240:2185–2186, 1978

Kinzel AF: Body buffer zone in violent prisoners. Am J Psychiatry 127:99–104, 1970

Lion JR: Evaluation and Management of the Violent Patient. Springfield, IL, Charles C Thomas, 1972

McCulloch LE, McNeil DE, Binder RL, et al: Effects of a weapon screening procedure in a psychiatric emergency room. Hosp Community Psychiatry 37:837–838, 1986

Marten S, Munoz RA, Gentry KA, et al: Belligerence: its frequency and correlates in a psychiatric emergency room population. Compr Psychiatry 13:241–248, 1972

Monahan J: The prediction of violent behavior: toward a second generation of theory and policy. Am J Psychiatry 141:10–15, 1984

Phelan LA, Mills MJ, Ryan JA: Prosecuting psychiatric patients for assault. Hosp Community Psychiatry 36:581–582, 1985

Rofman EF, Askinazi L, Fant E: The prediction of dangerous behavior in emergency civil commitment. Am J Psychiatry 317:1061–1064, 1980

Rosenbaum CP, Beebe JE: Psychiatric Treatment. New York, McGraw-Hill, 1975, p 75

Rossi MA, Jacobs M, Montelcone M, et al: Violent or fear inducing behavior associated with hospital admission. Hosp Community Psychiatry 36:643–647, 1985

Skodol AE, Karasu TB: Emergency psychiatry and the assaultive patient. Am J Psychiatry 135:202–205, 1978

Tardiff K, Sweillam A: Assault, suicide, and mental illness. Arch Gen Psychiatry 37:164–169, 1980

Telintelo S, Kuhlman T, Winget C: A study of the use of restraint in a psychiatric emergency room. Hosp Community Psychiatry 34:164–165, 1983

Yesavage J, Werner P, Becker J, et al: Short-term commitment and the violent patient. Am J Psychiatry 139:1145–1149, 1982

Chapter 12

Delirium and Dementia

O. Thienhaus, M.D.

Delirium and dementia each refer to symptom constellations that can be due to a large variety of underlying physical problems. They are not diseases sui generis but global organic mental syndromes. Just as cyanosis and anemia are symptom complexes that can necessitate emergency room admission, so are delirious or demented conditions often seen by emergency room psychiatrists. Delirium is an emergency by definition. Dementias can result in emergencies because of complicating problems. Table 12-1 compares features of delirium and dementia.

DELIRIUM

Assessment and Diagnosis

The diagnostic assessment of the delirious patient involves mental status evaluation, physical examination, and laboratory tests. On mental status examination, reduced attention span and a pervasive formal thought disorder are distinguishing features of delirium. Communicative exchange with the immediate environment is grossly impaired due to these

---

Shaded sections indicate areas of legitimate diversity of professional opinion in the literature. See Preface for further discussion.

Table 12-1. Differential features of delirium and dementia

Feature	Delirium	Dementia
Onset	Acute, often at night	Insidious
Course	Fluctuating, with lucid intervals during day; worse at night	Stable over course of day
Duration	Hours to weeks	Months to years
Awareness	Reduced	Clear
Attention	Lacks direction and selectivity, distractibility, fluctuates over course of day	Relatively unaffected
Orientation	Usually impaired for time, tendency to mistake unfamiliar for familiar place and persons	Often impaired
Memory	Immediate and recent impaired	Recent and remote impaired
Thinking	Disorganized	Impoverished
Perception	Illusions and hallucinations usually visual and common	Often absent
Speech	Incoherent, hesitant, slow or rapid	Difficulty in finding words
Sleep-wake cycle	Always disrupted	Fragmented sleep
Physical illness or drug toxicity	Either or both present	Often absent, especially Alzheimer's disease

Source. Adapted from Lipowski 1987.

symptoms. This impairment is further accentuated by the associated fluctuating state of consciousness, which may span the entire range from coma through full alertness to hypervigilance (Table 12-2). Recording

Table 12–2. Stages of impaired level of consciousness

Stage	Characteristics
Somnolence or lethargy	Drowsiness with delayed or incomplete response to ordinary stimuli
Obtundation	Drowsiness with response only to rigorous stimuli
Stupor	Loss of consciousness with arousal only in response to vigorous stimuli
Coma	Loss of consciousness and loss of all psychological and motor responses

Source. Adapted from Plum and Posner 1980.

the level of alertness over time is essential to differentiate delirium from acute psychotic states of other etiology, especially psychosis superimposed on a dementing illness (see below).

Disorientation is another characteristic symptom of delirium. Orientation to time is most vulnerable; orientation to place and person is lost with more severe impairment. Often, again, nature and extent of disorientation change over time so that serial examinations are needed. Other cognitive functions also are often impaired, especially short-term memory.

Associated mental status findings include perceptual phenomena. Visual, tactile, and olfactory misperceptions, illusions, and hallucinations are most characteristically of organic origin. Auditory symptoms, while less specific, can also be part of a delirious disorder.

Delusional ideation can be found. Delusions can be of any variety, but are typically less systematized than in schizophrenia or delusional disorder. Affective symptomatology presenting with such manifestations as anxiety, hostility, euphoria, or tearfulness is almost always present. Agitation is common and waxes and wanes depending on the level of consciousness and the intensity of other associated symptoms. To facilitate clinical differential diagnosis, Table 12-3 lists leading symptoms of delirium in order of their specificity.

Beyond the mental status examination, we recommend the following management for every patient with suspected delirium.

- Obtain a full physical examination including vital signs and neurological status (see Chapter 1).
- Obtain complete blood count and renal panel, including blood sugar.
- Obtain vital signs (along with mental status assessments) serially every 15 minutes.

Table 12-3. Symptoms of delirium in approximate order of specificity

1. Instability of all mental status findings over time
2. Nonauditory hallucinations
3. Misperceptions and illusions
4. Impaired attention span
5. Disorientation
6. Impaired level of consciousness
7. Auditory hallucinations
8. Other cognitive impairment
9. Delusional ideation
10. Affective symptoms

As the range of suspected causative factors (see below) is being narrowed down, additional tests need to be ordered. A summary is provided in Table 12-4.

Causes

Conditions resulting in delirium are numerous. Instead of a list of specific causes, a number of general causative classes will be presented. Within each category, various potential specific etiologies exist that can lead to delirious symptomatology.

Lack of oxygen. Cerebral anoxia can be a result of insufficient blood supply or inadequate oxygenation. In the latter case, respiratory obstruction or toxic oxygen displacement at the hemoglobin carrier site are possible underlying problems. Insufficient blood supply to the brain can be due to acute blood loss, circulatory collapse, or vascular obstruction. In any case, the decrease of oxygen available to central neurons must occur over a brief time span to manifest itself as delirium. If the causative condition persists longer, either the patient will die, or the brain will adapt to chronic undersupply of oxygen.

Metabolic disturbance. Generally speaking, metabolic causes of delirium are due to renal, endocrine, or hepatic pathology, or they are induced by exogenous toxins. The neuronal membrane reacts sensitively to changes in the body's internal milieu. Deviation from the physiological pH and osmotic pressure, abnormal electrolyte ratios, and temperature changes result in mental status alterations. Again, an acute disturbance is more likely to cause delirium. A classic example is the

Table 12-4. Classes of delirium

Pathophysiology	Associated clinical features	Vital signs	Additional diagnostic tests
Cerebral anoxia			
Circulatory	Tachypnea	BP low, PR up	Arterial blood gases
Respiratory	Dyspnea, cyanosis	BP up, PR low	Arterial blood gases
Metabolic cause	Variable, depending on nature of disturbance	Variable	Arterial blood gases
Increased intracranial pressure	Headaches, emesis	BP up, PR low	Neuroradiological imaging
Neurotoxicity	Variable, depending on nature of toxic substance	Variable	Toxic screen (blood and urine)
Inflammation	Opisthotonos	Temp and PR up	Lumbar puncture
Systemic infection	Leukocytosis, left shift	Temp and PR up	Blood culture, urinalysis
Delirium tremens	Tremor	BP and PR up	

Note. BP = blood pressure. PR = pulse rate. Temp = temperature.

developing ketoacidotic coma of diabetic patients.

A gross undersupply of blood glucose will result in cerebral impairment and, typically, delirious states as glucose is the almost exclusive source of metabolic energy available to the central nervous system. Hypoglycemia, especially diabetogenic hypoglycemia, is often associated with complicating electrolyte abnormalities.

Increased intracranial pressure. Headaches, vomiting, impaired alertness, and unequal pupil size or reactivity are the textbook features of acutely increased intracranial pressure. This is commonly caused by concussion after a closed head injury. Acute subdural hematomas (venous bleed) or an epidural hemorrhage after rupture of the meningeal artery can be complicating features, aggravating the rapid rise of intracranial pressure.

Neurotoxins. Directly neurotoxic substances such as various alcohols (including ethanol) and other solvents can cause delirium. Such substances can be ingested with suicidal intent or as an accidental overdose, especially in the context of chronic substance abuse. Psychoactive substances known to cause delirium include amphetamines, cocaine, and phencyclidine (PCP). Prescribed medications that cross the blood-brain barrier, e.g., theophylline, diphenylhydantoin, digoxin, lithium, or antidepressants, can also cause delirium at toxic serum concentrations.

Even at nontoxic blood levels, side effects of certain drugs can cause delirious symptomatology. A case in point is the anticholinergic delirium, especially in more susceptible elderly individuals, which can occur on therapeutic doses of psychotropic medications. The combination of tachycardia, hot dry skin, and large pupils should alert the clinician to the differential diagnosis of anticholinergic overload.

Inflammation. Encephalitis and meningitis are conditions that can present as delirium. They can be either infectious or aseptic. Heat-induced encephalitic reactions (heatstroke) should be included as a differential diagnosis.

Systemic infection. Septicemia is a condition that can be associated with delirium. However, infectious causes may not be as fulminant in order to present that way. Especially in the older patient, a seemingly more localized infection (e.g., urinary tract infection) can be associated with delirious symptomatology.

Delirium tremens. Withdrawal from alcohol, barbiturates, benzo-diazepines, and other sedating substances can cause, in some patients, a fairly specific syndrome of generalized adrenoceptor hyperactivity, gross tremor, and delirium with prominent perceptual symptoms (see Chapters 13 and 14).

Any condition that decreases the body's inherent adaptive flexibility to maintain homeostasis represents a predisposing factor rendering the person more likely to develop delirium in response to noxious stimuli. Thus, the very young and the elderly are at particular risk among the patients coming to the emergency room. Every new onset of mental symptoms or any acute qualitative change in existing mental illness in geriatric patients should raise the differential diagnosis of a delirious state until disproved.

Treatment

Untreated delirium can result in brain damage or even death (Rabins and Folstein 1982). Treatment is largely targeted at correction of the underlying causative condition. Generally, this requires referral to a medical or surgical service, if not admission to an intensive care unit. Intravenous therapy for restitution of fluid and electrolyte balance, circulatory stabilization, cardiac monitoring, cranial checks, peritoneal dialysis, and neurosurgical evacuation of intracranial bleeds are all indications for the attention of medical specialists. In our experience, the emergency room psychiatrist's task, beyond the diagnosis of a delirium, lies primarily in consultative advice regarding supportive symptomatic management of delirious patients.

Management of delirious patients should as much as possible be confined to environmental interventions. The goal is to keep the patient and the care providers safe without obscuring clinically important symptoms. Both excessive sensory stimulation and complete sensory deprivation should be avoided. Dazzling lights and loud noises are common in every emergency room, but can further agitate a delirious patient. On the other hand, a completely dark and very quiet private room may aggravate psychotic symptoms. We recommend that, if at all possible, a delirious patient be maintained in a semidark room with continuous or intermittent supervision.

If psychomotor agitation or combativeness are problems, physical restraints may be required. Psychotropic medications should be used with caution. They should only be introduced after the cause of the delirium has been determined, and if causative correction is not immediately possible or fails to result in expeditious symptom resolution. In such situations, neuroleptics can serve to achieve symptomatic relief in the case of prominent psychotic features. Benzodiazepines can calm nonpsychotic agitation by specifically alleviating the anxiety that often accompanies delirium. In the case of delirium tremens, systematic treatment with benzodiazepines is in fact the definitive therapy of choice (see Chapter 14).

DEMENTIA

Uncomplicated dementia does not represent an emergency and does not require hospitalization unless on an elective basis for a more convenient etiologic workup.

The symptom complex of dementia is characterized by pervasive cognitive impairment, particularly of memory function, but also of abstraction. Associated features include impaired judgment and evidence of other cortical disturbances, e.g., constructional apraxia or word-finding problems. Often a person's personality is changed, and invariably there has been interference with social or occupational functioning. In contrast to delirium, the other global organic mental syndrome, there is no rapid fluctuation of symptoms, and consciousness remains quite clear.

Demented patients reach the psychiatric emergency service primarily for two reasons. A change occurs in an existing support system, which then fails to compensate for the patient's functional disability, and a different placement is sought. Alternatively, superimposed, complicating symptomatology has led to behavioral features that cause an acute crisis in the patient's continued tenure in the original setting.

Emergency Room Presentations: Differential Diagnosis

Demented patients are typically brought to the emergency room by family, neighbors, caretakers, police, or life squad. In our own facility, we found that only 15% of patients with dementia were self-referred, compared to 46% of patients in general (Thienhaus et al. 1988). Demented patients are brought in, in most instances, because of an observed sudden deterioration. This deterioration manifests itself in decreased self-care, hazardous behaviors (e.g., forgetting to turn off the gas), agitation, or combativeness.

Careful examination of the patient and exploration of the situational circumstances surrounding the reported "sudden change" will differentiate between the following three pathogenetic alternatives. These pathogenetic alternatives are not mutually exclusive. The demented individual who loses an important social support factor still has an increased risk of developing delirium or may sustain thrombotic occlusion of a cerebral vessel.

Acute cerebral trauma. The most frequent case in our experience is the patient with a known history of multi-infarct dementia. An additional cerebrovascular accident, whether thrombotic or embolic, has resulted in perceptible clinical changes. These changes can comprise an abrupt worsening of cognitive deficiency, newly added mental status symptoms such as hallucinosis or delusions, or a superimposed delirium. The previous history of infarcts, the presence of associated conditions (e.g., hypertension, diabetes, atrial fibrillation), and focal findings on neurological status examination should clarify the situation. A neurological consultation is the appropriate next step to be taken. Noninvasive neuroradiological imaging techniques are generally not helpful in diagnosing recent infarcts, but can serve to rule out the presence of other cerebral trauma.

Delirium. The vast majority of demented patients are elderly. Elderly people are at higher risk of delirium (see Chapter 25). If a dementing process has already compromised cognitive processing under baseline conditions, any of the previously listed delirium-causing traumata can all the more easily lead to additional acute impairment. Thus, in any demented patient with a sudden change in mental status, a superimposed delirium must be ruled out.

Environmental change. A demented patient's community tenure depends on a match between the extent of the individual's cognitive-functional disability and the support, redirection, and supervision provided by the immediate environment. Change in environmental factors can include a daughter's vacation, staff change in a nursing home, or a broken-down elevator in a senior high-rise building. The mental status changes and behavioral complications in response to perceived sudden decrease in environmental support or orienting cues are similar to what Goldstein (1942) termed "catastrophic reaction" in brain-injured individuals. It can take the form of an anxiety reaction, psychomotor agitation, or positive psychotic symptomatology. Pseudodementia (McAllister 1982) is discussed in Chapter 25.

Treatment

The potential danger of added mental status changes in the demented patient must not be underestimated. The elderly woman who suddenly starts "sundowning" (i.e., nocturnal restlessness and agitation due to sensory deprivation) is at high risk for a hip fracture. And we know of a demented man in an unsecured nursing home who began to wander at night, walked out onto a balcony, climbed over the rail, and died from the ensuing fall.

The emergency room psychiatrist cannot hope to cure a dementing illness. The goal is to initiate appropriate treatment for optimal control of excess disability. To this end, we concentrate on evaluation and, to the extent possible, correction of the event causing the superimposed impairment, and begin symptomatic therapy. The causative interventions obviously depend on the nature of the etiologic factor that is responsible for the additional pathology. As far as a complicating delirium is concerned, the principles delineated in the first section of this chapter apply.

In addition, assessment of the environmental situation is crucial. Simple changes can be beneficial. For instance, leaving a bedside lamp on throughout the night or moving an institutional resident into a room closer to the nursing station may eliminate or alleviate "sundowning" symptomatology. In many cases, however, alternative disposition will be the most important therapeutic measure to be taken.

Causative treatment for behavioral complications of dementing illness may not be available, may be only partially effective, or may not work fast enough. In these cases, symptomatic therapy is required. The most frequent target symptoms are delusional ideation, psychomotor agitation, day-night disturbance, violence, verbal outbursts, tearful episodes, hallucinations, and anxiety (Reisberg et al. 1987).

Empirically, antipsychotic medications are the mainstay of psychopharmacological intervention. The research support for this indication of neuroleptic medications is not very robust (Helms 1985), but two randomized studies found that antipsychotics had a significantly greater impact on some symptoms of behavioral disturbance than did placebo, if only in a small number of patients (Barnes et al. 1982; Petrie et al. 1982). It is generally agreed that low-dose regimens are indicated. The rationale is outlined in Chapter 25, "Geriatric Patients."

Controversy surrounds the choice of neuroleptic (see Chapter 3). The spectrum of available neuroleptics ranges from low-antidopaminergic-potency drugs such as chlorpromazine or thioridazine to high-potency drugs such as butyrophenones. Drugs at either end of the spectrum have their own risks. We recommend caution regarding the orthostatic and anticholinergic properties of chlorpromazine and thioridazine, respectively, and the propensity for extrapyramidal side effects associated with haloperidol. If there is no clearly decisive precedent of an effective drug for a patient, we tend to use neuroleptics that occupy a middle position on the spectrum of antidopaminergic potency (see Chapter 3).

The efficacy of neuroleptic medications appears to be a function of the nature of the target symptom. If there is no detectable delusional or hallucinatory component to the behavior disorder, benzodiazepines are a possible alternative to control acutely disruptive symptoms. The controversy of whether short- or long-acting anxiolytics are preferable is briefly outlined in Chapter 3.

For more sustained behavioral adjustment, nonpharmacological modalities must complement, and can often replace, the use of benzodiazepines and occasionally of neuroleptics as well. Such modalities include environmental interventions as mentioned above, but also behavior modification strategies.

REFERENCES

Barnes R, Veith R, Okimoto J, et al: Efficacy of antipsychotic medications in behaviorally disturbed dementia patients. Am J Psychiatry 139:1170–1174, 1982

Goldstein K: After-effects of Brain Injuries in War. New York, Grune & Stratton, 1942

Helms PM: Efficacy of antipsychotics in the treatment of the behavioral complications of dementia: a review of the literature. J Am Geriatr Soc 33:206–209, 1985

Lipowski ZJ: Delirium (acute confusional states). JAMA 258:1789–1791, 1987

McAllister TW: Overview: pseudodementia. Am J Psychiatry 140:528–533, 1982

Petrie WM, Ban TA, Berney S, et al: Loxapine in psychogeriatrics: a placebo-

and standard-controlled clinical investigation. J Clin Psychopharmacol 2:122–126, 1982

Plum F, Posner JB: The Diagnosis of Stupor and Coma, 3rd Edition. Philadelphia, PA, FA Davis, 1980

Rabins PV, Folstein MF: Delirium and dementia: diagnostic criteria and mortality rates. Br J Psychiatry 140:149–153, 1982

Reisberg B, Borenstein J, Salob SP, et al: Behavioral symptoms in Alzheimer's disease: phenomenology and treatment. J Clin Psychiatry 48 (suppl):9–15, 1987

Thienhaus OJ, Rowe C, Woellert P, et al: Geropsychiatric emergency services: utilization and outcome predictors. Hosp Community Psychiatry 39:1301–1305, 1988

Chapter 13

Emergency Psychiatric Aspects of HIV Infection

George W. Lackemann, M.D.

There are several important reasons for including the psychiatric manifestations of acquired immunodeficiency syndrome (AIDS) and AIDS-
related disorders in this manual of emergency psychiatry. It is estimated
that between 1 and 2 million Americans have been exposed to human
immunodeficiency virus (HIV-1). These individuals, whether symptomatic or not, are assumed to be carriers of the virus and capable of
disseminating it to others. Because the virus is neurotropic as well as
lymphotropic, nearly 70% of patients will have clinically apparent
mental changes, mostly due to HIV itself, at some point in the course of
infection, and 90% will show neuropathological abnormalities
(McKhann 1988). The magnitude of the problem approaches that of
schizophrenia or bipolar affective disorder in prevalence, if not in
severity or chronicity. A much smaller number of infected persons
develop opportunistic infections and/or malignancies that directly involve the brain and produce significant psychiatric and neurologic
problems. In addition to these neuropsychiatric manifestations, the
psychosocial aspects of the epidemic are protean and affect virtually
every segment of the population. These include infected persons and
their families, friends, and sexual partners; persons at high risk of
infection; and persons at low risk of infection, including most health-

care workers, who are often misinformed and develop unjustified fears that can lead to discriminatory actions. Because no psychiatrist, regardless of locale, can expect to remain apart from these issues, it is essential that all psychiatrists become familiar with the American Psychiatric Association's position statement on AIDS (1987a) and position statement on HIV-related discrimination (1987b), which outline responsibilities in the areas of education, treatment, confidentiality, and research. Nowhere is the need for self-education more acute than in the emergency evaluation of patients and in crisis intervention.

THE EPIDEMIC

AIDS and AIDS-related conditions are caused by a retrovirus (HIV) that also has properties associated with the lentiviruses, including a long incubation period and relatively slow onset of symptoms and disease. Previously called lymphadenopathy-associated virus (LAV) and human T-cell lymphotropic virus (HTLV-III), the virus is thought to have originated in central Africa, possibly as a mutation of an endemic human retrovirus. HIV maintains the ability to mutate rapidly from person to person, and apparently even within a single individual. It is transmitted as free viral particles and within helper T (T4) lymphocytes and macrophages, which are transferred from person to person in body fluids. The virus must have direct access to the bloodstream of the recipient to cause infection. Although HIV has been isolated from blood, semen, vaginal secretions, saliva, and tears, its concentration in saliva and tears is low enough to suggest these fluids do not constitute a significant infective risk. The virus infects and destroys helper T (T4) lymphocytes, which disrupts cell-mediated immunity and allows opportunistic infections and certain malignancies to develop. The presence of these infections, neoplasms, significant dementia, or bodily wasting results in a diagnosis of AIDS. To date, AIDS has been nearly uniformly fatal. There is general disagreement over what percentage of infected persons will go on to develop AIDS, but recent studies suggest it may approach 100%.

In Africa, the virus has spread heterosexually, possibly through open lesions of concurrent sexually transmitted diseases and via unsterilized needles and frequent transfusions of unscreened blood products for the treatment of malarial anemia. It is hypothesized that travel from the endemic area to Haiti and then to the East and West Coasts of the United States and to Europe established the infection in these areas (Shilts 1987). The first cases of Kaposi's sarcoma and Pneumocystis carinii pneumonia were reported in homosexual men in New York in 1981.

HIV has subsequently spread to all 50 states and to at least 148 countries. The epidemiology of infection and transmission varies largely according to socioeconomic factors: in affluent and industrialized countries, the virus remains mostly confined to homosexual men and intravenous-drug users and their sexual contacts, with transmission via anal and, less frequently, vaginal intercourse and sharing of unsterilized needles; in poor and Third World countries, the male-to-female ratio approaches 1:1, with transmission via vaginal and anal intercourse, transfusions, and unsterilized health-care products (Piot et al. 1988).

As of December 1988, more than 150,000 cases of AIDS worldwide had been reported to the WHO, but due to underreporting, especially in Third World countries, WHO estimates that over 300,000 cases of AIDS had occurred and as many as 10 million people were infected by the end of 1987 (Piot et al. 1988). In the United States, over 90,000 AIDS cases and over 50,000 deaths had been reported by the spring of 1989 (Centers for Disease Control 1989). Because of the long incubation period, now considered to be a median of 9 years, most of the current infections were probably acquired before the discovery of HIV as the causative agent. In spite of modest educational efforts and modification of behavior in high-risk groups, most notably by homosexual men, the Centers for Disease Control (CDC) projects 270,000 cumulative AIDS cases in the United States by the end of 1991 (Elder and Sever 1988).

RISK GROUPS AND HIGH-RISK ACTIVITIES

The evaluation and treatment of any patient presenting with HIV-related psychiatric symptoms includes a thorough history of high-risk behaviors as well as education about the modification of such behaviors to prevent the spread of infection to others and to minimize the transmission of possible viral cofactors or additional HIV to the patient. Familiarity with the epidemiology of infection in the high-risk groups is essential. The percentages of total United States cases by risk group are presented in Table 13-1.

Because of infection prevalence rates ranging from 10 to 70% in homosexual and bisexual men, any unprotected receptive anal intercourse, especially with unknown or multiple partners, is extremely risky. The efficiency of transmission through other specific practices is as yet unknown, although a decrease in the number of sexual partners, the avoidance of mucous membrane contact with highly infectious body fluids (blood, semen, urine, feces), abandonment of any traumatic sexual practices ("fisting," douching, sharing of sexual devices), and

Table 13-1. Percentage of total AIDS cases by risk group

Risk group	Percentage
Homosexual or bisexual men without history of intravenous-drug abuse	65
Homosexual or bisexual men with history of intravenous-drug abuse	8
Women and heterosexual men with history of intravenous-drug abuse	17
Recipients of blood transfusions[a]	2
Hemophiliacs	1
Heterosexuals without history of intravenous-drug abuse	4
Persons with undetermined routes of infection	3
Pediatric cases[b]	1

[a]Mostly prior to 1985.
[b]Pediatric cases are in addition to the total adult cases.

consistent and proper use of latex condoms all appear to decrease the risk of transmission. Abstinence or a truly monogamous relationship with a known long-term seronegative person eliminates the risk.

Prevalence of HIV infection in the estimated 1,100,000 intravenous-drug abusers in the United States ranges from 0 to 70% depending on location, with the highest rates in and around New York City. Any sharing of unsterilized needles must be considered an extremely high-risk activity. A 1:10 dilution of household bleach in water will inactivate the virus. A better solution is entry into a drug treatment program with abstinence or methadone maintenance; unfortunately, less than 20% of intravenous-drug abusers are currently in treatment (Curran et al. 1988).

The risk of infection following transfusion of HIV-infected blood or blood products is extremely high, about 90%. Almost all infected transfusion recipients and patients with hemophilia received infected products before blood screening began in 1985 (Curran et al. 1988). Prevalence among patients with hemophilia ranges from 0 to 90% and is solely dependent on the amount of factor VIII received before 1985. Some infected hemophilia patients and transfusion recipients show overt or repressed anger toward other high-risk groups for "causing" their illness. The current risk of transfusion infection is low but not insignificant, especially in high prevalence areas, and is due to blood donations by infected persons who have not yet seroconverted. Any high-risk individuals should be strongly discouraged from donating blood, especially as a means of being tested for HIV.

Over half of the cases attributable to heterosexual transmission occurred in persons with sexual contact with individuals with documented

HIV infection (70% of index partners were intravenous-drug abusers, 18% of index partners for cases in women were bisexual men). The remainder of heterosexual cases were born in countries where heterosexual contact is the major route of infection. At present, the ratio of male-to-female heterosexual transmission cases is 1:3. It is unknown whether this reflects the larger pool of infected men or the higher efficiency of male-to-female transmission (Curran et al. 1988). In many of the 2,059 cases with undetermined routes of infection, the sexual or drug-use history was incomplete or unobtainable; risk factors were ultimately identified for a large number, and of the remaining 281, 38% reported sexually transmitted diseases and 34% of the men reported prostitute contact (Castro et al. 1988).

This information is important because much public concern arises over the issues of casual spread and the risk of infection in low-risk heterosexual populations. There is currently no evidence for casual or vector spread of the virus, and although the proportion of heterosexual cases has increased modestly since 1982, it appears that most cases can be traced to sexual contact with high-risk individuals or unreported intravenous-drug use. The risk of male-to-female transmission with unprotected vaginal intercourse over an extended period appears to be about 50%. Thus, cautious reassurance with emphasis on safe sex practices including the use of condoms with unknown partners, obtaining a sexual and drug-use history from potential sexual partners, avoidance of prostitutes, and monogamy is the proper response to concerns of low-risk individuals. Information in the popular press over- and underestimating the extent of risk should be discounted.

As of December 1987, 737 cases of AIDS in children under 13 years old had been reported, with an increase in new cases of 64% over the previous year. Most of the cases showed perinatal acquisition; the risk of perinatal infection from an infected mother may be as high as 50%. Most of the remaining infections were acquired through blood or blood-product transfusions (Curran et al. 1988).

Of major concern in health-care settings is the risk of infection due to needle-stick injury or other parenteral exposure. In a CDC-sponsored surveillance project, 3 of 351 health-care workers with documented exposure developed HIV infection (CDC 1987a). In all, there have been approximately 20 cases of infection due to needle-stick injury, exposure to contaminated blood, or contact with concentrated virus in laboratories. The small but not insignificant risk can be further diminished by strict adherence to CDC recommendations for prevention of transmission, including the use of gloves during phlebotomy and during examination when fluid or mucous membrane contact is possible (CDC 1987b). In the psychiatric setting, an additional concern is the agitated or psychotic seropositive patient who might spit at or bite a care giver. Although the risk of infection from such injuries is extremely low, all patients should be assumed to be infected and the usual precautions and proper use of restraints should be employed without exception. Health-care workers who cannot overcome irrational fears of infection or their negative countertransference toward homosexuals and drug addicts should be strongly encouraged to withdraw from the evaluation and care of these patients.

Problematic in any setting but particularly complex in the emergency room are the issues of confidentiality, ability to detain, duty to warn, notification of third parties, and disclosure to third parties when an infected patient refuses to change behavior that places other persons at risk of infection or refuses to notify identifiable individuals who may be at continuing risk of exposure. Because of the importance of these issues, the American Psychiatric Association's policy statements on confidentiality and disclosure (1988a) and on guidelines for inpatient psychiatric units (applicable to emergency settings) (1988b) are included in appendixes to this chapter.

HIV ANTIBODY TESTING

After the isolation of HIV in 1984, an antibody test to detect contact with and presumed infection by the virus was developed in 1985. Although HIV can sometimes be cultured from infected persons, there is as yet no marketed antigen test. The enzyme-linked immunosorbent assay (ELISA) is used for initial screening of individuals and blood products. This test is about 99% sensitive and specific, and if a result is positive or equivocal, the more accurate and expensive Western blot test is run for confirmation. Unfortunately, neither test will demonstrate infection until the individual produces antibodies (seroconversion). The incubation period between infection and seroconversion varies between several weeks to more than 1 year. The length of this interval is the reason the safety of blood products cannot be guaranteed, and the reason seronegativity is not proof of lack of infection.

Because test results are usually not immediately available, it does not make sense to test high-risk individuals indiscriminately in the emergency setting. If treatment or diagnosis is dependent on testing, it should be initiated on consultation with the patient's primary physician and only after informed consent is obtained and documented in the permanent record, along with documentation that the meaning and ramifications of the test have been fully discussed with the patient. If a decision to test is based on a patient's request or on the assumption that the result will assist the patient in modifying behavior, it is often best to refer the individual to an anonymous testing site, often a public health facility. These sites usually require pre- and posttest counseling, and test results are not recorded on the permanent medical record where the possibility exists for improper disclosure and discrimination.

The decision to be tested, the waiting period between testing and result, and the result itself can precipitate exceptional anxiety and/or depression in high-risk and low-risk individuals. Suicides and suicide attempts during this critical period have been documented. Whether adequate counseling, education, and evaluation of suicide risk and support systems could have altered these results is unknown, but such services should always be provided. A study has shown that AIDS patients are at much increased risk of suicide compared with the general population, compared with age-matched controls without the diagnosis, and compared with patients with other chronic illnesses (Marzuk et al. 1988). Psychosocial stresses that may precipitate suicide include the stigma of the disease, guilt, loss of family and peer support, deaths of friends from AIDS, diminished functioning, fear of prolonged terminal illness, and misinformation. Biological stressors include poor physical health, preexisting psychiatric illness, and the direct effect of HIV on the central nervous system (CNS). Many of these stressors can be present in patients with AIDS-related complex as well as in asymptomatic seropositive individuals, reinforcing the need for careful psychiatric evaluation at all stages of infection. Symptoms are intensified by pessimistic thinking in the weeks following a positive test result, and many calls and visits to psychiatric emergency centers occur at this time, especially from patients who were offered no counseling, or who were informed of results by telephone or mail. Suicidal ideation and adequacy of support systems must be actively pursued by interviewers.

COURSE OF ILLNESS

Medical and Neuropsychiatric Factors

Infected but seronegative persons are medically asymptomatic but may show signs of reactive psychiatric illness if suspicions about possible infection are harbored. When seroconversion takes place, a mononucleosis-like illness may occur with resulting depression. At the time of seroconversion or in the latent phase of infection, when the immune system usually controls but does not eliminate the virus, headaches, encephalitis, aseptic meningitis, ataxia, and myelopathy can occur but are unusual. These early manifestations are often indistinguishable from other acute viral infections and probably represent entry of HIV into the meninges and into the CNS. This stage of infection can be accompanied by delirium, although all symptoms usually resolve within days to several weeks (Price et al. 1988a).

Early asymptomatic infection of the CNS and meninges during the latency or incubation stage of HIV infection is common. Cerebrospinal fluid shows inflammatory cells and viral antibodies; imaging studies are normal. During the latency stage, which may vary from months to more than 10 years, the virus is at first held in check by the immune response, but either gradually or more suddenly destroys enough T4 lymphocytes to compromise the immune system, and the patient becomes physically symptomatic. This syndrome has been called AIDS-related complex (ARC) and includes weight loss, fevers, night sweats, generalized lymphadenopathy, chronic fatigue, oral leukoplakia, and oral candidiasis. Patients may have all or part of this symptom complex; many will complain of a cold that will not go away.

In a similar fashion, HIV begins to cause increasing neuropathology in the CNS, especially in the central white matter, the basal ganglia, thalamus, brain stem, and spinal cord, with relative sparing of the cortex; histopathology includes pallor of the white matter, multinucleated cell encephalitis, and vacuolar myelopathy (Price et al. 1988a). Cerebral atrophy and ventricular enlargement may be observed with computed tomography and nuclear magnetic resonance, whereas white matter vacuolization is seen with the latter. The pathology most likely arises not from direct infection of neurons by HIV, but rather from infection of glial cells with resulting abnormal metabolic products that are toxic to neurons. The course of CNS disease may parallel the immune deficiency, precede it, follow it, or never occur at all; however, at the time of AIDS diagnosis (usually the occurrence of opportunistic infection, Kaposi's sarcoma, or lymphoma), one-third of patients show overt and one-quarter show subclinical signs of this process. About 10% of patients will demonstrate significant CNS symptoms without any other sign of disease.

The symptom complex was first described and attributed to HIV rather than to opportunistic infections in 1985 (Navia et al. 1986); it is most commonly called the AIDS dementia complex. In 1987, the CDC revised the criteria for diagnosis, and included HIV encephalopathy

(AIDS dementia complex) as sufficient by itself, without opportunistic infections, neoplasms, or wasting syndrome, to indicate AIDS in a seropositive patient with no other explanation for the findings (CDC 1987a). The symptoms must be "disabling." Psychiatrists and neuropsychologists thus became responsible for diagnosing a significant segment of this patient population.

AIDS dementia complex is a subcortical dementia with a variable constellation of cognitive, behavioral, and motor disturbances. The cognitive dysfunction includes difficulty with concentration, with complaints of inability to follow written or verbal material; inability to carry out daily activities without lists; and general slowing and loss of precision in mentation. Forgetfulness and memory loss relate mostly to more complex tasks requiring concentration; orientation and simple object recall on mental status examination may be unimpaired, whereas serial 7s, reversals, or sequential mental and physical tasks will be slowed or broken down into component steps. Neuropsychological tests involving time pressure, problem solving, visual scanning, and alternation between two or more performance rules are often required to make the diagnosis.

Behavior changes most often include apathy and withdrawal from work and social and recreational activities, loss of spontaneity, and subtle changes in personality. Although these signs and symptoms appear to mimic depression, dysphoria is often absent. Less commonly seen are anxiety, hyperactivity, and regressed, inappropriate or "acting out" behavior. Organic psychoses with manic, paranoid, or nihilistic features have been reported and are often difficult to distinguish from schizophreniform disorder, bipolar disorder, psychotic depression, and reactive or drug-induced psychoses. A complete history of prior psychiatric problems, drug and alcohol abuse, and current medications and stressors is essential.

Motor symptoms usually lag behind. Complaints include loss of balance, gait disturbance, leg weakness, tremor, loss of fine motor control including deteriorating or small handwriting. Neurological examination reveals slowing of rapid alternating movements of the eyes and extremities; hyperreflexia, especially in the lower extremities; and pathological release phenomena including glabellar and snout (Navia et al. 1986; Price et al. 1988a, 1988b). HIV-induced peripheral neuropathy with numbness and pain is also a frequent occurrence.

Progression of the AIDS dementia complex is usually gradual but can accelerate in some individuals. It is also common for symptoms to fluctuate considerably from day to day. Psychomotor slowing, apathy, and mental impoverishment can evolve into mutism, severe dementia, or psychosis, while weakness and gait unsteadiness can progress to paraparesis, hypokinesia, and incontinence. Because the signs and symptoms at any stage are often indistinguishable from neoplastic and subacute opportunistic CNS pathology, high-risk patients, whether known to be seropositive or not, should be referred to their primary-care physician as quickly as possible. Consultation with the medical emergency room, with an AIDS-related disorders clinic, or with an infectious disease specialist should be obtained, with consent, if the patient is not in treatment. A summary of AIDS-related CNS diseases is presented in Table 13-2.

Psychosocial Factors

Receiving the diagnosis of AIDS is a catastrophic event, but for seropositive, high-risk, and even low-risk persons, the specter of the disease can also be overwhelming. Adaptation at all stages of illness results from a complex interplay of biological, psychological, and social factors. Biological factors include the illness itself with its fluctuating and irregular symptoms and relentless course; its debilitating and disfiguring consequences including the dementia complex; its invariably fatal outcome; the current lack of definitive treatment, cure, or vaccine; and any preexisting or concurrent disease, particularly major psychiatric disorders.

Psychological factors include the individual's personality structure, coping and defense mechanisms, prior functioning, interpersonal style, and social supports. These shape the response to the disease: anxiety about illness, doctors, and treatment; obsessions about new physical symptoms; anger and suspiciousness toward past sexual and blood contacts, toward high-risk groups, and toward an uncaring society; fears of isolation, reduced support, increasing dependency, and death; and depression with sadness, helplessness, lowered self-esteem, guilt, shame, worthlessness, hopelessness, suicidal thoughts, withdrawal, and anticipatory grief (Holland and Tross 1985). Another way of organizing this maze of affects, as with any fatal illness, is through the Kubler-Ross (1969) stages of denial, anger, bargaining, depression, and acceptance. The degree of a patient's denial must be carefully noted because, although helpful in moderation, a pathological excess can lead to ongoing high-risk activity.

Social and cultural factors include the stigma attached to the disease because of its associations with sex, blood, and death; the alienation of

Table 13-2. AIDS-related central nervous system diseases

- HIV syndromes
  AIDS dementia complex
  Atypical aseptic meningitis
  Vacuolar myelopathy
- Opportunistic viral illnesses
  Cytomegalovirus
  Herpes simplex virus, types 1 and 2
  Herpes varicella-zoster virus
  Papovavirus (progressive multifocal leukoencephalopathy)
  Adenovirus type 2
- Nonviral infections
  Toxoplasma gondii
  Cryptococcus neoformans
  Candida albicans
  Aspergillus fumigatus
  Coccidioides immitis
  Mucormycosis
  Rhizopus spp
  Acremonium alabamensis
  Histoplasma capsulatum
  Mycobacterium tuberculosis
  Mycobacterium avium
  Mycobacterium intracellulare
  Listeria monocytogenes
  Nocardia asteroides
- Neoplasms
  Primary central nervous system lymphoma
  Metastatic systemic lymphoma
  Metastatic Kaposi's sarcoma
- Cerebrovascular disorders
  Infarction
  Hemorrhage
  Vasculitis
- Complications of systemic AIDS therapy

Source. Adapted from Levy et al. 1988.

members of some high-risk groups by families of origin, by health-care providers, and by society in general; and the notion of innocent versus guilty victims.

Persons in specific risk groups and in specific stages of illness can present with similar symptoms. Low-risk individuals in the emergency room are often misinformed, phobic, obsessive, or somatic. High-risk persons can be obsessed with daily body scanning or looking for any suspicious lesion; or they can be ambivalent about whether to be tested. Not every high-risk person may benefit from knowing the result of antibody testing, particularly if the dangerous behavior has already been abandoned. The anxiety and risk of suicide of the recently tested individual has been discussed previously. After the acute anxiety subsides, the antibody-positive person, whether asymptomatic or with ARC, may develop body-scanning rituals and chronic anxiety or depression, waiting for the first sign of AIDS. There is often a gradual shift from anxiety to depression after the diagnosis of AIDS is made, and occasionally there is a brief period of relief. In the later stages, the physician will be challenged with distinguishing the dementia complex from depression (Fenton 1987; Lomax and Sandler 1988; Perry and Jacobsen 1986; Perry and Markowitz 1986).

EVALUATION

The interviewer must be flexible, empathic, nonjudgmental, and knowledgeable about the disease, about modes of transmission, and about specific behaviors and practices of the high-risk groups in order to form an alliance with the patient and to suggest appropriate treatment and referral. Questions about sexual and drug habits must be direct, and the interviewer should first use common names of body parts (e.g., penis, vagina, anus) and drugs (e.g., heroin, cocaine), resorting to slang only if the patient does not seem to comprehend. Medical jargon should be avoided. If suspicious physical symptoms constitute the chief complaint, the interview will proceed more smoothly if there is a gradual transition from medical to psychological issues. Even if the chief complaint is unrelated to HIV infection, any acute or chronic mental status change described by the patient should prompt the interviewer to include HIV disease in the differential diagnosis and pursue this with gentle questioning. Particular attention should be paid to the possibility of AIDS dementia complex superimposed on reactive or functional illness; a careful mental status examination is invaluable. If warranted, a neurologic examination can be performed to further assist with diagnosis. A summary of the evaluation of patients at high risk for HIV infection is found in Table 13-3.

TREATMENT AND REFERRAL

A significant part of any psychotherapeutic intervention should already

Table 13-3. Evaluation of patients at high risk for HIV infection

Factors that increase suspicion of infection, especially in the absence of drug or alcohol ingestion, prior major psychiatric problems, or preexisting cognitive impairment:

HISTORY
- *Physical*: Recent mononucleosis-like episode, aseptic meningitis or delirium, weight loss, chronic fevers, night sweats, lymphadenopathy, fatigue, chronic sore throat, cold or flu symptoms that linger
- *Cognitive*: Difficulty concentrating especially under pressure, slowed or inaccurate thinking, difficulty remembering what was seen on TV or read, memory loss when stressed, inability to accomplish tasks without lists, problems shifting from one task to another
- *Behavior*: Apathy, withdrawal from work and pleasurable activity often without feelings of depression, lessened spontaneity, unexplained anxiety or hyperactivity, unexplained regressed behavior, sudden onset of mania or psychosis
- *Motor*: Poor balance, gait disturbance, leg weakness, tremors, loss of fine motor control, handwriting smaller or more difficult to read, erratic visual scanning, unexplained numbness or tingling

EXAMINATION
- *Mental status*: Usually fully oriented and able to recall simple objects given enough time, digit spans and serial 7s decrease in accuracy with time constraints, serial mental and physical tasks performed slowly and broken down into component steps, difficulty shifting back and forth when performance rules are changed
- *Neurological*: Slowing of rapid alternating movements of extremities and eyes, lower extremity hyperreflexia, frontal release signs, glove and stocking sensory loss or paresthesias, loss of motor control as listed above

---

have occurred in an empathically conducted interview, by way of establishing a sense of trust in a possibly frightened and alienated patient. If the patient is without a primary-care physician or HIV specialist or is misinformed or uninformed about the disease, the most helpful initial course is to truthfully yet reassuringly educate the patient about HIV infection. This can include options about whether antibody testing is warranted, where the test can be obtained, the current stage of illness, the reasons for referral to an HIV specialist or clinic, and the need for immediate physical examination, laboratory tests, or hospitalization. Also useful is a summary of how the patient can best take care of himself or herself: proper diet, adequate sleep, avoidance of immune-depressant drugs and alcohol, and cessation of risky sexual and/or intravenous-drug activities. If ongoing behavior that is dangerous to others is anticipated, the limitations of confidentiality need to be explained. A review of the patient's support system can be followed with suggestions about who to tell about the crisis and when. Assistance with this difficult task can be offered; however, many psychiatrists and therapists who work with seropositive, ARC, and AIDS patients feel that significant supportive or insight work should only be undertaken by someone willing and able to stay with the patient throughout the course of the illness (Lomax and Sandler 1988).

In a similar fashion, psychopharmacologic interventions should be made cautiously. Just as in any other emergency psychiatric situation, adequate follow-up is not always possible. In addition, persons with systemic or CNS infection are particularly sensitive to dosage and side effects of psychotropic medication, much like the geriatric population. Acute anxiety or insomnia can be treated with low-dose, short-acting benzodiazepines such as lorazepam, alprazolam, or oxazepam. It is unlikely that any other types of medication would be initiated in the emergency setting unless the patient were being stabilized before psychiatric admission or transfer. Depression is best treated with low-dose, low-anticholinergic antidepressants such as desipramine, nortriptyline, trazodone, or fluoxetine, or with stimulants. Preexisting functional psychoses, concurrent reactive and drug-induced psychoses, or HIV-caused psychoses are best treated with low-dose, low-anticholinergic neuroleptics such as haloperidol, perphenazine, or trifluoperazine. Extrapyramidal side effects must be treated cautiously to avoid delirium. Some patients are more sensitive to extrapyramidal than anticholinergic side effects and can be treated with low-dose thioridazine. Lithium must be used with caution due to renal impairment during later stages of AIDS. The psychomotor slowing of the AIDS dementia complex can be partially ameliorated with the use of methylphenidate or amphetamine; the response is immediate but subjective improvement can exceed objective change (Fenton 1987; Lomax and Sandler 1988; Perry and Jacobsen 1986; Perry and Markowitz 1986). In some cases, azidothymidine (AZT) has been shown to gradually lessen the severity of the dementia.

Proper referral is a critical aspect of the psychiatric evaluation. As stated previously, consultation with physicians in the medical emergency area can expedite the need for comprehensive care, which is mandatory with this disease. If the patient is already in ongoing treatment, that physician or clinic should be notified as quickly as consent can be obtained, or without consent if necessary. Unless the private physician is expert in the management of HIV infection, the patient and physician should be tactfully encouraged to seek consultation from an AIDS-related disorders clinic or a specialist. Referral to a clinic is optimal, as consultants in infectious diseases, immunology, hematology, pulmonary medicine, neurology, psychiatry, dermatology, ophthalmology, and social work are generally available to the patient. This also solves the need for ongoing psychiatric management. Otherwise, referral should be made to psychiatrists or psychiatric clinics with willingness and experience to treat these complex problems.

The patient should also be given information about local AIDS organizations and volunteers who can assist with activities of daily living, transportation, applications for disability, and legal matters. Supportive group therapy has been shown to be of enormous value to patients in various stages of HIV infection; the patient should be referred to the leader or coordinator of such groups, if available in the area.

Seropositive intravenous-drug abusers and persons dependent on alcohol should be considered for admission to inpatient detoxification and/or rehabilitation programs (even moderate alcohol consumption has been shown to seriously dampen the immune response to HIV in vitro). Psychotic or suicidal patients should be admitted voluntarily or involuntarily to psychiatric units with an accepting staff and expert medical consultation available.

CONCLUSION

As the epidemic relentlessly gains momentum, psychiatrists will find themselves ever more involved in the diagnosis and care of persons with AIDS and HIV infection. Whether we view this as a challenge or a burden will depend on how well we apply all aspects of our biopsychosocial knowledge against this "great imposter" of our age.

REFERENCES

American Psychiatric Association Task Force on Psychiatric Aspects of AIDS: Position statement on AIDS. Am J Psychiatry 144:1122, 1987a

American Psychiatric Association Task Force on Psychiatric Aspects of AIDS: Position statement on HIV-related discrimination. Am J Psychiatry 144:1122, 1987b

American Psychiatric Association: AIDS policy: confidentiality and disclosure. Am J Psychiatry 145:541, 1988a

American Psychiatric Association: AIDS policy: guidelines for inpatient psychiatric units. Am J Psychiatry 145:542, 1988b

Castro RG, Lifson AR, White CR, et al: Investigations of AIDS patients with no previously identified risk factors. JAMA 259:1338–1342, 1988

Centers for Disease Control: MMWR 36 (suppl 1):1S, 1987a

Centers for Disease Control: MMWR 36 (suppl 1):2S, 1987b

Centers for Disease Control: MMWR 38 (suppl 1):1S, 1989

Curran JW, Jaffe HW, Hardy AM, et al: Epidemiology of HIV infection and AIDS in the United States. Science 239:610–616, 1988

Elder GA, Sever JL: AIDS and neurological disorders: an overview. Ann Neurol 23 (suppl):S4–S6, 1988

Fenton TW: AIDS-related psychiatric disorder. Br J Psychiatry 151:579–588, 1987

Holland JC, Tross S: The psychosocial and neuropsychiatric sequelae of the acquired immunodeficiency syndrome and related disorders. Ann Intern Med 103:760–764, 1985

Kubler-Ross E: On Death and Dying. New York, Macmillan, 1969

Levy RM, Bredesen DE, Rosenblum M: Opportunistic central nervous system pathology in patients with AIDS. Ann Neurol 23 (suppl 1):S7–S12, 1988

Lomax GL, Sandler J: Psychotherapy and consultation with persons with AIDS. Psychiatric Annals 18:253–259, 1988

McKhann GM: Research relative to AIDS. Ann Neurol 23 (suppl 1):S208–S209, 1988

Marzuk PM, Tierney H, Tardiff K, et al: Increased risk of suicide in persons with AIDS. JAMA 259:1333–1337, 1988

Navia BA, Jordan BD, Price RW: The AIDS dementia complex, I: clinical features. Ann Neurol 19:517–524, 1986

Perry S, Jacobsen P: Neuropsychiatric manifestations of AIDS-spectrum disorders. Hosp Community Psychiatry 37:135–136, 1986

Perry SW, Markowitz J: Psychiatric interventions for AIDS-spectrum disorders. Hosp Community Psychiatry 37:1001–1006, 1986

Piot P, Plummer FA, Mhalu FS, et al: AIDS: an international perspective. Science 239:573–579, 1988

Price RW, Brew B, Sidtis J, et al: The brain in AIDS: central nervous system HIV-1 infection and AIDS dementia complex. Science 239:586–592, 1988a

Price RW, Sidtis J, Rosenblum M: The AIDS dementia complex: some current questions. Ann Neurol 23 (suppl 1):S27–S33, 1988b

Shilts R: And the Band Played On: Politics, People, and the AIDS Epidemic. New York, St. Martin's Press, 1987

Appendix 13-1. **American Psychiatric Association AIDS policy: Guidelines for inpatient psychiatric units**

Patient Care

In the medical setting, all available evidence indicates that AIDS is a disease of low transmissibility. Education and counseling regarding HIV transmission continue to be needed and should be available to physicians and other medical personnel. Historically, physicians and other medical personnel have been exemplary in the treatment of patients, even in situations of personal risk, and it is expected that this tradition will continue.

- All psychiatric patients shall be treated based on their clinical conditions; neither HIV infection nor serologic status shall, in and of itself, impede the delivery of appropriate medical-psychiatric treatment.
- HIV serological testing should be performed on a case-by-case basis with informed consent when medically indicated. HIV serological testing should not be performed solely for the purpose of routine screening or staff awareness.
- Regardless of HIV serologic status, all inpatients should be considered potentially at risk for transmitting or receiving HIV infection. A minimal standard of care should include

  - Implementation and monitoring of infection control procedures as outlined by current CDC standards
  - Appropriate management of affective, cognitive, and behavioral disturbances to ensure risk reduction for both patients and personnel
  - Appropriate education and supportive services for patients, families, and staff

- If a patient known to be HIV infected engages, or threatens to engage, in behavior that places other individuals at risk, the responsible physician shall assure that appropriate clinical steps are taken to control the behavior, and, if necessary, isolate and/or restrain the patient.

Disclosure

Once a patient has been hospitalized on a psychiatric unit and responsibility for the patient's care has been assumed, a need to protect other patients and staff from foreseeable dangerous behavior arises. In the situation where a particular patient is known to be HIV positive, the following additional guidelines are recommended.

- Deciding whether to disclose a patient's HIV infection to other staff is a delicate clinical question. The responsible physician should disclose the information to appropriate staff only after discussions with the patient when the physician determines that appropriate treatment of the patient requires such disclosure.
- If the patient engages in behavior likely to transmit the virus and there is a significant risk that such behavior cannot be controlled by other measures, then disclosure of a patient's infectious condition to other patients at risk is permissible. Disclosure is not a substitute for adequate clinical care, and it is usually inappropriate for the physician or staff to disclose a patient's HIV infection to other patients.

Discharge

At the time when discharge is otherwise clinically appropriate, and the patient represents a substantial risk of danger to others by virtue of behavior known to transmit the virus, and this danger is not related to a specific mental condition, it is inappropriate to retain the person in the hospital solely for the purposes of quarantine or preventive detention.

Source. Reprinted from American Psychiatric Association 1988b. Copyright 1988, The American Psychiatric Association. Reprinted by permission.

Appendix 13-2. American Psychiatric Association AIDS policy: Confidentiality and disclosure

Introduction

The AIDS epidemic presents difficult and perplexing issues, many of which involve conflicts between the rights of infected individuals and the society's interest in containing the epidemic. Because these questions are highly controversial, and because so many important scientific questions about the disease remain unanswered, a definitive public health strategy has not yet emerged.

Physicians have an important role to play in controlling HIV infection. However, for physicians, the care and treatment of individual patients are of the utmost importance. Patients must be confident that issues discussed with their physicians are private and will not be unnecessarily divulged. Certainly any breach of confidentiality should be a last resort, only after scrupulous attention has been given to all other alternatives.

At the present time, the operational public health strategy promotes voluntary testing while eschewing programs of contact tracing, surveillance, segregation, and other measures that could discourage people from seeking testing. Many troublesome ethical and clinical questions arise in the context of dealing with individual patients, and the purpose of this document is to provide some guidance to members of the profession as they struggle to honor their duty to preserve the confidences of their patients while taking adequate precautions to protect other persons who may be at risk of contracting the disease.

Physicians should be aware that state laws may restrict some of the actions recommended in these guidelines. Where conflict exists, attempts should be made to modify laws in accordance with the principles expressed herein.

Confidentiality

Physicians have an ethical obligation to recognize the rights to privacy, to confidentiality, and to informed consent of all patients. During the initial clinical evaluation, the physician should usually make clear the general limits of confidentiality. If the physician has reason to suspect the patient is infected with HIV (i.e., is seropositive) or is engaging in behavior that is known to transmit HIV disease, the physician should notify the patient of the specific limits of confidentiality. Further, if the physician intends to inquire specifically about a patient's HIV status, the physician should, in such instances, notify the patient about the limits of confidentiality in advance of asking such questions.

Notification of Third Parties

In situations where a physician has received convincing clinical information (based on the patient's own disclosure of test results or on documented test records) that the patient is infected with HIV, the physician should advise and work with the patient either to obtain agreement to terminate behavior that places other persons at risk of infection or to notify identifiable individuals who may be at continuing risk of exposure. If a patient refuses to agree to change behavior or to notify the person(s) at risk, or the physician has good reason to believe that the patient has failed to or is unable to comply with this agreement, it is ethically permissible for the physician to notify an identifiable person who the physician believes is in danger of contracting the virus.

Disclosure to Third Parties

Most states now require physicians to report cases in which they diagnose AIDS to a public health agency, while only a few require the reporting of cases in which individuals test positive for HIV. It is ethically permissible for a physician to report to the appropriate public health agency the names of patients who are determined by convincing clinical information (based on the patient's disclosure of test results or documented test records) to be HIV infected and whom the physician has good reason to believe are engaging in behavior which places other persons at risk of HIV infection. Although we recognize that public health agencies have varying responses to the problem at the present time, provision of this information will allow them to take whatever measures they regard as appropriate.

Source. Reprinted from American Psychiatric Association 1988a. Copyright 1988, The American Psychiatric Association. Reprinted by permission.

Chapter 14

Alcohol

Paulette Gillig, M.D., Ph.D.

"When you hear hoofbeats, bet on horses, not zebras." With this pearl of house staff wisdom, a senior resident instructs a new intern: "Common things are common." Alcohol intoxication is the most common cause of acutely altered mental status. A study of emergency department patients with a depressed level of arousal found that 82% of them had a positive blood alcohol level (Holt et al. 1980). Alcohol has been identified as "part of the current problem" in 24–38% of psychiatric emergency service visits (Gillig et al. 1989). Alcoholism is a disorder that affects at least 10% of men and 3–5% of women in the United States (Schuckit 1987) and, as such, 14 million people in this country (West et al. 1984); yet alcoholism often is not diagnosed in the psychiatric emergency setting. Can we do better?

A recent study of the effectiveness of routine screening questions used to detect alcoholism in an ambulatory medical clinic found the pair of questions with the highest sensitivity to be "Have you ever had a drinking problem?" combined with "When was your last drink?" Questions with low sensitivities were "How much do you drink?" and "How often do you drink?" (Cyr and Wartman 1988). The definition of alcoholism that is probably most useful to clinicians is based on whether the patient is suffering from serious social or health problems related to alcohol (Schuckit 1984), so questions on these matters must also be part of history taking.

ALCOHOL INTOXICATION

Alcohol intoxication is a condition in which a patient displays impaired judgment, impaired social or occupational functioning, and disinhibition of sexual or aggressive impulses or mood lability, in the context of recent ingestion of alcohol. These changes are accompanied by slurred speech, incoordination, unsteady gait, nystagmus, or flushed face (DSM-III-R [American Psychiatric Association 1987]). Many of the above symptoms and signs can also be caused by other medical conditions and vice versa. For example, in a series of patients later diagnosed as having a concussion, 40% also had a positive blood alcohol level (Rutherford 1977). Before making the diagnosis of alcohol intoxication in a psychiatric emergency setting, it is important to ascertain whether the patient has ingested enough alcohol to cause the degree of apparent intoxication that is displayed clinically. Is there another substance, in addition to alcohol, that is contributing to the patient's symptoms? Is there a coexisting medical condition that is contributing to symptoms?

Evaluation

Initial evaluation in a psychiatric emergency setting of a patient presumably intoxicated with alcohol should include the following.

Vital signs. Accurate measurement of vital signs, including temperature, is essential to assist in evaluating possible coexisting medical conditions, such as encephalitis, pneumonia, diabetes, cardiomyopathy, etc., or impending delirium tremens.

Neurological checks. During the preliminary evaluation, the psychiatric nurse can determine whether the patient's pupils are dilated or constricted, whether nystagmus or ocular paralysis is present, and whether there is gross asymmetry of facial or limb movement.

Breathalyzer. The Breathalyzer alcohol level is useful because it enables staff to rapidly and inexpensively determine whether the degree of apparent clinical intoxication is consistent with the alcohol level. Although there is some variability in how a given patient may respond clinically to a particular alcohol level, depending in part on how chronically exposed the patient has been to alcohol, some estimates can be made (Adams and Victor 1981; Gibb 1986). A blood alcohol level of 20–50 mg/dl usually results in diminished fine motor control. At a level of 50–100 mg/dl, judgment and coordination are impaired. Difficulty with gait and balance is experienced at levels of 100–150 mg/dl. When the blood alcohol level reaches 150–250 mg/dl, the patient experiences lethargy and difficulty sitting upright. A level of 300 mg/dl can produce coma in the novice drinker, and respiratory depression results from levels above 400 mg/dl. A level of 500 mg/dl is potentially fatal.

The Breathalyzer has been found to be sufficiently accurate for clinical use (Gibb et al. 1984), with a high correlation to serum alcohol levels in cooperative patients and a significant correlation with serum levels in uncooperative patients. A Breathalyzer alcohol level (or blood alcohol level, if the Breathalyzer is unavailable) should always be obtained when there is significant alteration in mental status.

Medical history. Ideally, a psychiatrist or another physician on duty should obtain a medical history from the patient or collateral sources at the time of admission to a psychiatric emergency area. When staffing patterns do not permit this to be done, a triage nurse may take this history and determine whether to request that a physician see the patient.

Physical examination. Ideally, a brief general physical examination should be done at the time of admission for acutely intoxicated patients, particularly for patients who will remain the responsibility of the service for a number of hours. When vital signs or neurological checks are abnormal, the psychiatrist on duty should evaluate the patient further.

Toxicology screens. Patients who are psychotic or who develop significant alterations in level of consciousness despite relatively low alcohol levels, or who develop unstable vital signs, should have such a screen, especially for stimulants such as phencyclidine (PCP) and amphetamines. Drug quantification studies are needed only in cases where blood levels guide therapy (Gibb 1986).

Other laboratory tests. Determination of serum electrolytes, glucose, calcium, and magnesium levels is indicated if the patient is unstable or has a history of severe withdrawal symptoms.

Treatment

If the initial evaluation reveals no other abnormalities, the treatment of alcohol intoxication is supportive. One hundred milligrams of thiamine should be administered. The alcoholic patient may also be deficient in folic acid and niacin (Schuckit 1987); therefore, the patient should be prescribed oral multivitamins for several weeks after initial treatment.

Repeat alcohol levels are not mandatory in terms of the patient's safety, although sometimes they are helpful as a rough guideline for staff in determining when it is likely that the patient will become sober enough for a complete psychiatric interview. On an empty stomach, alcohol is absorbed within 30–60 minutes, so the alcohol level is likely to be at maximum when the patient presents to the psychiatric emergency service. Alcohol is metabolized by liver enzymes that can be induced by the chronic use of alcohol. In the novice drinker, alcohol is metabolized at a rate of 12 mg/dl per hour; in the chronic alcoholic, it is metabolized at a rate of 30 mg/dl per hour (Gibb 1986).

As indicated in the above discussion, it is possible to misdiagnose coexisting medical conditions (e.g., diabetes) as simple alcohol intoxication. Also, as the alcohol level drops, the patient may go into withdrawal. It is therefore essential to make regular checks on the patient. Staff are sometimes torn between a desire to assure that there has been no deterioration in mental status and not wanting to awaken the sleeping patient. A fair compromise, in the patient whose initial evaluation has shown no other abnormalities but who, because of staffing patterns, has not yet had a physical examination by a physician, is to repeat vital signs, neurological checks, and brief mental status testing at 1 and 3 hours after admission to the psychiatric emergency service. If the patient is stable or improving, he or she can probably be allowed to sleep for up to 6 hours. If the patient remains awake or awakens within this period, vital signs, etc., should be retested, because the patient may have awakened because of alcohol withdrawal symptoms or some other discomfort.

If during subsequent evaluations the patient develops psychosis, a significant alteration in level of consciousness especially in the face of a relatively low alcohol level, or has unstable vital signs or neurological checks, a physician on duty must examine the patient, and serum electrolytes, a complete blood count, and additional testing, such as a toxicology screen, will be necessary.

Psychiatric Evaluation

Being intoxicated with alcohol obviously does not protect an individual from other medical conditions, nor does it prevent the patient from having another psychiatric problem (Freed 1975). When a patient is admitted to the psychiatric emergency service, it becomes the responsibility of the staff to determine whether there is a coexisting psychiatric disorder, and if so, whether the patient requires further emergency treatment for this disorder. Patients with antisocial personality disorder and affective disorders (Schuckit 1984), as well as schizophrenia, have a high rate of secondary alcoholism. It is not possible to make a reliable diagnosis of these psychiatric conditions while the patient is intoxicated. Decisions sometimes must be made regarding whether to release an involuntary patient with incomplete information. Our position is that when intoxicated patients demand to leave a psychiatric emergency service and are probably not otherwise mentally ill, and the patients have a reliable person willing to assume responsibility and transport them home or to a care unit, we may consider allowing patients to leave. If patients desire to leave alone, they must wait until staff feel they will not be in danger from their impaired functioning, such as being too incoordinated to walk or having judgment too poor to cross the street. Staff should not release car keys to an individual who intends to drive while still clinically intoxicated. The decision-making process in such a case is similar to that faced by the general emergency room physician, who must decide whether to allow an intoxicated patient to leave on the basis of "medical safety."

On the other hand, when an intoxicated patient demands to leave but a third party (family, friends) gives a history of the patient's behavior that leads the staff to believe the patient may be mentally ill and a danger to self or others, or police or other delegated officials have signed a statement of belief of mental illness that the patient is a danger to self or others, a complete psychiatric evaluation must be done before the patient is allowed to leave.

PATHOLOGICAL INTOXICATION

This controversial diagnosis is characterized by a marked behavior change or behavior that is atypical for the patient when not drinking, such as blind, unfocused aggressiveness (Frances and Franklin 1987). It is thought to be due to the recent ingestion of alcohol, in quantities insufficient to induce intoxication in most people, resulting in amnesia for the period of intoxication. Persons with brain damage are thought to be especially at risk for this condition, having lost "tolerance" for alcohol. The differential diagnosis of this condition includes severe intoxication, epilepsy, compromised brain function from trauma, and histrionic behavior (Frances and Franklin 1987). Patients presenting to the psychiatric emergency service with symptoms of this disorder need to be evaluated by the psychiatrist as soon as possible.

ALCOHOL WITHDRAWAL

Alcohol is a central nervous system depressant. It can cause tolerance and physical dependence, and when heavy alcohol intake is stopped or decreased, withdrawal symptoms can occur that are the opposite of the acute effects of the drug (Schuckit 1987). Alcohol withdrawal can occur within several hours of a reduction in alcohol consumption in a person who has been drinking daily for a period of days to weeks. It is characterized by

- Hyperactive reflexes
- Reduction in the seizure threshold
- Coarse tremor of hands, tongue, or eyelids
- Nausea and vomiting
- Malaise or weakness
- Headache
- Insomnia with "bad dreams"
- Tachycardia
- Diaphoresis
- Elevated blood pressure
- Dry mouth
- "Puffiness" of the skin

Alcohol withdrawal can also be accompanied by transient psychiatric symptoms such as depressed mood, anxiety or irritability, and transient hallucinations.

Evaluation

A medical history and physical examination of the patient undergoing alcohol withdrawal is very important. These patients can become dehydrated and suffer an electrolyte imbalance, can suffer a hemorrhage of the gastrointestinal tract, and also are subject to infections such as pneumonia, causing hypoxia. Laboratory testing for these possible complications includes a complete blood count with differential, determination of glucose, blood urea nitrogen, electrolytes, bicarbonate, creatinine, serum calcium, and magnesium, and urinalysis. Chest X ray and electrocardiogram may also be indicated if the patient has a fever or has evidence of congestive heart failure.

In the patient with a long history of alcohol ingestion, the direct toxic effects of alcohol on various organ systems must be considered. The liver can be affected, with resultant hepatitis, cirrhosis, esophageal varices, and hepatic encephalopathy. The gastrointestinal tract may be involved, with peptic ulcer disease or pancreatitis. Cardiomyopathy may be present, resulting in chest pain, arrhythmia, and cardiomegaly. Finally, dementia, peripheral neuropathy, and cerebral degeneration may be present. Appropriate laboratory tests ordered in the psychiatric emergency room may include liver function tests, prothrombin time, serum amylase, and stool guaiac, in addition to the laboratory studies indicated above.

Complications

Table 14-1 compares features of three syndromes related to alcohol withdrawal.

Alcohol withdrawal seizures. Seizures during the alcohol withdrawal period are typically generalized and nonfocal, occur between 7 and 38 hours after cessation of drinking (Frances and Franklin 1987), and may occur in bursts of two to six generalized convulsions. Less than 3% of these patients develop status epilepticus (Adams and Victor 1981). Hypomagnesemia and hypoglycemia are associated with the development of seizures during alcohol withdrawal (Victor and Wolfe 1973). Approximately one-third of patients with alcohol withdrawal seizures go on to develop alcohol withdrawal delirium (also called delirium tremens), so seizures do have some prognostic value (Adams and Victor 1981). Seizures are usually a good indication for a medical, as opposed to a psychiatric, admission.

Alcohol withdrawal delirium. This disorder is characterized by delirium developing usually within 2–3 days after cessation of alcohol ingestion or a reduction in the amount ingested in alcoholic patients with 5–15 years of heavy drinking. Peak intensity is on the 4th or 5th day. Alcohol withdrawal delirium is characterized by marked autonomic hyperactivity, such as tachycardia and sweating. Terror, agitation, and primarily visual hallucinations or other perceptual distortions occur in about 50% of patients, although patients can also appear quietly confused. The level of consciousness may fluctuate widely (Victor and Adams 1953). Usually the delirium is short-lived, but can be character-

Table 14-1. Psychiatric emergency evaluation of alcohol withdrawal

Syndrome related to alcohol withdrawal	Time of onset	Physical signs	Other features	Possible complications	Recommended evaluation
Uncomplicated alcohol withdrawal	Several hours	Hyperactive reflexes, coarse tremor, tachycardia, hypertension, diaphoresis	Reduced seizure threshold, mood changes, transient hallucinations	Electrolyte imbalance, GI hemorrhage, pneumonia with hypoxia, seizures	CBC with differential, glucose, BUN, electrolytes, bicarbonate, creatinine, urinalysis, calcium, magnesium Consider chest X ray, ECG; liver function tests, prothrombin time, amylase, stool guaiac
Alcohol withdrawal delirium	2–3 days	Marked autonomic hyperactivity, tachycardia, diaphoresis	Terror, agitation, visual hallucinations and perceptual disturbances, fluctuating level of consciousness	Infections, pulmonary emboli, cardiac arrhythmia, secondary to electrolyte imbalance	As above
Alcohol hallucinosis	≥2 days	Clear sensorium, few autonomic changes	Lack of formal thought disorder	Coexistent seizures in early stages	CBC, electrolytes, calcium, magnesium (due to risk of coexistent seizures in early stages)

Note. GI = gastrointestinal. CBC = complete blood count. BUN = blood urea nitrogen. ECG = electrocardiogram.

ized by several relapses or can last as long as 5 weeks. Deaths during alcohol withdrawal delirium may be related to infections, pulmonary emboli, or cardiac arrhythmias associated with hyperkalemia, hyperpyrexia, poor hydration, or hypertension (Frances and Franklin 1987). Patients suffering from this disorder will probably require transfer to medical emergency services for a thorough physical examination to determine whether there is a concurrent medical condition, for administration of intravenous fluids, multivitamins, and folic acid, and for sedation with benzodiazepines or major tranquilizers (Schuckit 1987).

Alcoholic hallucinosis. This is an organic hallucinosis in which vivid and persistent auditory and visual hallucinations develop within 48 hours of cessation of or reduction in alcohol ingestion by a person dependent on alcohol. Typical patients are male and around the age of 40, with 10 or more years of heavy drinking. The disorder may last several weeks or months or may evolve into a chronic form, with severe impairment. In contrast to delirium, the hallucinations occur in an otherwise clear sensorium, and there are few, if any, autonomic symptoms. The symptoms may resemble schizophrenia, but there is a lack of formal thought disorder. If the risk of seizure is relatively low (i.e., 48 hours after onset of withdrawal), an attempt can be made to treat the patient with major tranquilizers while the psychosis persists, although the effectiveness of major tranquilizers in this setting is controversial (Victor and Wolfe 1973).

Treatment

Withdrawal symptoms are most dangerous when they take place in the context of other medical illnesses, and, therefore, a complete physical examination and appropriate laboratory testing are necessary before a decision can be made about inpatient versus outpatient management. Indications for hospitalization on a medical or surgical unit include a medical or surgical condition requiring treatment, such as infection, liver failure, arrhythmia, or abnormal vital signs (i.e., pulse greater than 110, blood pressure greater than 170 systolic or 110 diastolic, temperature greater than 99.5°F). Patients who are psychotic, encephalopathic, or delirious may be admitted to the psychiatry or medicine service, and patients suffering from a severe tremor or extreme agitation or seizures may be admitted to the neurology or psychiatry service. Finally, patients who have a history of severe withdrawal symptoms or of recent head trauma, who are abusing other substances in addition to alcohol, especially opiates, or who have no significant others to watch over them need to be in a protected environment for observation and treatment during alcohol detoxification. The goals of inpatient treatment during alcohol withdrawal include relieving symptoms, treating more serious complications, and preparing the patient for rehabilitation without introducing dependency on minor tranquilizers. On the other hand, 95% of alcoholic patients never experience severe signs of withdrawal (Schuckit 1987), and those with mild to moderate withdrawal symptoms can be treated initially in the psychiatric emergency service and then safely managed at home.

Outpatient management includes treatment with thiamine and multivitamins and may include treatment with benzodiazepines, which are the medications of choice for withdrawal symptoms (Frances and Franklin 1987; Jacob and Sellers 1977; Schuckit 1987). In patients who have severe liver diseases, a short-acting benzodiazepine, such as lorazepam, is useful because there is less of a problem of drug accumulation; however, a longer-acting drug, such as chlordiazepoxide or diazepam, is a better choice because it provides relatively smooth withdrawal.

If the psychiatrist in the psychiatric emergency service elects to undertake outpatient management of mild to moderate alcohol withdrawal, the patient must be seen daily to assure that sedation is adequate and to observe for complications. Chlordiazepoxide, which has a half-life of 30–36 hours but a relatively slow onset of action, can be given in doses of 25–50 mg po qid on the first day of treatment, with a 20% decrease in dose per day over a 5-day period. If a shorter-acting benzodiazepine is selected as the drug of choice because of compromised liver function, it must be given at shorter intervals and must be carefully tapered; for example, lorazepam 1–4 mg po q 6–8 hours.

APPROPRIATE REFERRAL

Once the psychiatrist makes a diagnosis of alcoholism in a patient who is in a state of denial about the condition, it is necessary to confront the patient to help him or her recognize the problem (Miller 1987). Schuckit (1984) recommends connecting the patient's area of concern (or chief complaint) with alcohol use and showing how they relate to each other. For example, the psychiatrist might say, "There is one way I have of pulling all of these findings together. I believe you have reached a point in life where alcohol is causing more trouble than it's worth." If the patient refuses to consider this possibility at that time, the psychiatrist should encourage the patient to come back at a future date when he or she has had more time to think things over. Psychiatric emergency staff sometimes become very frustrated and angry at the alcoholic patient who will not seek help or who does not improve, and these feelings can get in the way of trying to help the patient. For example, in a recent study of all patients presenting to two psychiatric emergency services, patients presenting with intoxication with alcohol or other substances were perceived as "hardest to empathize with" and were "least liked" by staff (Gillig et al., in press). If staff become overly discouraged, they can transmit this feeling of defeat to the patient and inadvertently sabotage the very rehabilitation they desire to promote.

Outpatient Referral

For the patient who is diagnosed as alcoholic, who has no other psychiatric disorder, and who does not present to the psychiatric emergency service in a severely intoxicated state, outpatient rehabilitation is recommended if possible because it is less costly and teaches the patient to adjust to life in the "real world" (Schuckit 1984). In such a setting, group counseling is probably as effective as individual counseling, using paraprofessional staff who are supervised by people with more formal training in counseling. Medications are to be avoided. Disulfiram (Antabuse) may be a reasonable adjunct to ongoing outpatient treatment but should almost never be prescribed from an emergency setting.

Alcoholics Anonymous

Alcoholics Anonymous can be helpful in offering the patient support and guidance in maintaining sobriety, and it is free. Alcoholics Anonymous has as its primary objective the goal of helping its members remain abstinent from alcohol and drugs. Membership is confidential and voluntary. A basic tenet of the program is that alcoholism is a physical, mental, and spiritual disease affecting alcoholic patients and their families. Al-Anon is a support group for families affiliated with Alcoholics Anonymous and is helpful for concerned relatives and friends who have assumed the role of caretaker. They have been called coaddicts by self-help groups, as they often neglect their own personal needs and rights in their attempt to support the alcoholic patient. There is a higher recovery rate in alcoholic patients where significant others are concurrently included in treatment (Cocores 1987).

Inpatient Treatment

Inpatient rehabilitation is indicated for patients who have not responded to outpatient counseling, who have serious medical problems, who have major psychiatric disorders, or whose lives are so chaotic that they are unable to focus on rehabilitation goals in an outpatient setting. The best course of treatment involves 2–4 weeks of inpatient care, followed by a 6- to 12-month aftercare program (Cocores 1987; Mosher et al. 1975).

Dual-Diagnosis Inpatient Units

Patients suffering from a primary psychiatric condition with alcohol abuse related to this condition benefit from specialized inpatient and outpatient treatment programs. When alcohol or other substance abuse complicates psychiatric problems, these persons often become "revolving door" patients to the psychiatric emergency service. They can be difficult to engage in treatment, but need such treatment as indicated by their relatively high rate of suicide (Bachrach 1986–1987; Stein et al. 1975).

REFERENCES

Adams RD, Victor M: Principles of Neurology. New York, McGraw-Hill, 1981

American Psychiatric Association: Diagnostic and Statistical Manual of Mental Disorders, 3rd Edition, Revised. Washington, DC, American Psychiatric Association, 1987

Bachrach L: The context of care for the chronic patient with substance abuse. Psychiatr Q 58:3–14, 1986–1987

Cocores JA: Co-addiction: a silent epidemic. Fair Oaks Hospital Psychiatry Letter 5:5–8, 1987

Cyr MG, Wartman SA: The effectiveness of routine screening questions in the detection of alcoholism. JAMA 259:51–54, 1988

Frances RJ, Franklin JE: Alcohol-induced organic mental disorders, in The American Psychiatric Press Textbook of Neuropsychiatry. Edited by Hales RE, Yudofsky SC. Washington, DC, American Psychiatric Press, 1987, pp 141–156

Freed E: Alcoholism and schizophrenia: the search for perspectives: a review. J Stud Alcohol 36:853–881, 1975

Gibb K: Serum alcohol levels, toxicology screens and the use of the breath alcohol analyzer. Ann Emerg Med 15:349–353, 1986

Gibb KA, Yee AS, Johnson CC, et al: Accuracy and usefulness of a breath alcohol analyzer. Ann Emerg Med 13:516–520, 1984

Gillig P, Hillard JR, Bell J, et al: The psychiatric emergency holding area: effect on utilization of inpatient resources. Am J Psychiatry 146:369–372, 1989

Gillig PM, Hillard JR, Deddens J: Therapists' emotional reactions to psychiatric emergency patients. Hosp Community Psychiatry (in press)

Holt S, Stewart IC, Dixon JM, et al: Alcohol and the emergency service patient. Br Med J 281:638–640, 1980

Jacob MS, Sellers EM: Emergency management of alcohol withdrawal. Drug Therapy 28–34, 1977

Miller NS: A primer of the treatment process for alcoholism and drug addiction. Fair Oaks Hospital Psychiatry Letter 5:30–37, 1987

Mosher V, Dairs J, Mulligan D, et al: Comparison of outcome in a 9-day and 30-day alcoholism treatment program. J Stud Alcohol 36:1277–1281, 1975

Rutherford WH: Diagnosis of alcohol ingestion in mild head injuries. Lancet 1:1021–1023, 1977

Schuckit MA: Drug and Alcohol Abuse: A Clinical Guide to Diagnosis and Treatment. New York, Plenum, 1984

Schuckit MA: Guidelines for the treatment of alcohol withdrawal. Fair Oaks Hospital Psychiatry Letter 5:13–20, 1987

Stein LI, Newton JR, Bowman RS: Duration of hospitalization for alcoholism. Arch Gen Psychiatry 32:247–252, 1975

Victor M, Adams RD: The effect of alcohol on the nervous system. Res Publ Assoc Res New Ment Dis 32:526–573, 1953

Victor M, Wolfe SM: Causation and treatment of the alcohol withdrawal syndrome, in Alcoholism: Progress in Research and Treatment. Edited by Bourne PG, Fox R. New York, Academic, 1973, pp 137–166

West LJ, Maxwell DS, Noble EP, et al: Alcoholism. Ann Intern Med 100:405–416, 1984

Chapter 15

Drug Abuse

Paulette Gillig, M.D., Ph.D.

Increasing numbers of patients are being seen in psychiatric emergency settings due to symptoms of substance abuse. Some have developed or will develop other mental disorders, either having turned to street drugs to self-medicate their psychiatric symptoms (Hasin et al. 1985; Khantzian 1985) or having precipitated a psychosis or affective disorder by drug ingestion (Breakey et al. 1974; Treffert 1978; Tsuang et al. 1982). In today's climate of deinstitutionalization, young chronically mentally ill patients often experiment with street drugs (Bachrach 1986–1987), and studies of psychiatric inpatients show that one-third to one-half also are substance abusers (Alterman et al. 1982; Crowley et al. 1974; Fischer et al. 1975).

One of the challenges in diagnosing and treating patients in a psychiatric emergency setting, who may be substance abusers and who may also have another psychiatric disorder, lies in making a correct diagnosis of the psychiatric disorder while not overdiagnosing transient symptoms related to substance abuse alone. It is well known that different classes of drugs can produce different psychiatric symptoms (Table 15-1) and can be related to different psychiatric disorders (Table 15-2), and illicit drug use is in the differential diagnosis for almost every patient presenting to a psychiatric emergency service. One factor complicating the emergency diagnosis and treatment of substance-abusing patients is that the patient's report of ingested substances often is unreliable (Soslow

1981), and although a toxicology screen can be helpful, signs of withdrawal, organic brain syndrome, and psychosis can persist for up to 2 weeks after blood and urine screens become normal (Gibb 1986).

Another common error made in psychiatric emergency services is attributing all symptoms of intoxication to alcohol rather than considering the possibility that the patient may be intoxicated with other substances as well. When alcohol Breathalyzer or blood levels are low relative to the patient's degree of clinical impairment, the emergency psychiatrist must consider the possibility that the patient is intoxicated with or withdrawing from other substances (Gibb 1986). Also, the emergency psychiatrist must be able to evaluate the possibility of an organic brain syndrome caused by another medical condition (e.g., subdural hematoma).

INITIAL EVALUATION

The psychiatric nurse doing triage should determine vital signs, assess level of consciousness (alert, stuporous, fluctuating), observe pupil size and reactivity, and look for the presence of nystagmus or asymmetric

Table 15-1. Psychiatric emergency considerations for selected drugs of abuse

Amphetamines	Hypertension, risk of violence
Anabolic steroids	Hypertension, mood instability
Anticholinergics	Delirium, atropine-like effects
Cannabis	Paranoid ideation, adverse drug interactions
Cocaine	Agitation, hypervigilance, tachycardia, dilated pupils, myocardial infarction, delirium with autonomic instability
Hallucinogens	Hallucinosis; delusional, mood, or perception disorder; pupillary dilation; tachycardia; tremors (mescaline)
Inhalants	Euphoria, impulsiveness, dizziness, nystagmus, stupor, arrhythmia, respiratory depression
Opioids	Euphoria, lethargy, somnolence, characteristic withdrawal syndrome
Phencyclidine	Rotary nystagmus, hypertension, arrhythmias, facial grimacing
Sedatives, hypnotics, anxiolytics	Labile mood, impaired judgment, amnestic disorder, life-threatening withdrawal syndrome

Table 15-2. Psychiatric disorders related to substance abuse

	Intoxication	Withdrawal	Delirium	Withdrawal delirium	Delusional disorder	Mood disorder	Amnestic disorder
Amphetamines	X	X		X			
Cannabis	X				X		
Cocaine	X	X	X		X		
Hallucinogens	X				X	X	
Inhalants	X						
Opioids	X	X					
Phencyclidine (PCP) and related substances	X		X		X	X	
Sedatives, hypnotics, or anxiolytics	X	X		X			X

Source. Developed using DSM-III-R.

gait. Any abnormalities should be brought to the attention of the emergency psychiatrist. Any life-threatening abnormalities, such as severely depressed level of consciousness or grossly abnormal vital signs, need immediate attention, and the patient should be referred to an emergency medicine setting to be stabilized and so that an adequate airway can be established, artificial ventilation provided if necessary, circulation supported, and convulsions treated if present.

The initial evaluation of a presumably intoxicated patient in a psychiatric emergency service also should include a medical and psychiatric history, with third-party corroboration where possible. This can be done in collaboration with a social work therapist. Information may become available in a progressive manner as friends or relatives call or are called and charts appear, and the emergency psychiatrist must continually reevaluate the patient's condition and working diagnosis as information is added.

The psychiatrist working in a psychiatric emergency setting will need to decide which laboratory studies, if any, will be obtained. An electrocardiogram should be considered if 1) pulse rate exceeds 120 or the rhythm is irregular or 2) a cardiopulmonary examination (performed when medical history or vital signs are abnormal or the patient complains of chest pain) or the history suggests the possibility of a cardiac complication (e.g., a patient who has overdosed on cocaine [crack] or a nonbarbiturate hypnotic). If a presumably intoxicated patient 1) displays abnormal vital signs or neurological checks, 2) has a history of medical illness such as diabetes, or 3) remains confused (delirious) for 2 hours or more, the following laboratory tests should be considered:

- Complete blood count to rule out infection or anemia
- Liver function tests, elevated if hepatitis is present
- Serum glucose
- Blood urea nitrogen
- Creatinine
- Electrolytes

If a complete toxicology screen cannot be obtained on a "stat" basis, a clinical decision must be made as to whether it is more important to obtain partial information quickly, or to wait until the complete screen can be run. When the results of these laboratory studies become available, consultation with other medical services may be necessary, and a decision must be reached concerning whether the patient needs admission and, if so, whether to psychiatry or medicine. Patients who remain confused, who have a history of heart disease, withdrawal seizures or withdrawal delirium, or who have a fever or a significantly elevated pulse or blood pressure that does not return to normal after treatment in the psychiatric emergency service should be admitted.

MANAGEMENT OF SPECIFIC DRUG-INDUCED PSYCHIATRIC EMERGENCIES

Amphetamine- or Similarly Acting Sympathomimetic– Induced Organic Mental Disorders

Amphetamine-related substances (*d-l*-amphetamine, dextroamphetamine sulfate, methamphetamine, and methylphenidate) can be taken orally, intravenously, vaginally, rectally, or intranasally. Pseudoephedrine, phenylpropanolamine hydrochloride, and other decongestants have effects similar to amphetamines if taken in high-enough doses. Amphetamine users sometimes use these drugs as substitutes, either knowingly or unknowingly. They are absorbed rapidly from the gastrointestinal tract, reaching a peak plasma level in 1–2 hours (Slaby and Swift 1987). Acute intoxication with a mild to moderate dose (less than 30 mg of dextroamphetamine) is characterized by excessive sympathetic activity, dilation of the pupils, tremor, hypertension, restlessness, hyperthermia, tachypnea, tachycardia, and hyperactivity. At higher doses, anxiety, panic, and confusion can occur, accompanied by vasomotor disturbance and, ultimately, severe hypertension (Table 15-3). In addition, the patient can suffer an acute paranoid psychosis with auditory hallucinations that is indistinguishable from a delusional disorder or paranoid schizophrenia. A study of 86 psychiatric patients found that those patients whose drug screens were positive for amphetamines had usually been diagnosed as having schizophrenia (Rockwell and Ostwald 1968). The differential diagnosis of amphetamine intoxication includes myocardial infarction or hyperthyroidism, and simultaneous depressant withdrawal must be considered. Amphetamine abusers commonly attempt to antagonize various toxic symptoms with opioids.

In the case of a serious overdose, appropriate life-support measures and treatment with antihypertensives are necessary and should be done by the emergency medicine service. A patient presenting to the psychiatric emergency service who may be intoxicated with amphetamines should have a toxicology screen to confirm the diagnosis and help determine the likelihood of symptoms clearing if the patient is held overnight, rather than admitted. The patient should be placed in a calm

Table 15-3. Physical findings at initial nurse triage

	Blood pressure	Pupils	Tremor	Fever	Pulse	Respiration
Amphetamine intoxication	High	Dilated	Yes	Yes	Rapid	Rapid
Anticholinergic intoxication		Dilated		Yes	Rapid	
Cannabis intoxication					Rapid	
Cocaine intoxication	High	Dilated	Yes		Rapid (?arrhythmia)	
Anabolic steroid intoxication	May be high					
Hallucinogen intoxication		Dilated			Rapid	
Phencyclidine intoxication		Rotary nystagmus		Yes	Rapid	
Inhalant intoxication		Nystagmus				
Opioid intoxication		Constricted				
Opioid withdrawal	Mildly high	Dilated		Yes		
Sedative, hypnotic, or anxiolytic intoxication	Orthostatic	Slow to react				Depressed
Sedative, hypnotic, or anxiolytic withdrawal			Yes	Yes	Rapid	

Note. Empty cells indicate that findings are not affected by these drugs.

environment. Haloperidol (5 mg q 6 hours) usually will suppress paranoid delusions, but the patient may require a brief hospitalization because the psychosis may persist for approximately 1 week. Treatment with haloperidol, perphenazine, or thiothixene is preferable to treatment with chlorpromazine, which may increase the half-life of amphetamines, and is preferable to treatment with anxiolytics, which may increase the risk of violence (Angrist et al. 1974). Restraints may be needed in the psychiatric emergency service during the acute intoxication period, because the patient is at risk for acting out violently.

Marked depression, which can be long lasting and sometimes requires antidepressant treatment, can occur with cessation of use in chronic amphetamine users, and such patients may present to the emergency psychiatrist because of suicidal ideation. Such patients also experience sleepiness, anxiety, gastrointestinal distress, nightmares, headaches, dyspnea, muscle cramps, and malaise.

"Ecstasy." Methylenedioxymethamphetamine (MDMA) is known as "Ecstasy" on the street. It is biochemically related to the amphetamines and was originally synthesized as an appetite suppressant but never marketed. Users report that it causes elevated mood and feelings of enhanced intimacy. Unfortunately, it also can cause tachycardia, a nervous desire to be in motion, insomnia, tremor, nausea and vomiting, and, rarely, transient hallucinations (Climko et al. 1987).

Anabolic Steroid Abuse

Athletes, especially weight lifters and body builders, recently have coveted the anabolic steroids as stimulants of skeletal muscle growth. Some athletes also have claimed they subjectively experienced less fatigue during their workouts when taking these drugs (Lamb 1984).

Unfortunately, the anabolic steroids have been reported to cause mood instability, aggressive outbursts, and occasional psychotic episodes (Lamb 1984) and, when used chronically, have caused a suppression in endogenous testosterone production persisting for several months, resulting in testicular atrophy, decreased libido, decreased spermatogenesis, priapism, and gynecomastia (Alen et al. 1985). Medical complications include sodium and fluid retention resulting in sometimes severe hypertension and a decrease in blood levels of high-density lipoprotein cholesterol with an increase in low-density lipoprotein cholesterol leading to coronary artery disease (Alen et al. 1985; Webb et al. 1984). Finally, anabolic steroid use has been associated with liver function abnormalities, including hepatic malignancy.

Users of these drugs may not mention them spontaneously. The possibility of steroid abuse should be considered in any athlete presenting to the psychiatric emergency service with behavior or mood changes.

Anticholinergic Abuse

Patients presenting to a psychiatric emergency service because they "lost" their Cogentin (for example) prescription should be evaluated for the possibility of anticholinergic abuse, which is increasing among young psychiatric patients who are also prescribed neuroleptics (Dilsaver 1988). These patients often also use marijuana to "come down" from the mildly euphoric "high" induced by anticholinergic drugs such as benztropine mesylate (Cogentin), biperiden (Akineton), diphenhydramine hydrochloride (Benadryl), and trihexyphenidyl hydrochloride (Artane). Delirium may occur as well, associated with atropine-like effects such as dry, warm skin; dilated fixed pupils; fever; tachycardia; diminished peristalsis; and an atonic bladder (Preskorn and Irwin 1982). These effects last for about 8–12 hours.

Cannabis-Induced Organic Mental Disorders

Patients with schizophrenia, even if stabilized on neuroleptics, can experience an exacerbation of the psychosis after cannabis use and therefore present a psychiatric emergency (Preskorn and Irwin 1982; Treffert 1978). Also, cannabis use can precipitate adverse drug interactions, by prolonging the half-life of barbiturates, increasing serum lithium levels, and causing an increase in heart rate and intense psychological distress when used with alcohol. One case of a hypomanic reaction associated with disulfiram plus cannabis has been reported. When combined with tricyclic antidepressants, cannabis use can cause panic attacks, and cannabis has additive physiological effects with amphetamines. Tachycardia is the most likely cardiovascular effect of cannabis-opioid combinations (Hillard and Vieweg 1983; Knudsen and Vilnar 1984).

Cannabis can induce dependence characterized by daily, or almost daily, use. Psychiatric effects of cannabis intoxication, which occur immediately after smoking and peak in 3 hours, may include euphoria, anxiety, suspiciousness, or paranoid ideation. Cannabis use also can be associated with problems with short-term memory, impaired judgment, and social withdrawal. Depersonalization or derealization may occur, but hallucinations are rare except with very high blood levels. A delusional disorder also may develop, which usually remits within a day. If the delusions do not clear, this usually is indicative of a preexisting psychosis. Patients who are novice users or who have not developed tolerance to the drug may experience a panic episode (Rottanburg et al. 1982), dysphoria, or inappropriate laughter, although most users develop a pleasant, euphoric "high."

Physical signs of cannabis abuse include conjunctival injection, tachycardia, and tachypnea, often associated with an increase in appetite (often for "junk food") and dry mouth. Some persons experience nausea, headache, nystagmus, and either transient increase or mild orthostatic decrease in blood pressure (Benowitz and Jones 1981; Rottanburg et al. 1982).

Whether an actual withdrawal syndrome is associated with discontinuation of cannabis use in the chronic user is controversial. If it occurs, it is likely dose related and is characterized by nausea, lowered appetite, mild anxiety, and insomnia (Mendelson et al. 1984).

Cocaine-Induced Organic Mental Disorders

Cocaine is a highly addictive drug of abuse, in part because of its effect of producing a temporary feeling of intense euphoria. Because of this psychological effect, it is the drug of choice of patients with mood disorders who may be trying to medicate themselves (Khantzian 1985) and, as such, is often confronted in the management of dual-diagnosis patients seen in a psychiatric emergency setting. Unfortunately, in addition to its quick euphoric effects, cocaine can produce ischemic chest pains and myocardial infarction within minutes to hours of use (Smith et al. 1987). Arrhythmias and myocarditis have also been reported, as well as a life-threatening delirium. In the past, most cocaine was taken intranasally (snorted), but recently, cocaine has become available in smokable or injectable forms (free base). The popularity of freebasing is apparently linked to a shift in cocaine distribution patterns, with dealers switching to selling freebase extracted from cocaine produced in tiny chunks known on the street as "crack." Crack, when smoked, is rapidly absorbed into the pulmonary circulation and is transmitted to the brain in less than 10 seconds. The drug's euphoric effects are intensified and compressed into 3–5 minutes, followed by dysphoria and intense cravings for more of the drug.

Cocaine intoxication results in tachycardia, dilated pupils, elevated blood pressure, perspiration or chills, and sometimes nausea and vomiting. Transient signs of psychosis may occur, such as ideas of reference or the experience of hearing one's name called, and therefore, intoxicated patients may be brought to the psychiatric emergency service. Tactile or visual hallucinations may occur, especially feeling or seeing insects crawling on the skin. The patient may respond to these experiences by fighting and becoming very agitated and hypervigilant.

In addition to the usual syndrome of cocaine intoxication, an acute delirious state can occur in either the chronic or first-time user. The delirious state is accompanied by hypertension, hyperpyrexia, metabolic acidosis, and potentially by convulsions and cardiovascular collapse. Patients with any signs of this syndrome should be transferred to the emergency medicine service.

Neuroleptics may be used for frankly psychotic but medically stable patients, but it must be kept in mind that 1) chronic cocaine users may be very sensitive to the extrapyramidal side effects of neuroleptics and 2) neuroleptics may increase craving for cocaine in these patients (Perry 1987).

After the immediate effects of intoxication, a rebound phenomenon occurs during which the patient experiences depression and craving for cocaine, sometimes associated with anxiety, tremulousness, irritability, and fatigue. If no additional cocaine is ingested, recovery should occur within 48 hours. However, if the patient has used cocaine heavily for several days or longer, a withdrawal syndrome can occur. Cocaine withdrawal is characterized by symptoms persisting for more than 24 hours of dysphoric mood, insomnia, or hypersomnia or psychomotor agitation, which are associated with paranoid or suicidal ideation. The symptoms usually peak in 2–4 days, although depression and irritability may persist for months. Cocaine withdrawal should be treated on an inpatient basis because of the potential for impulsive suicide attempts. Ideally, the patient should then be transferred to a halfway house because relapse into further cocaine abuse is very common.

Chronic cocaine abuse can lead to a picture that is impossible to differentiate in a psychiatric emergency setting from a functional paranoid disorder, with personality changes characterized by a clear consciousness and minimal cognitive impairment, but with impaired judgment, impulsivity, aggressiveness, suspiciousness developing into fixed delusional beliefs, and anorexia with weight loss. Other features that can help in the differential diagnosis are insomnia, irritability, inflamed nasal mucosa from repeated inhalation, hyperreflexia, masked facies, and a parkinsonian tremor.

Hallucinogen-Induced Organic Mental Disorders

Several psychiatric syndromes related to the use of hallucinogens may be seen in the psychiatric emergency service (DSM-III-R [American Psychiatric Association 1987]). *Hallucinogen hallucinosis* occurs in the fully alert patient usually 1 hour after ingestion and, in the case of lysergic acid diethylamide (LSD), lasts 8–12 hours. The syndrome is characterized by a subjective intensification of perceptions, a sense of depersonalization or derealization, visual (usually) illusions or hallucinations, and synesthesias (such as seeing colors when one hears loud sounds). These perceptual experiences can be accompanied by severe anxiety or paranoid ideation, although patients may instead by euphoric. Patients may have insight that the perceptual changes are caused by the drug, but also may develop a *hallucinogen delusional disorder* in which they become convinced that the disordered perceptions conform to reality.

A patient may also present to the emergency psychiatrist with depression or anxiety, which may persist for more than 24 hours after hallucinogen use (*hallucinogen mood disorder*). The mood disorder is associated with restlessness and difficulty sleeping. These symptoms may be transient but may also develop into a long-lasting episode of depression.

Finally, a patient who in the past has used hallucinogens may experience "flashback" hallucinations (*posthallucinogen perception disorder*). These hallucinations or illusions can be triggered by psychological stress or by the use of various drugs, especially cannabis. Half of the patients who develop this disorder experience remission of symptoms within months, but others continue to have symptoms for several years. Reassurance is usually effective; benzodiazepines can be used if the patient is anxious.

The hallucinogens include two groups of psychoactive substances. The first group includes LSD, dimethyltryptamine (DMT), and similar substances all related structurally to 5-hydroxytryptamine. The second group, which includes mescaline, is related to the catecholamines. Because the latter group of drugs tend to have adrenergic effects, the physical examination will reveal pupillary dilation, tachycardia, diaphoresis, palpitations, tremors, and incoordination.

The treatment for hallucinogen intoxication consists of placing the patient in a calm environment and correcting misperceptions when they occur ("talking down the patient") (Perry 1987). Benzodiazepines can be used as needed if the patient is extremely nervous. Haloperidol (5 mg q 2–4 hours) or other antipsychotics can also be used during acute phases of intoxication if the patient does not respond to more conservative management. One complicating factor in treating patients intoxicated with hallucinogens is that these drugs frequently are contaminated with other drugs such as phencyclidine (PCP) and amphetamines.

Inhalant-Induced Organic Mental Disorders

Inhalants are sometimes used by groups of children as young as 9 or 10 years old, as well as by adolescents and adults. The substances placed in the class of inhalants are mixtures of aliphatic and aromatic hydrocarbons found in gasoline, glue, paint, paint thinners, and spray paints, or halogenated hydrocarbons found in cleaners, typewriter correction fluid, and spray-can propellants and other volatile compounds containing esters, ketones, and glycols. To inhale these substances, patients may use soaked rags held to the nose or mouth, or inhale directly from containers or from aerosol cans.

Intoxication can occur within 5 minutes of inhaling the substance. Cessation can occur 1–1.5 hours after inhaling, but chronic users can titrate the dose to maintain a constant level of intoxication. A patient mildly under the influence of an inhalant may become euphoric and behave similarly to one mildly intoxicated with alcohol, but is more likely to become aggressive, behave impulsively, or otherwise display impaired judgment, and this may bring the individual to the attention of the psychiatric emergency staff.

Moderate to severe intoxication with inhalants can produce feelings of dizziness, nystagmus, slurred speech, unsteady gait, lethargy with psychomotor retardation, depressed reflexes, tremor, light sensitivity, blurred vision, and stupor or coma. The mental status examination usually reveals delirium, although hallucinations and delusions can occur. Muscle destruction, with skeletal muscle weakness, has been reported especially after chronic toluene abuse, and chronic gasoline inhalation can result in a peripheral neuropathy. Because hepatitis with possible liver failure has been reported after chronic exposure to solvents, and kidney failure has been reported with chronic abuse of toluene and benzine, hepatic and renal functions should be tested in patients known to abuse inhalants. Also, potentially fatal aplastic anemia has also occurred in some of these patients.

A life-threatening respiratory depression, accompanied by cardiac arrhythmias, has been associated with severe inhalant intoxication with fluorinated hydrocarbon aerosols (e.g., Freon), the inhalants most often associated with arrhythmias (Goldsmith 1989). Patients showing signs of this syndrome should be transferred to the emergency medicine service because they require cardiac monitoring and may require artificial ventilation.

PCP- or Similarly Acting Arylcyclohexylamine–Induced Organic Mental Disorders

PCP and similar mind-altering drugs known as "dissociatives" can induce a variety of psychiatric disorders, including atropine-like intoxication, delirium, a delusional disorder, and a disorder of mood. It is sometimes ingested through marijuana cigarettes soaked in PCP, known as "clickers." Symptoms of intoxication with PCP begin 1 hour after oral use but can start within 5 minutes of intravenous administration or smoking. PCP is one of a few substances that can produce characteristic rotatory or vertical as well as horizontal nystagmus (Pitts et al. 1982). It has sympathomimetic effects and can induce hypertension, increased heart rate with arrhythmias, and hyperthermia. Therefore, vital signs must be monitored carefully (every 15–30 minutes). The patient will often be ataxic, may display bizarre facial grimacing, may have muscle rigidity with catatonic posturing (sometimes confused with schizophrenia), and may have seizures. PCP can also cause an individual to have diminished responsiveness to pain, resulting in serious physical injury (Giannini et al. 1987).

Patients intoxicated with PCP may be brought to the psychiatric emergency service because they have become belligerent and violent. They also can represent a suicide risk because their behavior is unpredictable and impulsive, and they are startled easily. Such patients require restraints during this period. If the patient is suffering extreme anxiety, 5–10 mg of diazepam every 4 hours can be prescribed, which does not worsen muscle rigidity or lower the seizure threshold, although low doses of neuroleptics may be added. Giannini et al. (1987) found high-potency neuroleptics to be more effective than low-potency drugs in treating PCP-induced psychosis and suggested that dopamine-2 postsynaptic blockers such as haloperidol and pimozide may be more effective because PCP affects dopamine receptors at the dopamine-2 receptor site. Intoxication with PCP lasts 3–4 hours, and the degree of intoxication is dose related. The drug is only detectable in the blood for several hours, but can be detected in the urine for a longer period.

There is no clearly elucidated withdrawal syndrome; however, up to 1 week after discontinuing PCP, a state of delirium may begin, which fluctuates in severity and can last up to 1 week. This possibly may be related to the fact that PCP is stored in large amounts in body fat, particularly brain lipids. Although a delusional disorder can develop soon after intoxication, it can emerge as long as 1 week after the overdose. It usually abates in a week or so, but can persist up to 1 year although neuroleptics are appropriate management. Finally, a patient who has ingested PCP can experience depression within 1–2 weeks after using PCP. The depressive episode may be transitory, but can be long lasting and difficult to differentiate from a mood disorder.

Opioid-Induced Organic Mental Disorders and Other Analgesic Abuse

The group of substances referred to as opioids includes heroin and morphine, codeine, hydromorphone, meperidine, methadone hydrochloride, oxycodone, and pentazocine. Dependence and abuse develop in some patients after they have been prescribed analgesics for pain control, and often such patients will be referred to the psychiatric emergency service by other physicians who later become frustrated with a concern about the patients' "drug-seeking behavior."

Opioids, when ingested intravenously, exert their effect within 2–5 minutes and produce symptoms for 10–30 minutes. The first effect, usually euphoria, is followed by several hours of lethargy and somnolence, which can be confused with depression or underlying physical illness. During this entire period of intoxication, judgment is impaired, but in contrast to intoxication with other substances, aggression and violence are rare. In contrast to dilated pupils seen in intoxication with cocaine, amphetamines, and hallucinogens, pupillary constriction is generally present during intoxication with opioids. Speech is slurred, and there is impairment of memory and attention. Constipation, nausea, and vomiting may also occur.

Discontinuation of opioids and related compounds after 1–2 weeks of continuous use can result in opioid withdrawal. Withdrawal from opioids is characterized by lacrimation, rhinorrhea, pupillary dilation, piloerection (the goose flesh of going "cold turkey"), sweating, nausea and vomiting, diarrhea, yawning, mild hypertension, tachycardia, fever, insomnia, and muscle spasms especially in the legs ("kicking the habit"). Notice that many of these symptoms also occur with influenza, which must be included in the differential diagnosis (DSM-III-R). The duration of symptoms and time of highest intensity varies depending on the drug (Table 15-4).

Patients presenting with symptoms of opioid withdrawal can be difficult to manage in the psychiatric emergency setting. In general,

Table 15-4. Withdrawal from opiate preparations

	Morphine or heroin	Meperidine	Methadone
1st onset of symptoms (anxiety, drug-seeking)	6–8 hours	2–4 hours	1–3 days
Peak withdrawal symptoms	2nd or 3rd day	8–12 hours	Gradual
Duration of withdrawal	7–10 days	4–5 days	10–14 days

opioids should not be prescribed by the emergency psychiatrist. If the patient cannot be readily admitted to a detoxification program, 0.1 or 0.2 mg clonidine po may provide some temporary symptomatic relief.

Abuse of "Ts and Blues"

Talwin (pentazocine) is the "T" and Pyribenzamine (a blue 50-mg tripelennamine tablet) is the "blue" in a combination of a synthetic narcotic and an antihistamine which is deliberately intended by abusers to achieve euphoria and hallucinations (Schnoll et al. 1987). Users inject varying ratios of the pentazocine and tripelennamine tablets until the desired effects are achieved. Immediately after intravenous injection, the user feels a "rush," similar to that produced by heroin, which lasts 5–10 minutes, followed by several hours of euphoria. Withdrawal symptoms are similar to mild narcotic withdrawal and can be managed in a similar manner.

The most serious adverse reaction caused by injection of Ts and blues is that of generalized convulsions, due to rapid injection of large quantities of antihistamines. Other adverse effects include headaches, vomiting, blurred vision, memory loss, chest pain, and palpitations. Pulmonary complications can occur from injection of particulate matter, which can obstruct small vessels of the lungs and cause damage reflected in abnormal pulmonary function studies.

Sedative-, Hypnotic-, and Anxiolytic-Induced Organic Mental Disorders

Sedatives, hypnotics, and anxiolytics (minor tranquilizers) are grouped together for the purposes of DSM-III-R diagnostic criteria because all substances in these categories can cause mood lability and impaired judgment. These drugs are often obtained "on the street" but also are some of the most commonly prescribed drugs (particularly the anxiolytics). Patients abusing such prescription drugs often do not view their drug use as "a problem" because the drugs were prescribed by a doctor. Confrontation of abuse of these drugs in the psychiatric emergency service often results in anger and defensiveness and also in continued "doctor shopping" by the patient to obtain a prescription for their "medicine." Sedatives, hypnotics, and anxiolytics are associated with a potentially life-threatening withdrawal syndrome, which can be complicated by delirium, and also with an amnestic disorder after prolonged and heavy use.

Intoxication with sedatives, hypnotics, or anxiolytics can cause disinhibition of sexual or aggressive impulses, but aggressive outbursts are not as common as with alcohol intoxication. Otherwise, the characteristic symptoms and signs of sedative, hypnotic, or anxiolytic intoxication are similar to those seen in intoxication with alcohol: slurred speech, incoordination, unsteady gait, and impaired attention or memory. Usually such patients appear sedated, but paradoxical hyperactivity and affective lability may occur, especially in children or the elderly, or in patients with preexisting brain injury. Most of the benzodiazepines tend to accumulate over time and in elderly patients can result in a subtle delirium or "sundowning" which can precipitate a psychiatric emergency visit.

Overdoses with benzodiazepines are common, in part because they are commonly prescribed and in part because they can accentuate a preexisting depression. Fortunately, such overdoses are usually not fatal (less than 1%), but they are serious, especially when taken in combination with alcohol. Barbiturate overdose can be potentially lethal, particularly in persons who have developed a tolerance to the drug's sedative effects, because tolerance to its brain stem depressant effects develops much more slowly.

Toxic reactions to sedatives, hypnotics, and anxiolytics usually develop over a period of hours after ingestion, and the patient may present to the emergency psychiatrist in a stuporous state. Complications can include congestive heart failure, positional or infectious pneumonia, and/or respiratory depression. Cardiac arrhythmias may occur, especially with the short-acting barbiturates such as thiopental or methohexital (Schuckit 1985). Such patients need careful physical examination. Vital signs may reveal an arrhythmia, respiratory depression, or orthostatic blood pressure changes. Reflexes will be depressed, and pupils are usually midpoint and slowly reactive, except in the case of intoxication with glutethimide (Doriden), where they are enlarged. If the patient is stuporous, a toxicologic screen should be done to determine the specific drugs ingested, because a longer half-life or increased fat solubility (such as with glutethimide or ethchlorvynol [Placidyl]) would necessitate a longer period of observation and treatment. Electrolytes, renal function tests, and a complete blood count should also be obtained.

If the cause of the patient's stuporous condition is not entirely clear, a thorough search for complicating medical conditions must be carried out, and either the patient should be referred to emergency medicine or a consultation obtained.

Sedative-hypnotic withdrawal, like alcohol withdrawal, (but unlike opiate withdrawal) can be life threatening. Withdrawal from sedatives, hypnotics, or anxiolytics occurs 2–6 days after cessation or reduction of moderate or heavy use. In the case of benzodiazepines, usually the patient has been taking a daily dose of at least 40 mg of diazepam or its equivalent, although withdrawal has been reported with daily doses as low as 15 mg. The symptoms of sedative, hypnotic, or anxiolytic withdrawal can be confused clinically with anxiety disorders or withdrawal from alcohol.

Signs of sedative, hypnotic, or anxiolytic withdrawal include tachycardia and sweating, sometimes nausea and vomiting, malaise and weakness, orthostatic hypotension, often a coarse tremor of the hands and even tongue and eyelids, and sometimes myoclonic jerks (which can look "put on" and lead the emergency psychiatrist to suspect malingering) and generalized convulsions. The patient feels dysphoric, anxious, and irritable and cannot sleep well.

The patient who has used sedatives, hypnotics, or anxiolytics for 5–15 years may experience a delirium up to 1 week after the cessation or reduction of sedatives, hypnotics, or anxiolytics. If the patient is going to have seizures while undergoing withdrawal, they will ordinarily precede the onset of this delirium. The delirious patient will experience tachycardia and sweating and a coarse tremor and may develop a fever. The patient will have vivid hallucinations, which can be visual, auditory, or tactile. The period of delirium usually lasts 2–3 days.

A patient undergoing moderate to severe withdrawal symptoms from sedatives, hypnotics, or anxiolytics should be transferred to emergency medicine and admitted because of the possibility of developing convulsions or delirium. The patient who is experiencing mild withdrawal symptoms (e.g., minor tremors that are not worsening) can be treated on an outpatient basis by the emergency psychiatric service if seen daily, so that symptoms and signs can be monitored daily and only small quantities of medication can be given to prevent further abuse. With regard to the anxiolytics, a high rate of severe withdrawal symptoms has been reported after treatment with alprazolam (Xanax), and very gradual tapering of the dose over 1–2 months is recommended (Fyer et al. 1987).

Finally, the user or abuser of sedatives, hypnotics, or anxiolytics can develop an amnestic syndrome, the essential feature of which is the relatively sudden impairment of short- and long-term memory (but not immediate recall, such as is tested by digit span). Events of the very remote past are better recalled than more recent events. Because of the presence of memory loss or amnesia, patients often confabulate to fill in the gaps in their memories and often lack insight into their problem. Apathy, lack of initiative, and emotional blandness can occur during this period. In the case of sedative, hypnotic, or anxiolytic amnestic disorder, age of onset is in the 20s. The course is variable, and in contrast to alcohol amnestic disorder, full recovery is likely.

REFERRALS FOR FURTHER TREATMENT

For those patients not admitted by the psychiatric emergency service directly to an inpatient substance abuse, psychiatric, or other medical facility, a decision must be made regarding follow-up. For patients whose lives are not chaotic, an outpatient treatment program actually is preferable because there patients can learn to cope with the "real world" without resorting to drug abuse. Even some patients with substance abuse plus mental illness can be treated on an outpatient basis (Kofoed et al. 1986). Unfortunately, because of long waiting lists for outpatient treatment, the psychiatric emergency service may need to schedule "return visits" to accommodate such patients. Psychiatrists and other physicians sometimes become discouraged about the prognosis for patients with substance abuse problems, but a study of employed patients found that about two-thirds of patients remained drug and alcohol free 1 year after entering an industrial rehabilitation program (Schuckit 1985). The best prognosis is for patients who are employed, who have completed school, and who are not involved in a criminal life-style to support their habit.

On the other hand, the emergency psychiatrist must modify treatment goals depending on the patient population being served. Only 10% of "skid row" patients will be abstinent 12 months after treatment in a detoxification program, so total abstinence after one pass through such a program is an unrealistic goal which will lead to discouragement on the part of both the psychiatric emergency staff and the patient. "Success," instead, may be helping that 10% become abstinent, remaining available for the other 90% in the future, providing good medical care, and beginning to educate each patient and his or her family about the potential effects of the drugs on their lives and health. Education has been shown ultimately to motivate many substance abusers to seek treatment, and abstinence is enhanced as patients begin to accept increasing responsibility for their actions. This education can begin in the psychiatric emergency setting.

Patients can receive peer support through chapters of Narcotics Anonymous. Some Alcoholics Anonymous chapters also will accept substance abusers into their fellowship. Also, many mental health centers have specific specialty clinics available to treat substance abusers and dual-diagnosis patients, and patients can be referred there for further treatment.

REFERENCES

Alen M, Rahkila P, Marnieini J: Serum lipids in power athletes self-administering testosterone and anabolic steroids. Int J Sports Med 6:139–144, 1985

Alterman A, Erdlen D, LaPorte D, et al: Effects of illicit drug use in inpatient populations. Addict Behav 7:231–242, 1982

American Psychiatric Association: Diagnostic and Statistical Manual of Mental Disorders, 3rd Edition, Revised. Washington, DC, American Psychiatric Association, 1987

Angrist MD, Less HK, Gershon S: The antagonism of amphetamine-induced symptomatology by a neuroleptic. Am J Psychiatry 131:817–821, 1974

Bachrach LL: The context of care for the chronic mental patient with substance abuse problems. Psychiatr Q 58:3–14, 1986–1987

Benowitz NL, Jones RT: Cardiovascular and metabolic considerations in prolonged cannabinoid administration in men. J Clin Psychopharmacol 21:214S–223S, 1981

Breakey W, Goddell H, Lorenz P, et al: Hallucinogenic drugs as precipitants of schizophrenia. Psychol Med 4:255–261, 1974

Climko RP, Roerich H, Sweeney DR, et al: Ecstasy: a review of MDMA and MDA. Int J Psychiatry Med 36:359–372, 1987

Crowley TJ, Chesluk D, Ditts S, et al: Drug and alcohol abuse among psychiatric admissions. Arch Gen Psychiatry 30:13–20, 1974

Dilsaver SC: Antimuscarinic agents as substances of abuse: a review. J Clin Psychopharmacol 8:14–22, 1988

Fischer D, Halikas JA, Baker JW, et al: Frequency and patterns of drug abuse in psychiatric patients. Journal of Diseases of the Nervous System 36:550–556, 1975

Fyer AJ, Liebowitz MR, Gorman JM: Discontinuation of alprazolam treatment in panic patients. Am J Psychiatry 144:303–308, 1987

Giannini AJ, Loiselle RH, Giannini MC, et al: Phencyclidine and the dissociatives. Psychiatr Med 3:197–217, 1987

Gibb K: Serum alcohol levels, toxicology screens, and use of the breath alcohol analyzer. Ann Emerg Med 15:349–352, 1986

Goldsmith J: Death by Freon. J Clin Psychiatry 12:36–37, 1989

Hasin D, Endicott J, Lewis C: Alcohol and drug abuse in patients with affective syndromes. Compr Psychiatry 26:283–295, 1985

Hillard JR, Vieweg WVR; Marked sinus tachycardia from the synergistic effects of marijuana and nortriptyline. Am J Psychiatry 140:626–627, 1983

Khantzian E: The self-medication hypothesis of addictive disorders: focus on heroin and cocaine dependence. Am J Psychiatry 142:1259–1264, 1985

Knudsen P, Vilnar T: Cannabis and neuroleptic agents in schizophrenia. Acta Psychiatr Scand 69:162–174, 1984

Kofoed L, Kania J, Walsh T, et al: Outpatient treatment of substance abusers with other co-existing psychiatric disorders. Am J Psychiatry 143:867–872, 1986

Lamb DR: Anabolic steroids in athletics: how well do they work and how dangerous are they? Am J Sports Med 12:31–38, 1984

Mendelson JH, Mello NK, Lex BW, et al: Marijuana withdrawal syndrome in a woman. Am J Psychiatry 141:1289–1290, 1984

Perry S: Substance-induced organic mental disorders, in The American Psychiatric Press Textbook of Neuropsychiatry. Edited by Hales RE, Yudofsky SC. Washington, DC, American Psychiatric Press, 1987, pp 157–176

Pitts FN, Allen RE, Aniline O, et al: The dilemma of the toxic psychosis: differential diagnosis and the PCP psychosis. Psychiatric Annals 12:762–768, 1982

Preskorn SH, Irwin HA: Toxicity of tricyclic antidepressants: kinetics, mechanism, intervention: a review. J Clin Psychiatry 43:151–156, 1982

Rockwell PA, Ostwald P: Amphetamine use and abuse in psychiatric patients. Arch Gen Psychiatry 18:612–616, 1968

Rottanburg D, Robins AH, Bon-Aire O, et al: Cannabis-associated psychosis with hypomanic features. Lancet 2:1364–1366, 1982

Schnoll SH, Chasnoff IJ, Glassroth JG: Pentazocine and tripelennamine abuse: T's and blues. Psychiatr Med 3:219–231, 1987

Schuckit MA: Drug and Alcohol Abuse. New York, Plenum, 1985

Slaby AE, Swift R: Diagnosing and managing drug-induced emergencies. Psychiatr Med 3:233–251, 1987

Smith HWB III, Liberman HA, Brody SL, et al: Acute myocardial infarction temporarily related to cocaine use. Ann Intern Med 107:13–18, 1987

Soslow AR: Acute drug overdose: one hospital's experience. Ann Emerg Med 10:18–21, 1981

Treffert D: Marijuana use in schizophrenia: a clear hazard. Am J Psychiatry 135:1213–1215, 1978

Tsuang MT, Simpson JC, Kronfol Z: Subtypes of drug abuse with psychosis. Arch Gen Psychiatry 39:141–147, 1982

Webb OL, Laskarzewski PM, Glueck CJ: Severe depression of high-density lipoprotein cholesterol levels in weight lifters and body builders by self-administered exogenous testosterone and anabolic-androgenic steroids. Metabolism 33:971–975, 1984

Chapter 16

Psychosis—Acute and Chronic

J.R. Hillard, M.D.

Acute psychosis is one of the most serious psychiatric emergencies. Patients with chronic psychotic disorders are one of the largest and most important subpopulations of psychiatric emergency patients. This chapter will discuss the assessment and management of new-onset acute psychosis and the appropriate assessment and management of patients with chronic psychosis in light of their phase of illness (chronic psychosis associated with mood disorders is covered in Chapter 10).

NEW-ONSET PSYCHOSIS

Assessment

Patients with new-onset psychosis are usually frightened and often terrified. Their families are also frightened and usually groping for some kind of explanation. These patients and families generally need a concrete medical doctor–like approach, focusing on specific problems and providing considerable feedback (e.g., "Of course that was frightening" or "No, I do not hear anybody else in the room" or "Yes, I do think that we can help you"). Therapist passivity and lack of therapist feedback can sometimes increase patient anxiety to a dangerous level. Acutely psychotic patients, particularly patients with new-onset psychosis, are, in many cases, easily threatened by seemingly innocuous

229

comments or physical contacts and should always be regarded as potential assault risks. The principles for minimizing assault risk outlined in Chapter 11 need to be kept in mind in dealing with this population.

Differential Diagnosis

It is not always necessary, or even possible, to make a precise psychiatric diagnosis of patients with acute new onset of psychosis. Acutely psychotic patients are not usually very good historians, and without adequate history, precise diagnosis is never possible. Acute symptomatology, if evident during the examination, may suggest a diagnosis of, for example, acute mania rather than acute schizophrenia (Solovay et al. 1987). But such a diagnosis can seldom be confirmed on the basis of a single contact with the patient. Particularly among adolescents, mania can present with symptoms that we usually think of as more characteristic of paranoid schizophrenia (Ballenger et al. 1982). New-onset schizophrenia may present with symptoms that we usually think of as more characteristic of mania (Docherty et al. 1978). Furthermore, emergency management and referral are more a function of severity of dysfunction and need for further evaluation than of the five-digit DSM-III-R (American Psychiatric Association 1987) code.

It is always important to assess 1) Is this really a new-onset psychosis? 2) Could this condition be due to substance abuse? 3) Could this condition be due to other organic disorders? 4) Is this patient acutely a danger to self or others? 5) Could this condition be factitious, malingered, or hysterical?

Is this really a new-onset psychosis?   New-onset psychosis is almost always an indication for psychiatric hospitalization. Many patients, however, have had psychotic symptoms for a considerable period of time before their first hospitalization. Gift et al. (1981), for example, found that 20% of first-admission psychotic patients had been symptomatic for more than 2 years before admission. For patients such as these, "diagnostic" hospitalization may not be as necessary as for those who have been symptomatic for a period of only weeks to months.

Could this condition be due to substance abuse?   Psychoactive substance intoxication or withdrawal must always be near the top of the list of differential diagnoses for any new-onset psychosis. The most frequent offenders are intoxication with lysergic acid diethylamide (LSD) or other psychotomimetics, phencyclidine (PCP), cocaine or amphetamines, and withdrawal from sedative-hypnotics. At times, intoxication with anticholinergics or "decongestant-type" sympathomimetics, such as pseudoephedrine and phenopropanolamine, may present with psychosis. Mental disorders associated with substance abuse are discussed further in Chapter 15. Whenever history, abnormal vital signs, or atypical symptoms lead to a suspicion of substance-induced psychosis, it is useful to observe the patient over a period of hours. Toxicology screens should probably be ordered in such cases to facilitate further treatment, although in most facilities, results are unlikely to be ready soon enough to help with emergency management.

Could this condition be due to other organic disorders? Any illness that can cause delirium (see Chapter 12) can cause psychosis in the sense of a loss of contact with reality. Organic illnesses may present with a picture more consistent with psychosis than with delirium, and functional psychoses may present with a degree of disorganization suggestive of delirium (e.g., "delirious mania" [Taylor and Abrams 1973]). Every patient with new onset of psychosis deserves a vigorous medical workup, usually on an inpatient basis. Emergency room workup should include enough medical assessment to catch illnesses requiring medical or surgical rather than psychiatric admission. This assessment should include, at a minimum, vital signs and a focused physical examination (see Chapter 2) and may include a complete blood count, electrolytes, and possibly a toxic screen. The following facts are particularly suggestive of an organic etiology for psychosis.

- Abnormal vital signs
- Onset at age over 40. DSM-III-R, unlike DSM-III (American Psychiatric Association 1980), allows a diagnosis of schizophrenia to be made in patients with onset after age 45. However, there is an increasing probability of an organic cause with increasing age at onset
- Visual hallucinations. These certainly are not rare among schizophrenic patients but are certainly more characteristic of organic brain syndrome, as are tactile, olfactory, or gustatory hallucinations.
- Decreased level of consciousness
- Disorientation to time, place, or person
- Presence of medical symptoms with a close temporal relationship to onset of psychiatric symptoms
- New medication started or stopped at about the time of symptom onset
- Rapid onset of symptoms without a prodromal period

For most organic psychoses, acute management will be the same as for a functional psychosis (i.e., hospitalization for protection, further assessment, and initiation of antipsychotic treatment). These principles are the same for psychosis that ultimately turns out to be due to paranoid schizophrenia or for an illness that ultimately turns out to be due to systemic lupus.

Is this patient acutely a danger to self or others? Patients with new onset of psychosis must generally be regarded as at increased risk for suicide or other self-destructive behaviors, and also for outwardly directed aggressive behavior. The degree of acute anxiety, paranoia, or past aggressive behavior may be associated with acute risk of suicide or violence, but estimation of risk of violence is probably even more difficult for psychotic patients than for other groups (see Chapters 8 and 11).

Hallucinations commanding violence or suicide are certainly ominous. Also ominous are severe paranoid delusions, particularly if patients believe their life is in danger and if they believe they may have to "strike first."

Could this condition be factitious, malingered, or hysterical? Patients, for conscious or unconscious reasons, or for some combination of the two, may act psychotic when, in fact, they are not. When such behaviors occur in prisoners, they are referred to as Ganser syndrome (Stone 1988) and are often accompanied by other manufactured symptoms, such as giving approximately correct answers to mental status questions (e.g., $5 + 5 = 11, 7 + 7 = 13$).

Other symptoms that suggest the possibility of factitious, malingered, or hysterical psychosis are

- A normal range of affect with little affective reaction to delusions. If patients do not have markedly blunted affect, they will usually show marked fear or anger in response to delusions.
- Unusual visual hallucinations (e.g., "little green men in my oatmeal").
- Clear-cut secondary gain (e.g., avoidance of incarceration).
- Willingness to admit almost any psychiatric symptoms suggested (e.g., "Do you believe that God has appointed you to teach the Zolan beliefs to all people that you meet?") (Beaber et al. 1985).

It should be kept in mind, however, that factitious (Pope et al. 1982) or hysterical (Gift et al. 1985) psychoses are probably rare and that many patients so diagnosed will ultimately turn out to have genuine psychotic illness (Hay 1983).

Treatment

Inpatient treatment is almost always indicated for new-onset acute psychosis. Newly psychotic patients deserve an extensive workup and are rarely able to cooperate with it on an outpatient basis. Most of these patients realize that something is seriously wrong and readily agree to hospitalization. Others may be afraid of psychiatric hospitalization but may be reassurable, especially if family members support admission. Sometimes a joint interview with a hesitant patient and the family can be useful in convincing the patient of the need to be admitted.

A small group of patients, usually paranoid, are unable to see that they may have a problem. If there is evidence of dangerousness to self or others, these patients must be hospitalized involuntarily. If there is no evidence of dangerousness, hospitalization must be "sold" to the patient. This may be accomplished by finding any symptom that is troubling the patient (e.g., nervousness or insomnia) and stating that the hospitalization is likely to help with that symptom (which it is, if the underlying psychosis is treated). At times, it is useful to emphasize the possibility of a physical disorder underlying the symptoms and the need for further assessment.

If a patient is going to be admitted, it is better to avoid giving high doses of antipsychotic medication in the emergency room. These medications will be in the patient's system for a long time and will complicate diagnostic assessment on the inpatient service. Benzodiazepines, such as lorazepam, 1–2 mg im, are usually preferable first-line drugs when a patient needs to be medicated for acute agitation (see Chapter 3).

If a patient refuses admission and must be treated as an outpatient, the physical and laboratory assessments that would be done on the inpatient service need to be carried out. The patient should have a relative or friend willing to provide transportation to and from the hospital or clinic. The patient should be started on a moderate dose of antipsychotic medication (e.g., 5–10 mg haloperidol at bedtime) and should return daily. Prophylactic anticholinergics (e.g., 1 mg benztropine bid) should be used because an acute extrapyramidal syndrome out of the hospital will probably lead to extreme fear and discomfort and may lead to permanent resistance to medication. Paradoxically, once patients have improved slightly, they may be willing to come into the hospital voluntarily.

CHRONIC PSYCHOSIS

Many patients with schizophrenia, schizoaffective disorder, and delusional disorder develop a chronic pattern of impaired functioning with periodic decompensation. They may request or be brought for emergency treatment not only at times of decompensation but also during the immediate postpsychotic phase, the period of adaptive plateau, and during "end states" (McGlashan 1986). The goals and techniques of management for these "emergencies" will be a function of the patient's stage of illness. Chapters 24 and 25 deal with the problems of some subgroups of chronically psychotic people.

Postpsychotic Phase

The return home after a psychotic episode, particularly after a first psychotic break, is difficult, for both the patient and the family. Conflicts with family or therapists are likely to precipitate emergency visits during this phase. In general, it is preferable to avoid hospitalization as much as possible at this time to facilitate reintegration into the community (Drake and Sederer 1986). Over the first year after hospitalization, clinical depression develops in a significant percentage of psychotic patients (House et al. 1987) and may be a cause for suicide (Drake et al. 1985). Such "postpsychotic depression" may be difficult to treat and may necessitate rehospitalization in some cases. Antidepressant medication may be useful for some patients but should not ordinarily be started from an emergency room setting.

Adaptive Plateau

During the adaptive plateau phase, the patient is relatively asymptomatic and relatively motivated for social skills training and some degree of vocational rehabilitation. Outpatient programs may be encouraging the patient to move to less structured living arrangements, to try more challenging vocational placements, or to reduce medication. During these periods, patients may be tempted to regress to the relative safety of the hospital. Emergency services need to be reassuring and optimistic and in close communication with the patient's ongoing care providers. The most important emergency differential diagnosis is whether the patient is near or well below usual level, or baseline, of symptomatology and of functioning.

Decompensation

Chronically psychotic patients may relapse, either while on maintenance medication or after discontinuing it. A part of the natural history of schizophrenia for many patients involves periodic attempts to stop their medication. When schizophrenic patients stop their medication after having been on it for some time, they have about a 10% chance of relapse each month, and therefore, there is about an 80% chance that they will have relapsed within a year (Deacker et al. 1986). A common reason for psychiatric emergency visits is relapse after medication discontinuation.

A rational outpatient pharmacologic management plan for schizophrenic patients involves maintenance on as low a dose of antipsychotics as possible (Carpenter 1986) or even use of antipsychotics only during periods of relapse (Kane 1987). Such approaches will minimize patients' lifetime exposure to antipsychotic medications but will increase the number of emergency visits due to decompensation or near decompensation.

Many patients and their family members, over time, come to understand what patients' early symptoms of relapse are. One prospective study of relapse found that 90% of patients had one of the following prodromal signs of relapse: hallucinations, suspiciousness, change in sleep, or anxiety. Other common prodromal symptoms of relapse included thought disorder, anger, somatic symptoms, disruptive behavior, or depression (Heinrichs and Carpenter 1985). Usually these prodromal symptoms of relapse can be treated on an outpatient basis with increased doses of medication. If a 24- to 72-hour holding area is available, a high percentage of decompensating patients may be medicated and returned to the community after beginning to relapse. In many cases, such patients can be helped to use such near-relapse experiences to learn some degree of self-control over psychotic relapse. Common self-control mechanisms include self-instruction (e.g., "I have to remember that these voices are not real"), reduced involvement in activity (e.g., "People are getting on my nerves, I should stay home awhile"), and increased involvement in activity (e.g., "If I stay busy, it will keep my mind off things") (Breier and Strauss 1983).

The main indication for hospitalization is violent or self-destructive behavior. Suicidal thoughts occurring during psychotic relapse need to be taken very seriously. Violent behavior, even if not life threatening, can disrupt placements enough that hospitalization is needed.

When restarting medication, choose a drug that the patient feels has helped in the past. Start with a dosage that is about the same as the past effective dose. It is tempting to try to get patients better faster by giving more medication, but as discussed in Chapter 3, that does not really work.

It is important to keep in mind that patients with chronic psychotic disorders may relapse due to intercurrent physical illness. At a minimum, chronic patients with relapse need vital signs checked and a review of medical problems. If any of the factors mentioned earlier to be associated with organic psychosis are present, or if the patient has a medical illness, further physical assessment is in order.

When patients are living with family, the needs of the family members must be carefully assessed and responded to. Family members usually know the patient very well, and when they believe the patient needs rehospitalization they are likely to be correct. Family members were the original "case managers" and need to be treated as such.

End Stages

After many years of chronic psychotic symptoms, some patients develop an "end stage" with specific biopsychosocial characteristics. Negative symptoms of schizophrenia, such as lack of pleasure, flat affect, lack of motivation, poor attention span, and social withdrawal (Andreasen 1982; Carpenter et al. 1988), may be prominent. Patients will, in many cases, have had multiple hospitalizations and may have come to view hospitalization as a ready solution to personal crises. Patients may often have lost contact with family members and have very sparse social networks made up largely of mental health support workers.

Many of these patients are operating at a baseline level of functioning just above the minimum level necessary for physical survival. Relatively small decrements in social functioning may necessitate inpatient or crisis residential treatment. With this group of patients, even more than with others, appropriate acute assessment requires input from a case manager or someone else familiar with the patient's baseline level of functioning. Familiarity with available community support resources is also required.

REFERENCES

American Psychiatric Association: Diagnostic and Statistical Manual of Mental Disorders, 3rd Edition. Washington, DC, American Psychiatric Association, 1980

American Psychiatric Association: Diagnostic and Statistical Manual of Mental Disorders, 3rd Edition, Revised. Washington, DC, American Psychiatric Association, 1987

Andreasen NL: Negative symptoms in schizophrenia: definition and reliability. Arch Gen Psychiatry 39:784–794, 1982

Ballenger JC, Reus VI, Post RM: The "atypical" clinical picture of adolescent mania. Am J Psychiatry 139:602–606, 1982

Beaber RJ, Marston A, Michelli J, et al: A brief test for measuring malingering in schizophrenic individuals. Am J Psychiatry 142:1478–1481, 1985

Breier A, Strauss JS: Self-control in psychotic disorders. Arch Gen Psychiatry 40:1141–1145, 1983

Carpenter W: Early, targeted pharmacotherapeutic intervention in schizophrenia. J Clin Psychiatry 47 (suppl):23–29, 1986

Carpenter WT, Heinrichs DW, Wagman AM: Deficit and nondeficit forms of schizophrenia: the concept. Am J Psychiatry 145:578–583, 1988

Deacker SJ, Malm U, Lepp M: Schizophrenic relapse after drug withdrawal is predictable. Acta Psychiatr Scand 73:181–185, 1986

Docherty JP, Van Kammen DP, Siris SG, et al: Stages of onset of schizophrenic psychosis. Am J Psychiatry 135:420–426, 1978

Drake RE, Sederer LI: Inpatient psychosocial treatment of chronic schizophrenia: negative effects and current guidelines. Hosp Community Psychiatry 37:897–901, 1986

Drake RE, Gates C, Whitaker A, et al: Suicide among schizophrenics: a review. Compr Psychiatry 26:90–100, 1985

Gift TE, Strauss JS, Harder DW, et al: Established chronicity of psychotic symptoms in first admission schizophrenic patients. Am J Psychiatry 138:779–784, 1981

Gift TE, Strauss JS, Young Y: Hysterical psychosis: an empirical approach. Am J Psychiatry 142:345–347, 1985

Hay GG: Feigned psychosis: a review of the simulation of mental illness. Br J Psychiatry 143:8–10, 1983

Heinrichs DW, Carpenter WT: Prospective study of prodromal symptoms in schizophrenic relapse. Am J Psychiatry 142:371–373, 1985

House A, Bostock J, Cooper J: Depressive syndromes in the year following onset of a first schizophrenic illness. Br J Psychiatry 151:773–779, 1987

Kane J: Low-dose and intermittent neuroleptic treatment strategies for schizophrenia. Psychiatric Annals 17:125–130, 1987

McGlashan TH: Schizophrenia: psychosocial treatments and the role of psychosocial factors in its etiology and pathogenesis, in Psychiatry Update: American Psychiatric Association Annual Review, Vol 5. Edited by Frances AJ, Hales RE. Washington, DC, American Psychiatric Press, 1986, pp 96–111

Pope HG, Jonas JM, Jones B: Factitious psychosis: phenomenology, family history, and long term outcome of nine patients. Am J Psychiatry 139:1480–1483, 1982

Solovay MR, Sheaton ME, Holtzman PS: Comparative studies of thought disorder, I: mania and schizophrenia. Arch Gen Psychiatry 44:13–20, 1987

Stone EM: American Psychiatric Glossary. Washington, DC, American Psychiatric Press, 1988, p 45

Taylor MA, Abrams R: The phenomenology of mania: a new look at some old patients. Arch Gen Psychiatry 29:520–522, 1973

Chapter 17

Anxiety Disorders

J.R. Hillard, M.D.

This chapter will focus on those disorders whose most prominent symptoms are anxiety or avoidance behavior and will discuss how to differentiate them from other disorders in which anxiety may occur as an associated symptom. Epidemiological studies have indicated that anxiety disorders are the most commonly occurring psychiatric disorders in the general population (Myers et al. 1984). Some anxiety disorders, although common in the general population (e.g., phobic and obsessive-compulsive disorder), are unusual primary diagnoses in psychiatric emergency settings and will be discussed only briefly. Stress reactions, panic disorder, adjustment disorder with anxious mood, generalized anxiety disorder, and posttraumatic stress disorder will be discussed in more detail.

Assessment of Disorders Involving Anxiety

"Anxiety is apprehension, tension, or uneasiness from anticipation of danger, the source of which is largely unknown or unrecognized" (Werner et al. 1980, p. 10). Anxiety can be experienced during discrete episodes with sudden onset and prominent physical symptoms (as in panic disorder) or over more extended periods with less prominent physical symptoms (as in generalized anxiety disorder). Anxiety is generally accompanied by some degree of behavior aimed at avoiding objects or situations associated with anxious feelings. The avoidant behavior may be the predominant symptom, as in phobia, or behavior designed to neutralize the anxiety may be prominent, as in obsessive-compulsive disorder. A specific traumatic event may have precipitated anxiety or other symptoms, as in posttraumatic stress disorder, or the precipitant may be impossible to discern.

In every case of anxiety the following should be assessed:

- Time course—When did the symptoms begin? What possible precipitants existed? What events have tended to make the anxiety better or worse? Patients often feel a significant degree of relief when they have succeeded in attaching their diffuse anxiety to specific events and times.
- Physical symptoms—Patients are often quite alarmed by their physical symptoms and may not be able to discuss anything else until they have been allowed to discuss and, if possible, have been reassured about their physical symptoms.
- Avoidant behaviors—Patients will sometimes neglect to discuss these due to embarrassment or preoccupation with anxiety.
- Presence of medications or physical disorders.
- Presence of other psychiatric disorders.

When interviewing anxious patients, it is even more important than with other patients to relate in a calm, relaxed manner. At times, it may be necessary to premedicate a patient before an interview is possible (e.g., with 1 mg lorazepam po). After anxious patients have been allowed to tell their story for awhile, the interviewer will often have to become directive and active to elicit the history needed to make treatment decisions. Anxious patients will commonly describe themselves as feeling confused.

PANIC DISORDER

Panic disorder is characterized by discrete, rapidly developing episodes of fear or discomfort with at least four physical symptoms, which may include 1) shortness of breath, 2) dizziness, 3) palpitations or tachycardia, 4) trembling or shaking, 5) sweating, 6) choking, 7) nausea, 8) depersonalization, 9) numbness or tingling, 10) flushes or chills, 11) chest pain, 12) fear of dying, and 13) fear of going crazy or losing control. To qualify for a DSM-III-R (American Psychiatric Association 1987) diagnosis of panic disorder, a patient must have had four or more attacks within a 4-week period or have had one or more attacks followed by at least a month of persistent fear of having another. At times in emergency settings, patients are seen after having had only one or two attacks, and a diagnosis of anxiety disorder not otherwise specified is appropriate.

Differential Diagnosis

Physical disorder. Many, perhaps most, patients with panic disorder at some time in their illness believe themselves to be suffering from a physical condition. It is also well documented that many patients seen in medical emergency rooms (Wulsin et al. 1988), cardiology clinics, or in cardiac catheterization labs are, in fact, suffering from panic disorder (Katon 1986). On the other hand, a real myocardial infarction or angina pectoris or a pulmonary embolus can certainly give rise to the symptoms of a panic attack. A patient whose chief complaint is chest pain should always receive a medical evaluation before receiving a psychiatric evaluation.

Medical illnesses can give rise to organic anxiety disorder that may present with either a panic or a generalized anxiety picture. Table 17-1 lists physical causes of organic anxiety syndromes that are mentioned in DSM-III-R, but the list is by no means exhaustive. McNeil (1987), for example, lists about 120 medications or diseases associated with anxiety symptoms.

Table 17-1. Organic causes of panic or anxiety symptoms listed in DSM-III-R

- Hyper- or hypothyroidism
- Pheochromocytoma
- Fasting hypoglycemia
- Hypercortisolism
- Intoxication with caffeine, cocaine, amphetamine
- Withdrawal from sedative-hypnotics
- Seizure of the diencephalon
- Pulmonary embolus
- Chronic obstructive pulmonary disease (COPD)
- Aspirin intolerance
- Collagen-vascular diseases
- Brucellosis
- Vitamin B_{12} deficiency
- Multiple sclerosis
- Heavy metal intoxication

A reasonable approach to differential diagnosis of patients with panic or anxiety symptoms begins with measurement of vital signs. Anxiety is associated with tachycardia, tachypnea, and hypertension, but cannot be used as an explanation for elevated temperature. Pulse rates over 120 beats/minute are a cause for some concern that a medical disorder is present; pulse rates over 140 beats/minute are a cause for greater concern. An irregular pulse rate deserves further evaluation, probably including an electrocardiogram. Tachypnea is so frequent in panic attacks or less severe anxiety attacks that "hyperventilation syndrome" is a venerable emergency room diagnosis (Waites 1978). Tachypnea can lead to respiratory alkalosis, which can make anxiety worse—a vicious cycle. Having a patient rebreathe into a paper bag can sometimes terminate a panic attack and can be of some diagnostic value.

A history of endocrine disorders, even if treated, or of medication use for a chronic medical disorder should be suspected as possible causes of anxiety. Particularly important and common medical causes for acute anxiety are hypoglycemia due to errors in insulin dosage, sedative-hypnotic withdrawal syndrome, postictal state, hypoxia, stimulant intoxication, and akathisia due to neuroleptics. When symptoms are atypical or new in onset, further physical evaluation is particularly indicated.

Agoraphobia. Agoraphobia is, according to DSM-III-R, "fear of being in places or situations from which escape might be difficult (or embarrassing) or in which help might not be available in the event of a panic attack" (p. 236). Agoraphobia commonly occurs in the context of panic disorder but may also occur with "limited-symptom panic attacks" (attacks with fewer than four of the physical symptoms listed or, in some cases, without any history of panic attack or panic at all). Agoraphobia without panic attacks may result from a major depressive disorder, from psychotic disorder with paranoid symptoms, or from an extremely avoidant personality. At times, a similar syndrome can arise gradually among patients suffering from chronic organic brain syndrome. The treatment for agoraphobia should be aimed at its underlying disorder.

Hypochondriasis. Patients with what internists refer to as a "diffusely positive review of systems" are likely to respond "yes" to enough symptoms to qualify for a diagnosis of panic disorder. In fact, in some instances, treatment of the panic disorder can significantly ameliorate the other hypochondriacal symptoms (Noyes et al. 1986). In other cases, treatment of the panic disorder is nearly as misguided as exploratory surgery. We would recommend treating hypochondriacal patients for panic disorder only when they are seen during a panic attack or have been seen for at least several visits.

Treatment and Referral

Panic disorder is often a very rewarding disorder to treat on an emergency basis. Patients are often reassured to have a name for their condition, and it is sometimes useful to read to them the diagnostic criteria from a book like this or from DSM-III-R to help convince them that they are not alone with their symptoms.

We advocate starting tricyclic antidepressants from the emergency room, after an appropriate physical examination, for patients with clear-cut panic disorder. We have found unmedicated patients to be unlikely to complete referrals to psychiatric outpatient facilities. If there is a component of anticipatory anxiety, short-term 2- to 4-week prescription of a benzodiazepine is reasonable (e.g., 0.5 mg of alprazolam tid). Short-term benzodiazepine use may also help alleviate some of the unpleasant sense of agitation sometimes reported by patients with panic disorder beginning tricyclic antidepressant therapy (Pohl et al. 1988). It is appropriate to make the patient aware that the tricyclic antidepressant will not have its full effect immediately and that the benzodiazepine will be necessary only until the tricyclic antidepressant starts working. Many patients with panic disorder will conceptualize their problem as medical rather than as psychiatric, and, in many cases, there is no reason to discourage such a conceptualization (Noyes 1987).

It is often useful to help patients with avoidance symptoms appreciate the "contagious" nature of their avoidance. Many initially started avoiding situations where panic attacks have occurred and then gradually began avoiding situations with increasingly remote similarity to panic situations. Patients should be helped to set an initial goal of not allowing avoidant behavior to escalate and, later, a goal of having increasing exposure to previously uncomfortable situations (Ghosh and Marks 1987). In some cases of recent onset of panic attacks, it is possible to help patients delineate recent stresses that are related to the onset of panic disorder and to help them take a more psychological view of their symptoms and the treatment for them (Roy-Byrne et al. 1986). Patients with panic disorder do not tolerate waiting lists very well. The longer they go without treatment, the more avoidant symptoms they develop and the more demoralized they become, and the less likely they are to follow up referrals. If mental health referral resources are not immediately available, it is worthwhile to have such patients return to the emergency room or to refer them to primary-care physicians who are knowledgeable about panic disorder.

Stress Reactions

Stress reactions in response to misfortune are frequent causes for emergency psychiatric visits. These reactions can range from mild, short-lived, and "in proportion" for the external stresses to extreme, protracted, and apparently quite out-of-proportion reactions.

Uncomplicated bereavement has been rather arbitrarily separated in DSM-III-R from other reactions to loss or stressors. Loss of a spouse through divorce or separation, loss of custody of a child, loss of a job, severe economic problems, or family conflicts can give rise to symptoms in practically anyone. Such cases of severe, but not exceptional, external stresses and severe, but not extreme, reactions to them should ordinarily be dealt with in a way similar to that described for uncomplicated bereavement (see Chapter 10). Referrals should be offered, but the normality of the response should be emphasized, and natural support systems should be mobilized.

Adjustment Disorder With Anxious Mood

An adjustment disorder is a reaction to identifiable psychosocial stressor(s) that occurs within 3 months of onset of the stressors and that has not persisted for more than 6 months. The diagnosis is made only if the reaction is "in excess of the normal and expectable reaction to the stressor(s)" (DSM-III-R, p. 330), has led to functional impairment, and is not the result of another mental disorder. Most frequently, adjustment disorders lead to symptoms of anxious or depressed mood, but they can, in some cases, lead to conduct disturbances, physical complaints, or social withdrawal.

Adjustment disorders with anxious mood in adults seldom require inpatient treatment, but almost always require outpatient referral. At times, referral to short-term residential crisis centers may be appropriate. Benzodiazepines to be used on an as needed basis, or on a regular basis for up to 2–4 weeks, may be reasonable in some cases. At times, patients' degree of anxiety may be such that they are unable to deal with the problems causing the anxiety. In such cases, short-term or intermittent benzodiazepines can help lower patients' anxiety into a range that permits better resolution of problems.

GENERALIZED ANXIETY DISORDER

Generalized anxiety disorder is characterized by unrealistic or excessive anxiety or worry about two or more areas of life (e.g., health, children, or finances) for at least 6 months and is accompanied by physical symptoms of motor tension, autonomic hyperactivity (similar to symptoms of panic disorder), and hypervigilance. This diagnosis should not be made if the symptoms are present only during the course of mood disorders or psychotic disorders, if the worries are related to Axis I disorders (e.g., anxiety about weight gain in a patient with anorexia nervosa), if the physical symptoms are present only during panic attacks, or if the disturbance was initiated or maintained by an organic factor. The organic factors to be considered are the same ones mentioned for panic disorder.

The distinction between generalized anxiety with depressive symptoms and major depression with anxiety is quite important. Suicide is more of a concern in the latter disorder, and treatment is different. Although there is evidence that tricyclic antidepressants are useful in the treatment of generalized anxiety (Kahn et al. 1986), they ordinarily should not be started on an emergency basis for that indication. Benzodiazepines are ordinarily not indicated for generalized anxiety disorder except, perhaps, in the context of an ongoing therapeutic relationship. Patients with generalized anxiety disorder often make psychiatric emergency visits seeking benzodiazepines and should ordinarily not receive them; they should instead be referred to ongoing outpatient treatment.

POSTTRAUMATIC STRESS DISORDER

Posttraumatic stress disorder (PTSD) is a fairly common reason for patients to seek mental health care on an emergency basis. About 1% of the general population is estimated to suffer from PTSD at any given time. About 3.5% of civilians exposed to physical attack and about 20% of veterans wounded in Vietnam are estimated to suffer from PTSD (Helzer et al. 1987). PTSD is characterized by development of symptoms lasting for at least a month and recurring in relation to a psychologically distressing event outside the range of usual human experience. Usually this will be an event involving serious threat of harm to the patient or to loved ones. The characteristic symptoms involve 1) repetitive intrusive reexperiencing of the event (e.g., in memories, dreams or "flashbacks"), 2) persistent attempts to avoid stimuli or feelings related to the trauma (e.g., by avoiding thoughts or activities related to it or by general emotional numbing), and 3) persistent symptoms of increased arousal (e.g., insomnia, irritability, hypervigilance).

Some common situations that can lead to PTSD include military combat, natural or manmade disasters, rape, physical abuse, or, at times, automobile accidents, house fires, or threats of physical violence. When patients are seen soon after a traumatic event, it is usually most appropriate to help them feel that they are experiencing a normal reaction to an abnormal event. Particularly in cases of physical or sexual abuse, it is important to help victims to realize that they are not the sick one. Referral to shelters for battered women or to rape counseling centers is often useful. Psychotherapy should also be offered because many people faced with victimization need more than simple supportive counseling (Rose 1986). People with severe injuries or losses initially need physical support (medical care, food, shelter) more than they need psychological counseling.

PTSD deserves vigorous treatment early in its course. If an individual continues to be symptomatic for a month or more, the disorder is unlikely to resolve on its own. Hospitalization may be indicated if the individual is unable to function at home. Individuals should be encouraged to talk about the traumatic event in question but initially should not be pressured to talk about it more than they feel comfortable doing. In the case of delayed onset of PTSD, some attempt should be made to identify events in the present that have precipitated the reaction. Legal issues are often complicating factors in cases of PTSD and should be clarified at the initial meeting with the patient.

PTSD that has lasted a year or more should be dealt with as a chronic condition. It is unlikely to respond dramatically to short-term intervention, either psychotherapeutic or chemotherapeutic. Exacerbations should be explored and the possibility of a major depressive disorder developing secondary to PTSD should be kept in mind. Collaboration with the patient's ongoing therapist is essential.

PHOBIAS

Two common mental health problems that are uncommon for emergency mental health consultation are simple phobias (persistent fear of a specific object or situation) and social phobia (fear of situations in which the person is exposed to possible scrutiny by others). Two specific phobias that may occasion emergency visits are

• Needle phobia—This is a vexing problem for medical emergency services that is often escalated to a major power struggle between doctor and patient before referral. Usually it turns out that blood drawing is not absolutely essential anyway, and the major therapeutic problem may turn out to be finding a face-saving way out of the standoff for both the doctor and the patient. Needle phobia can sometimes lead to vasovagal syncope when phlebotomy is attempted. The syncope can, at times, be accompanied by some rhythmic movements of extremities (so-called convulsive syncope) giving rise to concern about a possible seizure disorder.

- Claustrophobia—This may complicate some medical procedures (e.g., involving a computed tomography or a hyperbaric oxygen chamber). Sedation with benzodiazepines (e.g., 2 mg lorazepam po or im) may be necessary to permit the procedure.

OBSESSIVE-COMPULSIVE DISORDER

Obsessive-compulsive disorder is frequent among patients seeking emergency mental health care but is infrequently a chief complaint. This disorder is characterized by persistent thoughts or action that a patient feels are senseless, intrusive, and uncontrollable. Recent research suggests that pharmacotherapy can be markedly beneficial for some patients with obsessive-compulsive disorder (Perse 1988), but such treatment ordinarily should not be initiated from an emergency setting.

The most important differential diagnostic consideration in an emergency setting is between obsessive-compulsive disorder and schizophrenia or delusional disorder. An obsessive thought sometimes may be described as a "voice." At times, an obsession may be elaborated to the point that it can be expressed in a similar manner to a delusion. Patients with an underlying obsessive-compulsive disorder may develop a reactive paranoid disorder (Insel and Akiskal 1986). Useful questions to help make this differential diagnosis include, "Is the voice inside your head or outside your head?" or "Is there maybe some possibility that this belief might turn out not to be true?"

When a patient does present an obsession or compulsion as a chief complaint, it is very important to search for other Axis I disorders, such as affective psychotic or anxiety disorders.

ANXIETY SECONDARY TO OTHER PSYCHIATRIC DISORDERS

Nearly all psychiatric disorders can present with anxiety as a chief complaint or as an associated finding. Personality disorders frequently present with anxiety as a chief complaint in response to the specific sorts of threat to which each is most vulnerable (e.g., criticism for a narcissistic personality or threat of abandonment for a dependent personality). In fact, it is probably appropriate to think of there being a continuum rather than a dichotomy between patients with anxiety disorders plus personality trait disturbances and patients with personality disorders plus anxious symptoms. The emergency treatment of each is probably similar (see Chapter 19).

Schizophrenia and delusional disorder frequently lead to extreme anxiety usually related to delusions or hallucinations. Particularly in the case of paranoid disorders, patients may be afraid to reveal the cause of their anxiety when it is at its worst. These patients, however, will usually have a degree of suspiciousness, hostility, and vigilance out of proportion to that normally observed in primary anxiety disorders.

Mania may present with anxiety as patients' poorly thought-out schemes begin to collapse or when consequences of impulsive actions begin to be unavoidable. Although full-blown mania is difficult to miss, early mania in previously well-functioning patients may go unrecognized. Cases of this sort may require hospitalization for diagnosis and for containment of self-destructive behavior. Major depressive disorder with marked anxiety is a dangerous combination, as noted in Chapter 8. The anxiety may be more acutely uncomfortable than the depression, especially if the depression has been going on for some time. As noted in the beginning of this chapter, depression should be searched for in every case of anxiety.

References

American Psychiatric Association: Diagnostic and Statistical Manual of Mental Disorders, 3rd Edition, Revised. Washington, DC, American Psychiatric Association, 1987

Ghosh A, Marks IM: Self-treatment of agoraphobia by exposure. Behav Ther 18:3–16, 1987

Helzer JE, Robins LN, McEvoy L: Post-traumatic stress disorder in the general population: findings from the epidemiologic catchment area survey. N Engl J Med 317:1630–1634, 1987

Insel TR, Akiskal HS: Obsessive-compulsive disorder with psychotic fantasies: a phenomenologic analysis. Am J Psychiatry 143:1527–1533, 1986

Kahn RJ, McNair DM, Lipman RS, et al: Imipramine and chlordiazepoxide in depressive and anxiety disorders, II: efficacy in anxious outpatients. Arch Gen Psychiatry 43:79–85, 1986

Katon W: Panic disorder: epidemiology, diagnosis and treatment in primary care. J Clin Psychiatry 47 (suppl 10):21–27, 1986

McNeil GN: Anxiety, in Handbook of Psychiatric Differential Diagnosis. Edited by Soreff SM, McNeil GN. Littleton, MA, PSG Publishing, 1987

Myers JR, Weissman MM, Tischler GL, et al: Six-month prevalence of psychiatric disorders in three communities. Arch Gen Psychiatry 41:959–967, 1984

Noyes R: Is panic disorder a disease for the medical model? Psychosomatics 28:582–586, 1987

Noyes R, Reich J, Clancy J, et al: Reduction in hypochondriasis with treatment of panic disorder. Br J Psychiatry 149:631–635, 1986

Perse T: Obsessive compulsive disorder: a treatment review. J Clin Psychiatry 49:48–55, 1988

Pohl R, Yeragani VK, Balon R, et al: The jitteriness syndrome in panic disorder patients treated with antidepressants. J Clin Psychiatry 49:100–104, 1988

Rose DS: "Worse than death": psychodynamics of rape victims and the need for psychotherapy. Am J Psychiatry 143:817–824, 1986

Roy-Byrne PP, Geraci M, Uhde TW: Life events and the onset of panic disorder. Am J Psychiatry 143:1424–1427, 1986

Waites TF: Hyperventilation: chronic and acute. Arch Intern Med 138:1700–1701, 1978

Werner A, Campbell RJ, Frazier SH, et al: A Psychiatric Glossary, 5th Edition. Boston, MA, Little, Brown, 1980

Wulsin L, Hillard JR, Geier P, et al: Screening emergency room patients with atypical chest pain for depression and panic attacks. Int J Psychiatry Med 18:315–323, 1988

Chapter 18

Somatoform Disorders

Lawson R. Wulsin, M.D.

Patients with somatoform disorders usually challenge, and sometimes frustrate, the skills and goodwill of emergency room physicians. In this chapter, I will review the approach that meets this challenge. More than most other psychiatric emergencies, the management of the somatoform emergency hinges on the psychiatrist's effective collaboration with medical staff.

The somatoform disorders raise difficulties in the emergency room in several ways. First, diagnosis is often complicated by the possibility of true organic disease and of a medical emergency. Second, diagnosis is often complicated by other psychopathology. Third, strong feelings and misunderstandings between medical and psychiatric staff about patients with somatoform disorders intensify the process of assessment and management. Finally, patients often do not want to hear that they have a somatoform disorder, so the approach must be angled indirectly rather than head-on.

Patients with somatoform disorders present to psychiatric emergency rooms in a limited number of ways. Conversion disorders commonly include motor and sensory deficits, pseudoseizures, and amnesias (Lazare 1981). Somatization disorder presents after a long history of multiple complaints in multiple organ systems, often with increasing urgency. Patients with hypochondriasis come to the psychiatric emergency room after several visits to medical emergency rooms have failed to establish a medical basis for the patient's concern about a particular symptom or disease. The somatoform pain disorder presents as a pain crisis often complicated by depression. Body dysmorphic disorder rarely presents as an emergency.

Assessment and treatment focus not on the disorder of the soma but on the disorder of interpretation. Patients with somatoform disorders often misinterpret the benign meaning of their symptoms and take them as evidence of physical disease (Kellner 1987). In addition to establishing the diagnosis of somatoform disorder, the dynamic formulation of each patient's misinterpretation provides the emergency psychiatrist with a useful basis for the development of the individual treatment plan.

ASSESSMENT GUIDELINES

Several principles of assessment will help decrease diagnostic uncertainty and point toward specific interventions.

- Understand the medical history and recent medical evaluations. Whenever possible, speak directly with the patient's primary medical physician or whomever performed the medical evaluation. Develop your own opinion about the adequacy of the medical evaluation to rule out organic disease or to relate the somatoform disorder to an established medical diagnosis.
- Take a careful psychosocial history with attention to family psychiatric history, models of illness behavior, the social context of the current disorder, and the patient's understanding of medical and psychological dimensions of the current disorder. Make sure your legible psychosocial history becomes a part of the medical chart. This longitudinal overview may serve as an intervention against misguided medical investigations in the future (Brown and Vaillant 1981).
- Because patients with somatoform disorders may amplify somatic and psychological symptoms (Barsky and Klerman 1983), it is best not to rely solely on the patient's reports. Obtain multiple points of view from old charts, recent and past sources of medical care, longtime family members, and current members of the household.
- The somatoform disorders are often associated with other current or past DSM-III-R (American Psychiatric Association 1987) Axis I diagnoses. Look carefully for these associated disorders because they may strengthen the diagnosis of a somatoform disorder and they may require treatment.
- Consider use of formal screening measures as an aid to identifying

associated psychopathology in the context of multiple somatic complaints: the Beck Depression Inventory (Beck 1978) or the Center for Epidemiologic Studies Depression Scale (Radloff 1977) for depression, the screening test for somatization disorder (Othmer and De-Souza 1985), and the Mini-Mental State Exam for differentiating the cognitive deficits of depression from dementia (Dick et al. 1984; Folstein et al. 1975).

MANAGEMENT GUIDELINES

Ford (1983; Ford and Smith 1987) has developed three rules for the management of somatoform disorders. First, "invasive diagnostic and therapeutic procedures should be initiated only on the basis of objective evidence of pathophysiologic dysfunction, not solely on subjective complaints" (Ford and Smith 1987, p. 206). Echoed by many recent authors, this rule can be helpful when deciding in the emergency room whether to request further evaluation of physical symptoms, and when arguing for restraint with medical colleagues bent on yet another comprehensive evaluation. The dilemma for the emergency psychiatrist is how to ensure adequate medical evaluation without reinforcing the patient's dysfunctional illness behavior. The answer lies in understanding the patient's medical history and current differential diagnosis.

Second, keep the primary physician involved in the care of the patient. For the emergency psychiatrist, this means contacting the primary physician from the emergency room, collaborating with him or her about follow-up plans, and at times reviewing together the outpatient management of somatoform disorders. For example, recent work has reaffirmed the clinical and economic value of regular appointments with the primary physician (Ford 1983; Smith et al. 1986) that involve brief physical examinations focused on the current complaint as well as some time for talking. The primary physician's degree of interest will increase if the emergency psychiatrist can begin arrangements for regular collaboration between the primary physician and a psychiatrist.

The third rule is that "arguing with a patient about the reality of a physical symptom is not only fruitless—it is antitherapeutic in that it denies the personal experience of the patient" (Ford and Smith 1987, p. 207). Allying with the patient's experience is the essential first step to helping the patient reframe the symptoms in a way that allows a combined medical and psychological approach. Make a point of telling patients their symptoms are real, you believe them, and they are not crocks or hypochondriacs or whatever pejorative word may have been said or implied. Shift the focus away from the amplification of symptoms and toward the management of physical and psychological distress. Most people find it less damning to view their stress as a normal consequence of physical illness, rather than as the only source of their symptoms. The psychiatric emergency room visit can, in the hands of a skilled clinician, become the pivot point for shifting the patient's view of the symptoms from a narrow physical context to a broader biopsychosocial context. The psychiatrist's response to the somatizer's insistence on the physical nature of his or her experience is "Yes, and . . ." rather than "Yes, but. . . ."

One additional point addresses the possibility that a somatoform disorder is actually a factitious disorder (see Chapter 20). Emergency psychiatrists are often asked to "unmask the crock" by puzzled colleagues in medicine. But rarely, if ever, does the emergency psychiatrist have both the information and the alliance with the patient necessary to effectively challenge the deceitful behaviors of those with factitious disorders. Good care of the patient suggests that the emergency psychiatrist resist the invitation to such dramatic challenges in favor of carefully communicating with the referring physician about the differential diagnosis and ways to approach the possibility of factitious disorders with the patient over several visits.

SPECIFIC DISORDERS

Conversion Disorders

Conversion disorders may present in three ways: 1) "pure" conversion disorder, 2) conversion disorder mixed with organic disease, and 3) undetected organic disease mistakenly diagnosed as conversion disorder. From 13 to 30% of patients with "conversion disorders" in four follow-up studies later developed organic disease that could explain the original symptoms labeled conversion (Lazare 1981). For this reason and because the implications of the diagnosis for treatment are dramatic, the psychiatrist should initiate the diagnosis of conversion disorder in the emergency room only after careful evaluation and while remaining open with the patient about the possibility of undiagnosable early organic disease.

Perhaps as much as half the time, conversion symptoms will present in patients with known physical illness that does not explain the conversion symptoms (Lazare 1981; Smith et al. 1986). For example, the presence of multiple sclerosis does not account for glove anesthesia, nor does epilepsy eliminate the possibility of pseudoseizures. On the contrary, the patient's experience of illness may serve as the unconscious model for the conversion reaction. Teasing the conversion symptoms apart from the known physical illness requires a clear understanding of the physical illness as well as the psychology of conversion reactions.

"Pure" conversion disorder, though pure of organic disease, is often not pure of other psychopathology. One-third to one-half of patients with conversion disorders have another current diagnosis, the most common being depression, somatization disorder, schizophrenia, and personality disorders (Lazare 1978). In the presence of these more pervasive disorders, the diagnosis of conversion disorder should not be made (DSM-III-R), but conversion symptoms should be noted as a feature of the more pervasive disorder.

Lazare's (1981) review of studies of conversion disorders has led to the development of several psychological criteria that strengthen the diagnosis when present in addition to the DSM-III-R criteria. Prior somatization or conversion disorder argues in favor of a symptom being part of a conversion disorder rather than an organic disorder. Serious current or past psychopathology also argues in favor of conversion disorder. Models for illness behavior and acute stress before the symptom may add significantly to the formulation of the dynamics of the symptom and indirectly support the diagnosis. A history of disturbed sexuality (e.g., abuse, paraphilias) is associated with conversion disorders. Other factors such as primary or secondary gain, hysterical personality, and la belle indifference are less helpful in distinguishing conversion disorders from organic disease.

In addition to treating concurrent psychopathology and providing adequate medical and psychiatric follow-up, the emergency psychiatrist must decide whether to attempt to relieve conversion symptoms in the emergency room. This decision relies on the specific psychosocial history and the psychodynamics of the conversion symptoms. Swartz and McCracken (1986) have identified three contraindications to uncovering work aimed at relieving conversion symptoms in the emergency room:

- Chronic conversion symptoms have persisted because they serve a necessary function (primary or secondary gain), and unless the patient has other resources that he or she can consciously enlist to serve that function, removing the symptoms may only destabilize a process that cannot be repaired during the brief emergency room visit.
- The enmeshed family system may depend on the illness behavior of

the patient with conversion symptoms. When the psychosocial history or the emergency room behavior of the family suggests enmeshment, the symptoms should be treated more gradually and in the context of outpatient family therapy.

• When one function of the conversion symptoms is to protect the patient against aggressive behavior, the uncovering work should be done in a secure setting where the patient will be followed up, such as an inpatient unit or a day hospital.

The decision to proceed with uncovering work rests on the assessment that the patient is now ready to bear previously unbearable feelings, perhaps because of the current crisis or the available professional help. The first step is a combination of support and suggestion: "You have been putting up with impossible demands from your family and the recent accident—more than anyone could bear alone. Now you are getting the help you need, and as you sit here, you will find some of the strength returning to your legs and it will feel safe to begin to move them again. You will continue to feel stronger over the next few days as you work with your doctor." The choice and extent of the suggestion are crucial to success. The suggestion should address not only the symptom but the patient's fears and hypothesized conflict. Intensely anxious patients will attend less well to suggestion and may benefit from the use of diphenhydramine or another mild sedative before the suggestion.

When support and suggestion fail to improve function, two options for further uncovering may be considered—hypnosis and the amobarbital (Amytal) interview. Of these, the simplest and safest is hypnosis. This technique capitalizes on a patient's ability to focus attention and respond to suggestion, and it is effective only in the hands of a clinician with training in hypnosis. Perry and Jacobs (1982) have reviewed the applications of the Amytal interview in the emergency setting (Tables 18-1 and 18-2). Psychological contraindications to the Amytal interview, in addition to those discussed above in the section on conversion disorders, include patient refusal and paranoia. Medical contraindications include 1) upper respiratory inflammation that impairs breathing, 2) severe liver or kidney impairment, 3) hypotension, 4) porphyria, and 5) barbiturate addiction (Perry and Jacobs 1982). These authors also recommend that a cardiopulmonary resuscitation cart be available.

Somatization Disorder

Somatization disorder is best diagnosed by a historical review of sys-

Table 18-1. Indications for the amobarbital (Amytal) interview

---

- Aid to diagnostic interview of mute or stuporous patients:
  - Catatonia
  - Hysterical stupor
  - Unexplained muteness
  - Differentiating depressive, schizophrenic, and organic stupors
- Therapeutic interview aid for disorders of repression and dissociation:
  - Abreaction of posttraumatic stress disorder (traumatic neurosis)
  - Recovery of memory in psychogenic amnesia and fugue
  - Recovery of function in conversion disorder

Source. Adapted from Perry and Jacobs 1982.

tems. The feature that distinguishes somatization disorder from other somatoform disorders is the history of multiple complaints in multiple organ systems over an extended period of time (beginning before age 30). DSM-III-R lists 35 possible symptoms in the diagnostic criteria. This list will often seem tedious to the busy emergency psychiatrist, who would do better first to screen using Othmer and DeSouza's (1985) screening test for somatization disorder, which has been incorporated into DSM-III-R:

- Have you ever had trouble breathing?
- Have you ever had frequent trouble with menstrual cramps?
- Have you ever had burning sensations in your sexual organs, mouth, or rectum?
- Have you ever had difficulties swallowing or had an uncomfortable lump in your throat that stayed with you for at least an hour?
- Have you ever found that you could not remember what you had been doing for hours or days at a time? (If yes) Did this happen even though you had not been drinking or taking drugs?
- Have you ever had trouble from frequent vomiting?
- Have you ever had frequent pain in your fingers or toes?

A positive response to two or more of these seven questions demands evaluation with the full symptom checklist from DSM-III-R.

The first step in the treatment of somatization disorder, and also hypochondriasis, is a clear and supportive explanation of the findings of the medical evaluations. Do not assume that the necessary information has been communicated to and understood by the patient. Ask the patient to paraphrase what you have just said to verify the patient's level

Table 18-2. Protocol for administering the amobarbital (Amytal) interview

---

1. Have the patient recline.

2. Explain again to the patient that medication should make him or her relax and feel like talking.

3. Insert narrow-bore scalp-vein needle.

4. Begin injecting a 50% solution of amobarbital sodium (500 mg dissolved in 10 cc of sterile water) at a rate no faster than 1 cc/minute (50 mg/minute) to prevent sleep or sudden respiratory depression.

5. Interview

   With a verbal patient, begin with neutral topics, gradually approaching areas of trauma, guilt, and possible repression.

   With an initially mute or verbally inhibited patient, continue to make the technical suggestion that soon the patient will feel like talking. Prompting with known facts about the patient's life may also help.

6. Continue the infusion until either sustained rapid lateral nystagmus is present or drowsiness is noted. Slight slurring of speech is common at this point. The sedation threshold is usually reached at a dose between 150 mg (3 cc) and 350 mg (7 cc), but can be as little as 75 mg (1.5 cc) in elderly patients or patients with organic illness. Prompts to talk should have their strongest effect from here on.

7. To maintain the level of narcosis, infuse the sodium amobarbital at a rate of about 0.5–1.0 cc every 5 minutes or so.

8. Conduct the interview as you would any other psychiatric interview, but with several caveats:

   Approach affect-laden or traumatic material gradually and then work over it again and again to recover forgotten details, their attendant feelings, and the patient's current reactions to them.

   In the initially mute or verbally inhibited patient, do not press too hard in areas that would normally be inhibited (e.g., murderous rage toward an important attachment) to prevent development of panic after the interview.

9. Terminate the interview when enough material has been produced (often 30 minutes in the verbally inhibited patient), or when therapeutic goals have been reached (sometimes an hour or so). Have the patient lie down for 15 minutes or so until he or she can walk with close supervision.

Source. Adapted from Perry and Jacobs 1982.

of understanding. Surprisingly often these repeated efforts succeed in reassuring patients labeled with somatization disorder. Their misinterpretation may have been due to misinformation.

When clear communication and reassurance by the emergency psychiatrist fail to diminish the somatizing behavior, more extensive psychological work is necessary, and the disposition should include psychotherapy in combination with routine medical care (Kellner 1987).

Hypochondriasis

Hypochondriasis requires an approach similar to that for somatization disorder. As defined by DSM-III-R, hypochondriasis differs from somatization disorder by being more focused on one symptom or one system or one disease and often has a briefer history (i.e., onset need not be before age 30). The distinction between hypochondriasis and delusional disorder, somatic type, lies in hypochondriacal patients' acknowledgment that their fears may be unfounded. The diagnosis of hypochondriasis should be considered only when hypochondriacal symptoms are not a feature of a more pervasive Axis I disorder such as schizophrenia or depression.

Although results are variable and the studies are few, there is some evidence that tricyclic antidepressants are effective in hypochondriasis without depression (Brotman and Jenike 1984). In some cases when the emergency psychiatrist and the physician who will follow the patient can agree on the plan, it may be helpful to begin the antidepressant trial in the emergency room. This response to the patient's request for action should be coupled with a clear discussion of the target symptoms and the plans for management.

Somatoform Pain Disorder

Somatoform pain disorder usually comes to the emergency psychiatrist via the medical emergency room for one of two reasons—either for the assessment and treatment of associated depression or for adjustment of psychotropic medications. Less often the psychiatrist must assess suicide risk during a pain crisis.

The first target of the evaluation is anxiety and fear that magnify pain. Much somatic behavior during a crisis can be calmed by careful attention to anxiety and fear through a combination of empathic interviewing and judicious use of minor short-acting tranquilizers in the emergency room setting only. Chronic use of benzodiazepines may exacerbate the pain and should be discouraged.

The second target is depression. The diagnosis of depression should rely less on the patient's report of mood or interpersonal problems, which are often denied in this disorder, and more on preoccupation with pain, anergia, anhedonia, insomnia, hopelessness, and a family history of affective disorder or chronic pain (Blumer 1982). Low doses of antidepressants are commonly prescribed for the management of chronic pain, but the presence of major depression warrants an increase to doses effective for depression.

The third target for evaluation in somatoform pain disorders is substance abuse. Alcohol abuse was a relatively common (38%) associated diagnosis in one study of 37 inpatients with chronic pain (Katon et al. 1985). Other common substances used in an attempt to dull the pain at the risk of dependence include benzodiazepines, narcotics, and barbiturates. Before prescribing medications or follow-up plans, the emergency psychiatrist must evaluate current and past dependences and the treatment history. In some cases, decreasing medication doses and referral to a drug or alcohol treatment program may be the most significant intervention for the reduction of somatoform pain.

Tell patients that they have a well-known pain disorder, that the pain is real or understandable, that the pain does not mean harm to their body, and that their task is to "learn to ignore the pain as much as possible while finding distractions and gradually become more active again" (Blumer 1982). Reliable follow-up is crucial to the effect of emergency room interventions.

REFERENCES

American Psychiatric Association: Diagnostic and Statistical Manual of Mental Disorders, 3rd Edition, Revised. Washington, DC, American Psychiatric Association, 1987

Barsky AJ, Klerman GL: Overview: hypochondriasis, bodily complaints, and somatic styles. Am J Psychiatry 140:273–283, 1983

Beck AT: Depression Inventory. Philadelphia, PA, Center for Cognitive Therapy, 1978

Blumer D: Psychiatric aspects of chronic pain: nature, identification and treatment of the pain prone disorder, in The Spine, 2nd Edition, Vol 2. Edited by Rothman RH, Simeone FA. Philadelphia, PA, WB Saunders, 1982, pp 1090–1117

Brotman AW, Jenike MA: Monosymptomatic hypochondriasis treated with tricyclic antidepressants. Am J Psychiatry 141:1608–1609, 1984

Brown HN, Vaillant GE: Hypochondriasis. Arch Intern Med 141:723–726, 1981

Dick JPR, Guiloff RJ, Stewart A, et al: Mini-Mental State Exam in neurological patients. J Neurol Neurosurg Psychiatry 47:496–499, 1984

Folstein MF, Folstein SE, McHugh PR: "Mini-Mental State": a practical method for grading the cognitive state of patients for the clinician. J Psychiatr Res 12:189–198, 1975

Ford CV: The Somatizing Disorders. New York, Elsevier, 1983

Ford CV, Smith GR: Somatoform disorders, factitious disorders, and disability syndromes, in Principles of Medical Psychiatry. Edited by Stoudemire A, Fogel BS. Orlando, FL, Grune & Stratton, 1987

Katon W, Egan K, Miller D: Chronic pain: lifetime psychiatric diagnoses and family history. Am J Psychiatry 142:1156–1160, 1985

Kellner R: Hypochondriasis and somatization. JAMA 258:2718–2722, 1987

Lazare A: Hysteria, in Massachusetts General Hospital Handbook of General Hospital Psychiatry. Edited by Hackett TP, Cassem NH. St. Louis, MO, CV Mosby, 1978

Lazare A: Conversion symptoms. N Engl J Med 305:745–748, 1981

Othmer E, DeSouza C: A screening test for somatization disorder (hysteria). Am J Psychiatry 142:1146–1149, 1985

Perry C, Jacobs D: Overview: clinical applications of the Amytal interview in psychiatric emergency settings. Am J Psychiatry 139:552–559, 1982

Radloff LS: The CES-D Scale: a self report depression scale for research in the general population. Applied Psychological Measurements 1:385–401, 1977

Smith GR, Monson RA, Ray DC: Psychiatric consultation in somatization disorder: a randomized controlled study. N Engl J Med 314:1407–1413, 1986

Swartz MS, McCracken J: Emergency room management of conversion disorders. Hosp Community Psychiatry 37:828–832, 1986

Chapter 19

Personality Disorders

J.R. Hillard, M.D.

Personality disorders are common among psychiatric emergency patients, just as they are among patients in all clinical populations. Personality disorders, however, are difficult to diagnose in emergency settings because the diagnosis implies an enduring pattern of maladaptive personality traits that 1) are characteristic of the patient's recent and *long-term functioning* and 2) are not limited to discrete episodes of illness (DSM-III-R [American Psychiatric Association 1987]). Seeing a patient on a one-time basis in the midst of an acute episode of illness certainly does not put the clinician in an ideal situation for evaluating such a disorder. Often the best that can be hoped for in an emergency setting is to be able to identify maladaptive personality traits that may be relevant to a patient's presentation or to be able to make a diagnosis of personality disorder not otherwise specified. Patients commonly have traits of more than one personality disorder and may, in fact, qualify for more than one personality disorder diagnosis (Morey 1988; Widiger et al. 1988).

Personality disorders complicate the diagnosis and treatment of any problem a patient may have. Most personality disorders, however, rarely lead to psychiatric emergency visits or hospital admissions, unless depression or psychoactive substance use, or other DSM-III-R Axis I disorders, are superimposed on them. The personality disorders that do frequently lead to psychiatric emergency visits, even without a superimposed Axis I disorder, are those with prominent borderline, antisocial, schizotypal, or paranoid traits. The emergency assessment and treatment of patients with these disorders will be discussed in this chapter. Other personality disorders are mentioned in other chapters as they relate to the disorders covered by each chapter.

BORDERLINE PERSONALITY DISORDER

Although patients with borderline personality disorder do not account for a large proportion of all psychiatric emergency visits, they do account for a large proportion of the "really hard cases"—the cases that tie up a lot of staff time, energy, and emotion (Beresin and Gordon 1981).

Assessment

Although a diagnosis of borderline personality disorder, as defined by intrapsychic structures, cannot be made without extensive longitudinal contact with the patient (Kernberg 1975), borderline personality disorder as defined in DSM-III-R can often be diagnosed, or at least strongly suspected, on the basis of history obtainable in a psychiatric emergency contact.

A history of the following symptoms characteristic of borderline personality disorder can be identified on the basis of a single interview:

- Intense unstable relationships
- Potentially self-damaging impulsiveness
- Mood fluctuations
- Inappropriate intense anger
- Recurrent suicidal or self-mutilative threats, gestures, or behavior
- Marked or persistent identity disturbances
- Chronic feelings of emptiness or boredom
- Frantic efforts to avoid real or imagined abandonment

A major obstacle to diagnosing these patterns under such circumstances, however, is that a patient's current state of mind will always affect recall of past events. Thus, a currently depressed patient may describe a lifelong feeling of emptiness which he or she would not have described when in a better frame of mind. It is generally a good idea to be conservative in diagnosing borderline personality because this is one of the most stigmatizing diagnoses in psychiatry. It is often most appropriate to diagnose borderline traits rather than disorder.

When a patient has made multiple psychiatric emergency visits, it is possible to be more certain of the diagnosis as the patient's pattern of behavior over time emerges. A common pattern of emergency room visits involves repetitive presentations with suicidal gestures or thoughts after problems in either personal relationships or psychotherapy relationships. (See Chapter 26 for more discussion of psychiatric emergency room "repeaters" currently in therapy.)

Regardless of current presenting symptoms, borderline patients always need to be assessed for the presence of 1) ongoing suicide risk, 2) superimposed major depressive disorder, 3) psychoactive substance use disorder, and 4) psychotic symptoms.

Assessing Suicide Risk in the Borderline Patient

A borderline patient's answer to a question like, "Have you been thinking about suicide lately?" is seldom a reliable guide in assessment of suicide risk. Mood fluctuations and impulsiveness make a negative answer suspect, whereas interpersonal manipulativeness may make a positive answer suspect. Even more than with other patients, a complete assessment of suicide potential, as outlined in Chapter 8, should guide treatment rather than simply the patient's self-report of suicidal feelings.

A particularly unpleasant problem arises in dealing with borderline patients who have prominent passive-aggressive traits. Such patients are often seen after an overdose and give the message, "I can't say I am not going to kill myself, but I am not going to let you put me in the hospital." The therapist is left with the unpleasant choice of, in effect, telling the patient either 1) "You are going to the hospital whether you like it or not" or 2) "I don't care whether you live or die." It is, of course, appropriate to hospitalize patients involuntarily if the overall evaluation suggests high risk of suicide. If the overall evaluation suggests low risk, it is also perfectly appropriate to discharge patients who are unwilling to say for sure that they will not kill themselves. Either way, patients need to receive the messages 1) I am bound to follow the state commitment law and 2) I do care about you.

It is important to remember that borderline patients are, in fact, at increased risk for completed suicide and that, among borderline patients, as among other patient groups, a past history of suicide attempts and suicidal behavior at the time of admission correlate with completed suicide (Kullgren 1988). Borderline patients with concurrent affective or substance use disorders are at higher risk for serious suicide attempts than are other borderline patients (Fyer et al. 1988).

Assessing Psychotic Symptoms in Borderline Patients

Although "brief psychotic episodes" are termed an "associated feature" of borderline personality, such psychotic episodes deserve further differential diagnosis and may be due to psychoactive substance intoxication or major depression or may be factitious (Pope et al. 1985). (See Chapter 16 for discussion of factitious psychosis.) Differentiation among these possible causes has clear-cut treatment implications. Identification of factitious symptoms in borderline patients is particularly important in that they generally imply the need for psychosocial, rather than biochemical, intervention.

Management of the Borderline Patient

Psychological. Just as these patients rapidly form intense, unstable relationships with other people in their lives, so they form such relationships with psychiatric emergency personnel. These relationships can alternate rapidly between idealization ("None of the other doctors have been able to help me, but I can tell that you're different") and devaluation ("You're just like all the rest; in fact, you're a lot worse than the rest"). This sort of "splitting" can give rise to intense feelings in the therapist, and, in fact, such countertransference reactions have been suggested as useful in diagnosing borderline personality disorder (Kernberg 1975). In addition, borderline patients have a tendency toward "projective identification," a particularly intense and primitive form of projection that involves the patient seeing his feelings in another ("I can see that you think my wife is right and that you think I am a worthless piece of garbage") and the patient simultaneously identifying with the feeling perceived in the other ("Well, if you hate me so much, then I hate you").

Psychological approaches to keep in mind are

- Minimize splitting between the emergency personnel and the patient's ongoing therapist. Calling the therapist is usually a good idea not only to gain clinical information, but also to emphasize that you are working together.
- Minimize splitting of psychiatric emergency personnel. Multidisciplinary staff, such as are common in psychiatric emergency settings,

often have various interpersonal and interdisciplinary conflicts that are just below the surface and that can be tapped into by a borderline patient's tendency to overvalue some individuals while devaluing others (e.g., "I know I can trust you. Do you think that I should report that nurse to the administration for the way she has been treating patients all night?").

- Don't let yourself be provoked, which is, of course, sometimes easier said than done.
- Attempt to promptly correct transference distortions, either positive or negative.
- Cultivate institutional transference (e.g., "If things get worse rather than better, feel free to come back. We never close."), letting the institution serve as a transitional object to help the patient get through periods of rejection.
- Help the patient see the current crisis as an acute manifestation of a chronic condition rather than as a de novo crisis that needs a solution right now. If possible, observe and interact with patients over a period of hours to see if they are able to calm down and regain self-control.
- Encourage patients who always come in after suicide gestures or impulsive actions to come in before, rather than after, making an attempt.
- Develop a consistent plan for use by both the emergency room and community personnel.

Biological.   Pharmacologic treatment of borderline personality disorder should be aimed at the symptoms the patient has (Cowdry 1987). An increase in paranoid symptoms or a brief reactive psychosis should be treated with antipsychotic medication on at least a short-term basis. Antidepressant medications should probably be started with even more caution in borderline personality patients than in other groups because borderline patients frequently suffer from short-lived affective disturbances which may resolve spontaneously and because borderline patients are prone to impulsive overdoses. One recent study has suggested that borderline patients with depressive symptoms may do better over a 1-year period on antipsychotic medication than on antidepressant medication (Frances and Soloff 1988; Soloff et al. 1986). Given the chronic nature of borderline distress and the tendency of borderline patients to abuse drugs, use of benzodiazepines should also be approached with caution and may be associated with episodes of behavior discontrol in this population (Gardner and Cowdry 1988). Short-term use after major

Table 19-1. Use of hospitalization for patients with borderline personality disorder or other severe personality disorders

---

Indications for admission
- The patient's ongoing therapist wants the patient admitted as part of an ongoing treatment plan or for reevaluation.
- Suicidal gestures are escalating.
- Secondary major depression or psychoactive substance abuse requires admission.
- Psychotic reaction that does not respond to emergency interventions (structured environment and/or antipsychotic medication) occurs.
- Severe losses or other stress occur.

Contraindications to admission[a]
- Repeating a treatment that has already failed.
- Using the hospital because nothing else works.
- Attempting to make major characterologic change.
- Attempting to try a new medication in the absence of any positive indication for its success.
- Trying to convince patients to change their living situations.
- Treating the patient's unwillingness to follow treatment plans.
- Sheltering malingerers or patients facing legal charges.

---

[a]Adapted from Glick et al. 1984.

external stresses may be appropriate for some patients, however. Table 19-1 summarizes the use of hospitalization for patients with borderline personality disorder or other severe personality disorders.

ANTISOCIAL PERSONALITY DISORDER

Antisocial personality disorder is characterized by a pattern of irresponsible and antisocial behavior starting in childhood or early adolescence and continuing into adulthood. Such individuals are frequently in the criminal justice system but may turn up in psychiatric emergency settings under a variety of circumstances.

Presentations of Antisocial Patients

Family wants "help" for the patient. The patient has been verbally or physically aggressive, abusing substances, and getting into trouble. Concerned family members bring the patient in, stating that there is clearly something wrong with him and that he needs help *now*. When the family is in the room, the patient is likely to say that he does want help. When the family is not in the room, the patient is likely to say that he doesn't really think that there is very much wrong with him.

Unless the patient has a superimposed affective, psychotic, or other DSM-III-R Axis I disorder, acute treatment is unlikely to be of much help (Gabbard and Coyne 1984). Unless the patient has some degree of motivation for substance abuse treatment, that is unlikely to be of much help either.

The main problem for the clinician is helping the family to approach the patient's situation realistically. Family members need to see themselves as allied with the therapist in dealing appropriately with the patient, rather than seeing themselves and the patient allied in asking for "help" which the therapist is withholding. It is important to inform the family if acute mental health treatment is not likely to help.

Often family members of antisocial individuals have been shielding them from the consequences of their actions for years. They may be quite resistant to letting the patients take the consequences of their actions from the criminal justice system, rather than having the mental health system absolve them of responsibility. Antisocial individuals clearly have "something wrong" with them, and it is useless to try to tell a patient's family that the patient is not mentally ill. A better approach involves educating the family about when hospitalization is or is not indicated and helping them to see criminal justice interventions as being the only therapeutic approach to some personality problems.

Patient facing criminal sentencing. Sometimes antisocial patients about to be sentenced for substance abuse–related crimes will ask to be admitted for substance abuse treatment. Sometimes they are quite explicit in stating that they desire treatment, hoping to get a reduced sentence. This is probably not the best possible motivation, but is probably better than no motivation. If a treatment resource is available, and the patient did not recently leave it against medical advice, inpatient substance abuse treatment is often reasonable under these circumstances.

A similar situation may arise when a patient has just been left by his wife or girlfriend and hopes that getting substance abuse treatment may help get her back. Patients with this type of motivation can frequently benefit from treatment.

Inpatient mental health treatment, however, for "intermittent explosive disorder" (see controversy in Chapter 11) or for dysthymia or adjustment disorder is seldom indicated under such circumstances.

Patients about to go to jail. Malingering has to be high on the list of differential diagnoses, although it is not necessarily the diagnosis, in every antisocial patient facing a jail term. Such patients certainly have the potential for major depressive disorder, or even for a brief reactive psychosis. Hospitalization should be avoided if at all possible. The jail should be informed that the patient may be a suicide risk if that appears to be the case.

Unless absolutely indicated, medication should not be prescribed for patients about to be incarcerated. In correctional settings, almost any drug is likely to be abused—even drugs like amitriptyline or thioridazine.

Patients currently in jail. Antisocial patients are sometimes brought from jail for psychiatric evaluation after suicidal gestures. After they have gotten appropriate medical treatment, patients should almost always be sent back to jail. Jails would often like to get rid of these individuals, but they are just as capable of putting them on suicide precautions as is an inpatient psychiatric unit. Psychiatric admission is ordinarily appropriate only if the patient is about to be discharged from jail. If the jail really needs to get a patient transferred to a hospital, that transfer is usually best handled through the judicial system.

Schizotypal and Paranoid Personalities

These are odd-appearing individuals who do not usually come to psychiatric emergency services on their own, but who may be brought in by others. The main emergency problem in differential diagnosis is not distinguishing between these and other personality disorders, but distinguishing them from schizophrenia or other psychoses. Particularly when under stress, people with these personality disorders can relate in a disorganized or hostile, suspicious manner, suggesting a psychotic illness (Jacobsberg et al. 1986). Hospitalization can be counterproductive, particularly in the case of an individual with a solid, but marginal, adaptation to the community. Hospitalization should generally be avoided unless the patient or others describe an increase in the patient's level of symptomatology. Even under these circumstances, prescription of antipsychotics plus outpatient referral may be most appropriate.

References

American Psychiatric Association: Diagnostic and Statistical Manual of Mental Disorders, 3rd Edition, Revised. Washington, DC, American Psychiatric Association, 1987

Beresin E, Gordon C: Emergency ward management of the borderline patient. Gen Hosp Psychiatry 3:237–244, 1981

Cowdry RW: Psychopharmacology of borderline personality disorder: a review. J Clin Psychiatry 48 (suppl 8):15–22, 1987

Frances A, Soloff PH: Treating the borderline patient with low-dose neuroleptics. Hosp Community Psychiatry 39:246–248, 1988

Fyer MR, Frances AJ, Sullivan T, et al: Suicide attempts in patients with borderline personality disorder. Am J Psychiatry 145:737–739, 1988

Gabbard GO, Coyne L: Predictors of response of antisocial patients to hospital treatment. Hosp Community Psychiatry 38:1181–1185, 1984

Gardner PL, Cowdry RW: Pharmacotherapy of borderline personality disorder. Arch Gen Psychiatry 45:111–119, 1988

Glick ID, Klar H, Braff P: When should chronic patients be hospitalized? Hosp Community Psychiatry 35:934–936, 1984

Jacobsberg LB, Hymowitz P, Barasch A, et al: Symptoms of schizotypal personality disorder. Am J Psychiatry 143:1222–1227, 1986

Kernberg O: Borderline Conditions and Pathological Narcissism. New York, Jason Aronson, 1975

Kullgren G: Factors associated with completed suicide in borderline personality disorder. J Nerv Ment Dis 176:40–44, 1988

Morey LC: Personality disorders in DSM-III and DSM-III-R: convergence, coverage and internal consistency. Am J Psychiatry 145:573–577, 1988

Pope HG, Jonas JM, Hudson JI, et al: An empirical study of psychosis in borderline personality disorder. Am J Psychiatry 142:1285–1290, 1985

Soloff PH, George A, Nathan RS, et al: Progress in pharmacotherapy of borderline patients: a double-blind study of amitriptyline, haloperidol, and placebo. Arch Gen Psychiatry 43:691–697, 1986

Widiger TA, Frances A, Spitzer RL, et al: The DSM-III-R personality disorders: an overview. Am J Psychiatry 145:786–795, 1988

Chapter 20

Other Emergencies

J.R. Hillard, M.D.

This chapter covers disorders that can lead to requests for emergency psychiatric care but that did not require chapters of their own. These are eating disorders, sleep disorders, sexual disorders, dissociative disorders, impulse control disorders, factitious disorders, and marital problems.

EATING DISORDERS

Eating disorders are common in the United States. It is reasonable to estimate the lifetime prevalence of bulimia nervosa at about 10% and anorexia nervosa at about 1% among women of reproductive age (Pope et al. 1984). Prevalence is much lower in men but does not appear to be lower in lower socioeconomic status patients (Pope et al. 1987). It is unusual for patients to bring themselves into psychiatric emergency settings for eating disorders because such disorders tend to have a gradual onset and tend to be at least somewhat ego-syntonic. Patients are most often brought in by friends or family members who have discovered and have been disturbed by the behavior. The most important differential diagnosis for eating disorders is major depression, which is

---

Shaded sections indicate areas of legitimate diversity of professional opinion in the literature. See Preface for further discussion.

frequently associated with abnormal eating behaviors (Herzog 1984), is treatable, and may be life threatening. If weight loss is the primary symptom, physical illness, such as malignancy, must also be considered. Patients with an extreme degree of self-induced vomiting (e.g., multiple episodes per day) may develop hypokalemia, and for that reason require a check of blood chemistries.

Recognition and identification of eating disorders among patients presenting with other problems can have positive consequences. Patients may have been engaging in extensive binge eating and purging behavior for years and kept it as a guilty secret even from their doctors. Once the behavior has been identified and labeled, patients may be more capable of seeking appropriate treatment. Binge eating and purging should probably be inquired about routinely among young women patients.

Ordinarily, outpatient referral should be the first-line treatment for eating disorders. Antidepressants should not be started from the emergency room for treatment of eating disorders, but only as part of an overall treatment plan. Table 20-1 lists indications for hospitalization of patients with eating disorders, on either an emergency or an elective basis. If weight restoration in anorexia is the only goal of hospitalization, a medical unit may be an adequate facility. Under most circumstances, however, a psychiatric unit is generally preferable. A specialized eating disorder unit should be considered if one is available.

SLEEP DISORDERS

The only sleep disorder that is a frequent cause for psychiatric emergency visits is insomnia. Among young or middle-aged patients, the primary differential diagnostic considerations are depression and substance abuse. Short-term use of benzodiazepines can be useful and humane for patients in this age group with acute onset of insomnia, as long as they do not suffer from major depression or substance abuse. The goal of these medications can be explained to patients as helping them break out of the vicious cycle of going to bed not expecting to go to sleep, thus making the likelihood of sleep lower, and thus making expectations of sleep even lower. For patients with chronic insomnia, acute pharmacotherapy is probably contraindicated.

Among patients with schizophrenia or manic-depressive disorders, sleep disturbance may be an early sign of relapse and may call for temporarily adding an antipsychotic or for raising the patient's dose of antipsychotic medication (Heinrichs and Carpenter 1985).

As people age, their sleep decreases in quantity and in quality, as

Table 20-1. Indications for hospitalization of patients with eating disorders

Emergency

- Weight loss >30% over 3 months
- Severe metabolic disturbance (pulse <40 beats/minute, temperature <36°C, systolic blood pressure <70 mmHg, serum potassium <2.5 nmol/L despite oral potassium
- Severe depression or suicide risk
- Psychosis
- Diabetes mellitus in poor control
- Failure of outpatient treatment elective

Elective

- Family crisis
- Complex differential diagnosis
- Need to confront patient or family denial

Source. Adapted from Herzog 1987.

measured by sleep latency (time until falling asleep) and by number of nighttime awakenings (Miles and Dement 1980). In addition, elderly patients are more sensitive to the sleep-disrupting effects of caffeine, nicotine, alcohol, and various prescription medications. In addition, they are more likely than younger individuals to experience confusional or amnestic reactions to benzodiazepines. For these reasons, benzodiazepines should not ordinarily be prescribed from the emergency room for elderly patients (those more than about 60 years old). Instead, these patients should be educated about 1) normal sleep changes with aging, 2) evening fluid restriction to decrease nocturia, 3) avoidance of daytime napping, and 4) avoidance of stimulating medication (Jenike 1985).

SEXUAL DISORDERS

Sexual disorders are a surprisingly uncommon reason for psychiatric emergency visits.

Paraphilias

Patients with exhibitionism and pedophilia are often brought for emergency psychiatric evaluation after having been criminally charged. It is usually not possible, or desirable, to shield them from the legal system, although patients and family members may very much wish you to do so.

When patients who have not been charged request treatment, there may be a duty to report them to children's protective service under state statute, and there may be a duty to protect a potential victim if one can be identified (see Chapter 6). Ordinarily, outpatient treatment is preferable to inpatient treatment for these problems.

Sexual Dysfunction

Male erectile disorder (impotence) and premature ejaculation are the most frequent dysfunctions that lead to emergency psychiatric visits. Although these disorders, when they have had a recent acute onset, have an excellent prognosis with appropriate treatment (Kaplan 1974), either can lead to acute distress and even to suicidal behavior. Suicidal behavior may be particularly common among patients with acute erectile failure while intoxicated.

Impotence of acute onset, such as is likely to present as an emergency, is usually related to substance abuse or to nonorganic causes (Spark et al. 1980). Outpatient referral is generally most appropriate, accompanied by appropriate optimism. If a patient is intoxicated and acutely upset about erectile failure, it is often best, if possible, to allow the patient to sober up before release.

DISSOCIATIVE DISORDERS

Dissociative disorders are a fairly rare but dramatic cause for psychiatric emergency visits.

Psychogenic Amnesia

A simple system for categorizing amnesia distinguishes between discrete, time-limited amnesia and persistent memory impairment and between organic and functional amnesia. Table 20-2 lists differential diagnoses of each type of amnesia. Kopelman (1987) noted that "in both discrete and persistent amnesia the differentiation of psychogenic from organic causation can be surprisingly difficult" (pp. 428–429). In the discrete, time-limited type, loss of personal identity suggests a psychogenic cause because it is rare in organic amnesia, except in the final stages of dementia. Unimpaired ability to learn new material also suggests a psychogenic etiology, as does onset at a time of acute stress, depression, or anxiety. In the persistent type, the factors noted in Chapter 12 as distinguishing between dementia and pseudodementia need to be explored.

Fugue

Psychogenic fugue is characterized by sudden, unexpected travel away from home or work with inability to recall one's past, accompanied by assumption of a new identity, complete or partial (DSM-III-R [American Psychiatric Association 1987]). The episode usually resolves in a matter of days, but may go on for years. These patients most often seek help upon resolution of the fugue state, having been left with a residual memory gap. Patients may, at times, go into a fugue state when suicidal and again be suicidal upon emerging from it (Kopelman 1987).

In a study of 30 patients seen in the Cincinnati Psychiatric Emergency Service, who presented unwilling or unable to give their name, we found that, interestingly enough, most appeared not to be suffering from amnesia (Parks et al., in press). The most common causes were psychosis with suspiciousness or substance abuse with uncooperativeness. Emergency service staff were able to identify, by name, 22 of the 30 patients after observation for between 1 and 12 hours. Within that time, patients either "gave in" and gave their name or else were identified by

Table 20-2. Differential diagnosis of amnestic states

Etiology	Discrete episode	Persistent impairment
Organic	Toxic confusional state Head injury Epilepsy Sedative-hypnotic "blackout" Hypoglycemia Post–electroconvulsive therapy	Drug toxicity Alcohol amnestic disorder Dementia, global
Psychogenic	Fugue states Psychogenic amnesia Multiple personality disorder Situation specific (e.g., for an offense) Factitious Malingering Psychosis	Pseudodementia Factitious Malingering Psychosis

Source. Adapted from Kopelman 1987.

possessions or through contacts with missing-persons agencies. About two-thirds of patients who presented this way were hospitalized, as opposed to one-third of all patients seen on the service. None of these patients required amobarbital interviews for diagnosis, but suspected psychogenic amnesia is one of the indications for this procedure. (See Chapter 18 for method of conducting an amobarbital interview.)

Multiple personality disorder, factitious disorders, and malingering, all discussed below, may also give rise to "memory gaps."

Multiple Personality Disorder

Multiple personality disorder is a disorder characterized by the existence within a person of at least two distinct personalities that recurrently take full control of the person's behavior (DSM-III-R). In few disorders do the estimates of prevalence vary so widely. Kluft (1987) stated that "one view is that the condition is rare to non-existent and that the apparent exponential increase in its reportage reflects iatrogenesis, cultural factors, loose diagnostic criteria, the personal agendas of a few individuals, and the efforts of misguided patients who search out clinicians who will sanction the diagnosis" (p. 364). Other researchers have estimated prevalences of 10% or above among inpatient and outpatient psychiatric populations (Bliss and Jeppsen 1985). Series of successfully treated multiple personality disorders have been reported (Kluft 1984), as well as series of patients who have gone untreated and remained unimproved (Kluft 1985a).

A key element in this debate is the extent to which searching for multiple personalities may tend to induce them. Some researchers believe that apparent multiple personalities can be induced in normal individuals by means of hypnosis (Kampman 1976). Others believe that they have demonstrated important differences between such hypnotically induced "multiples" and the spontaneously occurring variety (Kluft 1985b).

We have been impressed that few patients requesting emergency psychiatric evaluation and treatment spontaneously report multiple personalities. The few who do spontaneously report multiple personalities tend to be in treatment already with one of the clinicians in the community who treat a lot of patients as multiple personality disorder. On the other hand, we see a lot of patients with the sort of history of childhood physical and sexual abuse frequently reported among patients with multiple personality disorder (Putnam et al. 1986), and many of these patients give the impression of having a capacity to dissociate.

Without necessarily taking a position in the debate on the prevalence of multiple personality disorders, we would recommend against vigorously searching for "multiples" in the psychiatric emergency setting. This is consistent with the general policy of not opening up areas in the emergency setting that cannot be closed up in that setting. We would recommend outpatient referrals for the potential multiple personality disorders noted above, leaving a decision about the type of treatment to the outpatient therapists. If patients spontaneously exhibit or mention multiple personalities, we recommend referral to someone who is interested in treating them, assuming they are not already in treatment with such a person.

IMPULSE CONTROL DISORDERS

So-called intermittent explosive disorder is highlighted as a controversial issue in Chapter 11. Patients with kleptomania or pathological gambling occasionally present to psychiatric emergency services—often when they are starting to get into trouble with the law. Again, they should not be shielded from the consequences of their actions, but recent studies suggest that with appropriate treatment (which may include inpatient care and Gamblers Anonymous) there is reason for optimism about recovery (Taber et al. 1987).

Pyromania, as diagnosed in DSM-III-R, is rare in psychiatric emergency populations, but fire setting is common. Most fire setting by adult psychiatric patients is associated with schizophrenia, affective disorders, personality disorders, alcohol abuse, or mental retardation—additional diagnoses that usually fulfill exclusion criteria for a DSM-III-R diagnosis of pyromania (Geller 1987). Residential placement of such individuals is, understandably, difficult. Long-term hospitalization with a psychosocial rehabilitation focus may be indicated with the goal of teaching less destructive communication techniques.

FACTITIOUS DISORDERS

These conditions are frequently considered in the differential diagnoses of various presentations and are thus alluded to in various chapters of this book.

Factitious Disorder With Physical Symptoms (Munchausen Syndrome)

If emergency medicine physicians detect intentional production or feigning of a medical disorder, they are likely to refer the patient for mental health evaluation. Ordinarily, the patient will get angry and refuse to be seen by the psychiatrist. Such patients, when they do agree to be seen, are usually diagnosed as borderline (Nadelson 1979) or other personality disorder (Reich and Gottfried 1983). Confrontation of the dissimulation often leads to its cessation at least for that episode, but results of psychotherapeutic attempts have been almost uniformly negative. The most important consultative interventions involve helping emergency room staff to deal with their anger and to avoid cynicism.

Factitious Disorder With Psychological Symptoms and Malingering

These conditions are supposed to differ from each other in terms of the motivation of the patient. The patient with factitious disorder is supposed to be motivated by "a psychological need to assume the sick role, as evidenced by the absence of external incentive for the behavior, such as economic gain, better care, or physical well-being" (DSM-III-R, p. 319), whereas the malingerer is motivated by such external incentives. Pending legal charges, antisocial personality, or pending compensation claims may suggest the possibility of malingering, and lack of cooperation with the examination may also suggest that diagnosis. Some cases may be difficult to classify one way or the other. Chapter 16 suggests some methods for distinguishing true from factitious or malingered psychosis. Chapter 27 suggests some approaches to the patient who desires but does not require hospitalization. Care of patients who demand hospitalization for suicide threats is discussed in Chapter 8.

MARITAL CONFLICT

Marital conflicts frequently precipitate psychiatric emergency visits but are less frequently the chief complaint of either spouse. Most frequently, one spouse will have been designated as the patient after having developed symptoms. As discussed in Chapter 1, the spouse initially identified as the patient is not always the one needing help most immediately.

Times of acute marital conflict and particularly the threat of divorce or separation are a major stress for anyone. Such stresses can elicit suicide attempts or other maladaptive behavior from ordinarily well-functioning people. Such patients often benefit dramatically from a crisis intervention approach such as outlined in Chapter 4 or from referral to outpatient marital or individual therapy. Because the couple is such an important part of every married person's life, it is important to assess the strengths and weaknesses of the marriage in every psychiatric emergency case.

Spouse Abuse

A particularly important problem to search for actively is physical abuse of a spouse. Spouse abuse tends to be underrecognized by physicians and can give rise to a wide variety of symptoms in the victimized spouse (Hilberman 1980). Most cities in the United States now have shelters for abused women and children where they can be safe and can receive help in getting out of, or making a change in, the abusive relationship. Mental health referrals may be appropriate for patients who have developed a major depressive disorder secondary to ongoing physical abuse, but care must be taken that the patient does not come to regard herself as "the sick one" in the relationship.

REFERENCES

American Psychiatric Association: Diagnostic and Statistical Manual of Mental Disorders, 3rd Edition, Revised. Washington, DC, American Psychiatric Association, 1987

Bliss EL, Jeppsen EA: Prevalence of multiple personality among inpatients and outpatients. Am J Psychiatry 142:250–251, 1985

Geller JL: Firesetting in the adult psychiatric population. Hosp Community Psychiatry 38:501–506, 1987

Heinrichs DW, Carpenter WT: Prospective study of prodromal symptoms in schizophrenic relapse. Am J Psychiatry 142:371–373, 1985

Herzog DB: Are anorexic and bulimic patients depressed? Am J Psychiatry 141:1594–1597, 1984

Herzog DB: Advances in Psychiatry: Focus on Eating Disorders. New York, Park Row Publishers, 1987

Hilberman E: Overview: the "wife-beater's wife" reconsidered. Am J Psychiatry 137:1336–1347, 1980

Jenike MA: Insomnia: nonpharmacologic treatments. Topics in Geriatrics 3:25–28, 1985

Kampman R: Hypnotically induced multiple personality. Int J Clin Exp Hypn 24:215–227, 1976

Kaplan HS: The New Sex Therapy: Active Treatment of Dysfunction. New York, Brunner/Mazel, 1974

Kluft RP: Treatment of multiple personality disorder: a study of 33 cases. Psychiatr Clin North Am 7:9–29, 1984

Kluft RP: The natural history of multiple personality disorder, in Childhood Antecedents of Multiple Personality. Edited by Kluft RP. Washington, DC, American Psychiatric Press, 1985a

Kluft RP: Using hypnotic inquiry protocols to monitor treatment progress and stability in multiple personality. Am J Clin Hypn 28:63–75, 1985b

Kluft RP: An update on multiple personality disorder. Hosp Community Psychiatry 38:363–373, 1987

Kopelman MD: Amnesia: organic and psychogenic. Br J Psychiatry 150:428–442, 1987

Miles LE, Dement WC: Sleep and aging. Sleep 3:191–220, 1980

Nadelson T: The Munchausen spectrum: borderline character features. Gen Hosp Psychiatry 1:11–17, 1979

Parks J, Hillard JR, Gillig P: John and Jane Doe in the psychiatric emergency service. Psychiatr Q (in press)

Pope HG, Hudson JI, Yurgelun-Todd D: Anorexia nervosa and bulimia among 300 suburban women shoppers. Am J Psychiatry 141:292–294, 1984

Pope HG, Champoux RF, Hudson JI: Eating disorder and socioeconomic class: anorexia nervosa and bulimia in nine communities. J Nerv Ment Dis 175:620–623, 1987

Putnam FW, Guroff JJ, Silverman EK, et al: The clinical phenomenology of multiple personality disorder: review of 100 recent cases. J Clin Psychiatry 47:285–293, 1986

Reich P, Gottfried LA: Factitious disorders in a teaching hospital. Ann Intern Med 99:240–247, 1983

Spark RF, White RA, Connolly PB: Impotence is not always psychogenic. JAMA 243:750–755, 1980

Taber JI, McCormick RA, Russo AM, et al: Follow-up of pathological gamblers after treatment. Am J Psychiatry 144:757–761, 1987

PART III

SPECIAL POPULATIONS

Chapter 21

Children and Adolescents

M. Slomowitz, M.D.

Assessment and treatment of children and adolescents with emergency psychiatric needs present particular challenges. For the purposes of this chapter, children will be referred to as persons younger than age 13, adolescents as ages 13–21. Children and adolescents usually present in a clinical setting with a preponderance of behavior problems, rather than with intrapsychic distress. More often than their adult counterparts, they will be brought by a caretaker. The behaviors they manifest may be problematic for their families, but the patients themselves may not perceive the behaviors to be problems. The behavior disturbances may include aggressiveness, school problems, familial disruptiveness, running away, and threats or acts of self-destruction.

Unlike adults, many of whom present with acute exacerbation of symptoms of a preexisting and recognizable psychotic or affective illness, children and adolescents will most likely not have had such previous diagnoses of major mental disorders. For children and adolescents, the emergency visit may be their first experience with the mental health system. In addition, the symptoms bringing them to attention will often not fit easily into a DSM-III-R (American Psychiatric Association 1987) diagnostic category.

An additional difference between the two groups is the degree of relative autonomous functioning. Children and adolescents are truly dependent on adults for basic needs to an extent that most adults are not.

Their behavior must be seen in the context of a larger family system, and the emergency represents a family in crisis. There is an additional problem of defining who is the patient needing treatment: the child or the parent, or both.

Development issues, such as levels of cognitive, psychological, social, physical, and biological development, must also be taken into account when dealing with children and adolescents. These issues make diagnosis and treatment planning more complicated. Development does not progress uniformly for each individual. There may be tremendous variability between level of development in different areas for a given child or adolescent and between different children and adolescents of the same age.

Few communities have a large enough volume of child and adolescent emergencies to justify a full-time child emergency specialist, even if such a person were available. Furthermore, children and adolescents generally make up only a small percentage of all psychiatric emergencies seen by a given service. For this reason, services sometimes have a tendency to deal with such patients as though they were "small adults."

PRESENTING PROBLEMS: CHILDREN

There are only a relatively small number of problems that commonly lead to emergency psychiatric evaluation of children. The most important of these are school phobia, aggression, depression, suicidal behavior, and physical or sexual abuse.

School Phobia

A sudden onset of anxiety in relation to beginning grade school deserves immediate attention. Although the condition is called a school phobia, the child is not fearful of the school situation per se, but experiences distress on being away from caretakers, often with concerns that they might die or leave when he or she is not home. These children may have had no previous problems interpersonally or behaviorally. Using DSM-III-R diagnostic categorization, they may have a separation anxiety disorder. What is required in the emergency setting is an explanation of the child's fear and a behavior plan to quickly reintegrate the child into the classroom. Such a plan might include having an adult take the child to school and having family members telephone the child at school every day. Psychotherapeutic interventions to help the parents with their apprehensions about the child might be helpful. If the emergency service cannot provide this, then immediate referral to an outpatient psychiatric clinic is indicated. Hospitalization is usually contraindicated.

Aggression

Children may present with aggressive or hyperkinetic behavior. The evaluation of these children requires assessment of the specific problematic behaviors and the context. Questions to ask would include 1) Under what circumstances does the behavior occur at school, at home, or both? 2) How long-standing is the behavior? 3) Have there been recent events within the family that may have an influence on the behavior? 4) What is of immediate concern to both child and family? 5) Is the child's behavior disturbing to himself or herself, to his or her family, or both? 6) To what degree is the behavior impulsive? Some of these children will have an undiagnosed attention-deficit disorder and/or undiagnosed learning disorders contributing to behavior problems at school. Parental discord (e.g., separation, divorce, arguments) may be affecting the child's sense of stability in the world, leading to aggression. Families in which violence is an acceptable behavior may find children growing up with aggressive behavior. The possibility of coexisting mood disorders should be considered in all children presenting with a behavior disorder.

Occasionally, an aggressive child's reality testing may be poor. Although it is unusual for a child to be psychotic, psychosis must be considered as one possible reason for change in behavior. If the behavior is drastically different, disorganized, and confused, then a toxic ingestion must be considered. A complete child psychiatric evaluation including educational and neuropsychological testing and consultation with the school cannot be done during an emergency assessment. Such extensive evaluations and treatment recommendations can be done in outpatient facilities, assuming the parents feel they can help the child reasonably manage the behavior. If the parents do not feel they can contain the behavior, then hospitalization should be considered.

Depression and Suicide

Children can suffer from a depression similar to adults (Puig-Antich 1982). DSM-III-R diagnostic categories on mood disorder are applicable to children. The prevalence of major depressive disorders in 9-year-old children has been reported to be 1.8% (Kashani et al. 1983).

Children can also be at risk for suicide. Suicidal children will appear sad and depressed, will feel hopeless, and will talk about wanting to die when explicitly asked. It is rare for prepubescent children and children under age 15 to commit suicide (Shaffer and Fisher 1981), but suicidal behavior even in preschool children has been documented (Rosenthal and Rosenthal 1984).

Despite the relatively few suicides in children, suicidal intent in a child must be taken seriously. Particularly for children under age 6, death may not be recognized as final, or inevitable. They may continue some of the magical thinking of preschool years, believing they will wake up. The intent to die may be a plea to get attention from a parent, a revengeful desire for their hurts, or a wish to be with someone they loved who has died.

The emergency-setting intervention will depend on the child's developmental level, on the capacity to delay impulsive behavior, and on the ability of the parents to respond adequately and sufficiently to the child. Many suicidal children suffer from affective disorders, but some may become suicidal impulsively in response to anger or frustration (Pfeffer 1981). Should the child be seen as at risk of imminent suicide, hospitalization is necessary.

Physical or Sexual Abuse

If a child presents with evidence of being battered or sexually abused, state law ordinarily mandates that the psychiatrist contact the appropriate protective services. Hospitalization is indicated if there is risk of further harm to the child or if there is overwhelming immediate psychological distress experienced by the child. Counseling for the child and family about the acute trauma can be offered in the emergency setting. There is an excellent chapter on this subject in the *Manual of Clinical Child Psychiatry* (Sauzier and Mitkus 1986).

PRESENTING PROBLEMS: ADOLESCENTS

As with children, adolescents present to emergency settings with a relatively small number of chief complaints. Their problems tend to be more complex, however, due to their relatively older age and more complex social environment. Presenting problems include depression and suicide, aggression, running away, psychosis, substance abuse, and acute stress reactions. A significant number of adolescent patients seen as emergencies will have had some kind of inpatient or outpatient treatment and may constitute a prechronic category of patients.

Depression and Suicide

For adolescents, suicidal thoughts or behaviors are a major finding in psychiatric emergency settings. In a recent study, 40% of adolescents who presented to a general hospital psychiatric emergency service had a suicidal act or threat as their chief complaint (Hillard et al. 1987). A recent rise in teen suicides has been well documented (Brent et al. 1988). There are a variety of forms in which suicide-related problems may present, including threat of suicide, impulsive ingestion of a few pills, or planned ingestion of a large number of toxic agents. Often these patients may take an overdose in a state of anger or rage, to get back at someone, and may have little wish to die.

Adolescents who express suicide run the gamut of psychiatric disorders. The relationship between psychiatric disorder and suicide among adolescent patients is less clear-cut than among adult patients. However, adolescents with bipolar affective disorder or affective disorder with substance abuse are at particularly high risk for completed suicide (Brent et al. 1988). An evaluation of such an adolescent would require assessing the suicide attempt itself. The nature and circumstances of intent (e.g., planned or impulsive), perceived lethality, precipitant of attempt, motivation, and degree of hopelessness need to be ascertained. Changes in the adolescent's current life situation need to be addressed, both with the individual and the family. Changes in school performance, boyfriend or girlfriend relationships, or familial functioning or events that caused a drop in self-esteem must be looked for. Also, it is important to consider whether the suicide act or threat was propelled by intoxication with substances. The attitude of the family toward the threat or act must be assessed. A lack of concern for, or anger at, the adolescent would be of concern. A thorough assessment of the adolescent's mental status is indicated, to assess presence and extent of poor impulse control or disorganized thinking.

The decision to hospitalize an adolescent should take into account all of the above factors. The balance between risk factors for suicide and available social support determines the need for hospitalization for adolescents, as it does for adults. The impulsiveness of adolescents probably suggests a lower "threshold" for hospitalization for them than for older patients.

Aggression

Aggressive acts or threats are often crises that bring an adolescent and family for emergency interventions. A fight with peers, siblings, or parents may be the precipitant for seeking psychiatric treatment, as may a threat of serious harm to other adolescents or adults. On interview of the adolescent and family, the psychiatrist will need to assess the degree of impulsivity and anger in determining the most appropriate intervention.

The evaluation of this adolescent will address the precipitant to the aggressive act or threat, history of previous aggression, presence of intoxication at any time with aggressive acts, and other known use of substances. The psychiatrist will want to ask if there has been a change in overall behavior or functioning, and if this particular outburst is a new phenomenon or one of a series. If not new, the patient's family should be asked how this incident is different from past incidents and why the emergency setting was used at this time. The presence of a specific target for threats of harm must be elucidated because there may be a duty to warn the intended victims. The psychiatrist must distinguish between a disorganized feeling of intense anger and/or rage leading to the act and a thoughtfully planned act. One should consider whether there has been an episode resulting in an acute humiliation with a corresponding drop in self-esteem that makes the adolescent more vulnerable to feelings of rage and loss of control. Ascertaining acceptability of violence in the family or community is also helpful.

Adolescents who show patterns of aggressive behavior often have other symptoms of dysfunction: they may have school problems or attention-deficit or learning disorders, or they may come from families that are themselves disorganized, making it less likely that the family structure can safely protect the adolescent. Many of these adolescents may have psychotic experiences: although on mental status examination they may show no formal impairments in perception or thought process, they may describe episodes prior to the aggressive act in which they suddenly developed hallucinations in response to a rage. The reality testing may be quite poor, i.e., grandiose and dangerous, and fantasies may occur, often as an attempt to bolster a poor self-esteem.

The critical issue in deciding whether to hospitalize a violent adolescent is whether the aggressive impulses are under control by the adolescent. If there is serious doubt, the patient needs to be either hospitalized or incarcerated. If an adolescent has charges pending, incarceration is *usually* preferable to hospitalization unless there are specific indications for inpatient treatment. Such indications would include evidence of psychosis or affective disorder, recent onset of aggression, or need for further diagnostic evaluation. If an adolescent is returned to a police agency, recommendations (e.g., suicide precautions) should be made to the agency. Either in the inpatient unit or in the outpatient treatment, the etiology of contributing factors can be evaluated and appropriate treatments prescribed.

Should such an adolescent present to an emergency service in an acutely agitated state for which the etiology is not known, the immediate concern will be to provide for the patient's safety. This may mean restraints and medication to calm the patient, with hospitalization proceeding from there.

Running Away

The emergency psychiatrist may also be asked to see an adolescent with running away as the presenting problem. Interviewing the adolescent and family is essential to determine both the cause of the behavior and associated symptoms. Repeated running away is often symptomatic of a severely disturbed relationship between the adolescent and the family. The running away may occur as a final alternative to a bleak environment or as part of an oppositional stance in a maladaptive attempt to psychologically separate from parents. Aspects to question the adolescent about are 1) the precipitant to the actual runaway event; 2) degree of impulsivity or planning; 3) other infractions of family or societal rules, i.e., fighting, truancy, legal problems; 4) parental response to adolescent violation of family norms, e.g., overly rigid or permissive; and 5) presence of violence or abuse in the family. Usually there is a constellation of behavior problems associated with running away. The adolescent may also have an associated mood or substance use disorder. A combination of individual and family treatment on an outpatient basis is usually the initial treatment recommendation. If, however, such treatment has been attempted and has not been seen as useful, or if there is a suspected coexisting psychiatric disorder contributing to the running away, one would strongly consider using the hospital as the treatment choice.

A comment should be made about adolescents who chronically run away. Often these adolescents repeatedly run away because of intolerable living situations. They are sometimes referred to as "throw-away" children, as they are unwanted. Many of these adolescents become involved in drug use and prostitution, with very dismal outcomes (Hartman et al. 1987).

Psychosis

Psychosis is a relatively unusual presentation of adolescents in an emergency setting. Clearly, one would immediately want to ascertain whether the psychosis was of acute onset with possible organic etiology, or the result of a previously unrecognized gradual deterioration. With an acute onset, drug ingestion must be considered. These adolescents may appear acutely agitated with auditory, visual, and/or tactile hallucinations, disorientation, and confused thinking. In addition to drug ingestions as an etiology in an organically induced psychosis, one must also consider neurologic, metabolic, infectious, oncologic, and immunologic disorders. A toxic screen may be useful in determining the agents of a drug ingestion. The other possible etiologies may take longer to evaluate. In such a patient, hospitalization would be indicated to obtain a definitive diagnosis and to initiate treatment in a safe environment. Psychopharmacologic agents may be necessary in the emergency setting should the patient be acutely agitated. Medication should be prescribed generally following the guidelines established for adult patients, with the caveat that adolescents are particularly sensitive to developing extrapyramidal symptoms from neuroleptics, and routine use of an antiparkinsonian medication with the neuroleptic to prevent the side effects is suggested.

Adolescents may have psychotic symptoms due to a major mental disorder such as schizophrenia or bipolar affective disorder. These patients will usually have a less dramatic and acute onset. Often, there is a progressive worsening of school performance with isolation from family or friends. These patients may initially come to the emergency service after an academic or social failure, presenting with suicidal ideation or anxiety. Psychotic symptoms may not be mentioned spontaneously. Making a differential diagnosis of schizophrenia or bipolar affective disorder is difficult in this population, as the symptoms overlap. Hospitalization of newly psychotic adolescents is usually indicated because of the level of emotional distress and the severity of the confused thinking. Some adolescents may have a prepsychotic disorder. Although they may exhibit no formal thought disorder or presence of hallucinations, they may still show some eccentricities of thought and behavior. These are the patients who may fall into schizotypal personality disorder. Their reality testing may be shaky at best, with deterioration under stress. Hospitalization is usually indicated for first psychotic episodes and in cases in which adolescents' symptoms are sufficiently disturbing to themselves and their family, and seriously disrupt their function at home or school.

Substance Abuse

Substance use is a frequent phenomenon among adolescents with or without psychiatric disorders. As previously pointed out, psychiatric disorders often present with behavioral symptoms such as truancy, running away, school problems, and aggression. The psychiatrist must ask about use of alcohol, marijuana, and other illicit drugs in a straightforward manner, and about the disrupting effect of these substances in the individual's life. A family history of substance abuse should raise one's suspicion. It may be very difficult to ascertain if the substance abuse is a primary or secondary problem, or whether there are two or more problems coexisting. Addressing the seriousness of this potential problem with the adolescent and family is important in the emergency setting.

If an adolescent is heavily abusing substances, substance abuse is most often the primary problem, and the adolescent should be referred for substance abuse treatment before mental health treatment. Adolescent impulsiveness and peer presence often make inpatient substance abuse treatment preferable to outpatient. Inpatient programs geared specifically toward adolescents are usually preferable to programs geared primarily toward adults.

Acute Stress Reactions

Adolescents and their families may come to an emergency setting with an acute problem, but may have otherwise stable and uneventful lives. A death of a friend with acute grief, a breakup with a boyfriend or girlfriend with a drop in self-esteem, and other losses that may be experienced as overwhelmingly painful may be the impetus for a family to bring an adolescent to emergency attention. A trauma for the entire family may also bring them. At these times, attention to the nature of the loss and the trauma and helping the individual and family use their strengths can be very effective at ameliorating psychological distress. Referral to outpatient care can be made if there is not adequate resolution of symptoms.

COLLEGE STUDENTS

Emergency problems of college students often have to do with negotiating the developmental tasks between late adolescence and early adulthood. They may present with acute anxiety related to school or grades, or depression related to change in status in college or loss of significant relationships. Often away from home for the first time, they struggle to be independent and develop a new life for themselves, while still feeling frightened. The psychiatrist can be very helpful in clarifying for the student the nature of the distress and arranging for outpatient treatment, if warranted.

College students have special life-styles. Often living in dormitories, they must contend with roommates and peer pressure. Student advisors, if present, are often surrogate parents. Students are confronted with academic and social pressures. Experimentation with drugs or sex is common. On their own for perhaps the first time, they lack the experience to sort psychological upset from serious disturbance. A student may present to an emergency room experiencing subjective distress over a matter that may seem trivial to the psychiatrist. It is important to keep in mind that the college student's developmental level may make a problem (e.g., failing a test or breaking up with a girlfriend or boyfriend) more traumatic than it might be to an older person. The emergency room takes on the role of mother to these students, offering reassurance. Given the vicissitudes of peer pressure among students and the desire to be attractive, young women are vulnerable to developing bulimic symptoms. Also, a major mental disorder can arise during this phase of life. A first psychotic episode may occur while a college student.

TREATMENT CONSIDERATIONS

Biologic Therapies

The use of biologic therapies in children and adolescents requires judiciousness and care. The complexities of diagnosis, the developmental considerations, and the possibilities of substance use complicating the picture make it more difficult to prescribe based on known clinical disorders. Antidepressants, neuroleptics, and lithium are being used in children and adolescents for disorders that are counterparts to adult disorders in inpatient and outpatient settings.

Hospitalization

One of the major functions of a psychiatric emergency service is triage. The decision to hospitalize children and adolescents should not be taken lightly.

Despite these cautions, there are times when hospitalization is the treatment of choice. Children and adolescents will require hospitalization should they lack sufficient internal and/or external control to maintain their safety. In a recent study at one emergency setting, the factors most strongly associated with hospitalization of adolescents were suicidal tendencies, history of recent physical abuse, and a primary diagnosis of schizophrenia (Hillard et al. 1988). Other uses of hospitalization can be to reevaluate treatment strategy after a period of unsuccessful outpatient treatment and to obtain a thorough diagnostic assessment that would not otherwise be possible in an outpatient setting.

The meaning of hospitalization for children and adolescents is complex. Particularly for younger children, the staff of the hospital comes to be family for the time they are away from home. For adolescents, staff may be "as if" parents, but are, foremost, adults with whom to negotiate. For many, being in the hospital will be a relief, as the structure of the hospital can provide the containment the child or adolescent needs. There can be a different perceived meaning of hospitalization—i.e., that of the hospital as a punishment for their "bad" behavior, as a coercive and punitive measure over which they have no control. The experience of adolescents in the emergency setting can influence how they may view hospitalization. Not taking patients' feelings into account and gathering data primarily from parents will contribute to patients' sense of powerlessness in the process. Their wish for hospitalization because of their own recognition of their impulsivity will make hospitalization a much more attractive process, if it is necessary.

Often hospitalization is picked as the most reasonable solution for a problem because of a lack of suitable alternatives. Many communities offer limited outpatient care. Day programs are not common, and residential facilities tend to have long waiting lists. Because of the lack of intermediary way stations, hospitalization becomes the site of best treatment in the community.

LEGAL CONSIDERATIONS

The legal considerations in the emergency psychiatric treatment of children and adolescents center on the dependent nature and the duty by parents and society to protect. Each state has its own set of laws addressing the relationship of child or adolescent and guardian and the medical and mental health systems, and practitioners need to know the laws of their own state. The general considerations have to do with informed consent for treatment in the emergency setting, limits of confidentiality, the process of voluntarily or involuntarily hospitalizing a child or adolescent, and the emancipation of minors.

Children and adolescents are not capable of giving informed consent for treatment, as this, by definition, is a property of adults. They can, however, agree to treatment, or assent. Most states allow adolescents to obtain medical care in very narrow areas without parental consent, e.g., treatment for sexually transmitted diseases or receiving birth control. The law therefore recognizes that older adolescents have the capacity to make particular decisions about themselves in circumscribed areas. The age varies, but usually 16 is recognized as the age when adolescents can take more responsibility for themselves. In a true emergency situation, permission is not required to pursue treatment. Should an adolescent present to the emergency room alone, the psychiatrist can ask the adolescent for permission to contact the guardian for permission to treat. Without parental consent, the psychiatrist can evaluate, but not provide treatment, unless the situation is truly an emergency (see Chapter 6).

Confidentiality between patient and physician is another area to discuss. There are clear limits on confidentiality, i.e., there is the obligation to report physical or sexual abuse, or to warn an intended victim of potential harm. There is always a question of how much should the therapist tell the parents of the adolescent's disclosures.

A useful way of preventing "secrets" from emerging is to meet initially with all family members and address the visit as a crisis affecting each of them. If one person feels threatened by harm from another for revealing particular information, the psychiatrist will need to act as this person's advocate in obtaining safety.

The term *emancipated minor* refers to the recognition by the law that these persons fulfill the requirements for being an adult. Usually, the adolescent must be living away from parents, be self-supporting, and have completed legal documentation. Such teenagers have the rights and obligations of adults and need to be treated accordingly.

References

American Psychiatric Association: Diagnostic and Statistical Manual of Mental Disorders, 3rd Edition, Revised. Washington, DC, American Psychiatric Association, 1987

Brent DA, Perper JA, Goldstein CE, et al: Risk factors for adolescent suicide. Arch Gen Psychiatry 45:581–588, 1988

Hartman CR, Burgess AW, McCormack A: Pathways and cycles of runaways: a model for understanding repetitive runaway behavior. Hosp Community Psychiatry 38:292–299, 1987

Hillard JR, Slomowitz M, Levi LS: A retrospective study of adolescents' visits to a general hospital psychiatric emergency service. Am J Psychiatry 144:432–436, 1987

Hillard RJ, Slomowitz M, Deddens J: Emergency psychiatric hospitalization of adolescents: a comparison of admissions determinants for adolescent vs. adult patients. Am J Psychiatry 145:1416–1419, 1988

Kashani J, McGee RO, Clarkson SE, et al: Depression in a sample of 9-year old children. Arch Gen Psychiatry 40:1217–1223, 1983

Pfeffer CR: Suicidal behavior of children: a review with implications for research and practice. Am J Psychiatry 138:154–159, 1981

Puig-Antich J: Major depression and conduct disorder in prepuberty. J Am Acad Child Psychiatry 2:118–128, 1982

Rosenthal PA, Rosenthal S: Suicidal behavior by preschool children. Am J Psychiatry 141:520–525, 1984

Sauzier M, Mitkus C: Emergencies II: sexual abuse and rape in childhood, in Manual of Clinical Child Psychiatry. Edited by Robson KS. Washington, DC, American Psychiatric Press, 1986, pp 213–240

Shaffer D, Fisher P: The epidemiology of suicide in children and young adolescents. J Am Acad Child Psychiatry 20:545–565, 1981

Chapter 22

Mentally Retarded Patients

G.A. Barker, M.D.

Mentally retarded persons represent approximately 1% of our population. Furthermore, "the prevalence of other mental disorders is at least three or four times greater among people with mental retardation than in the general population" (DSM-III-R, American Psychiatric Association 1987, p. 29). These patients frequently present to emergency psychiatric centers after staff or family notice a change in functioning or observe an unacceptable behavior. The deinstitutionalization of mentally retarded patients has placed those unable to live independently in small community residential settings and has encouraged the use of mainstream community resources for treatment. The literature suggests, however, that, in general, most mentally retarded people are not receiving the ongoing psychiatric services that they need (West and Richardson 1981). Emergency services provide a very important support to staff and patients and their families.

BASIC CHARACTERISTICS OF PERSONS WITH MENTAL RETARDATION

According to DSM-III-R, a person is considered to be mentally retarded if, before the age of 18, they are found to have an IQ of 70 or below and demonstrate impairments in adaptive functioning. These impairments

299

result in the inability of the person to meet expected cultural standards in such areas as social skills, daily living skills, independence, responsibility, and self-sufficiency.

Mental retardation is further subclassified, by IQ and associated features, as either mild, moderate, severe, profound, or unspecified.

Mild Mental Retardation

People in this group represent 75–85% of the mentally retarded population. They have an IQ in the 50–55 to 70 range and were formerly classified as educable. They generally are able to acquire academic skills up to the sixth grade level and can acquire sufficient vocational skills to allow employment and independent or loosely supervised community living. In a mainstream society, they are at risk for decreased self-esteem as they compare themselves to their brighter peers. "Socioeconomic, nutritional and environmental, and cultural factors" likely contribute to the etiology (Valente 1989, p. 179). It should be noted that they are generally an underserved group, even by the mental retardation system.

Moderate Mental Retardation

People in this group have an IQ in the 35–40 to 50–55 range and are generally verbal. Formerly classified as "trainable," this group constitutes 10% of the mentally retarded population. They are generally able to achieve a second grade academic level and can contribute to their own support by doing supervised skilled and semiskilled work. They usually live in supervised group homes in the community or with family.

Severe Mental Retardation

Characterized by an IQ from 20–25 to 35–40, this form of mental retardation is usually diagnosed in the preschool period by delayed motor development and the failure to talk. With training, these individuals may learn to talk and to acquire the skills necessary to maintain their own personal hygiene. In the adult years, they generally live in highly supervised group homes or nursing homes, or with their families. The gross central nervous system impairment associated with severe mental retardation is evident in the high frequency of multiple handicaps. These include special sensory impairments and seizure disorders.

Profound Mental Retardation

These are individuals with an IQ below 20–25. With highly individualized training and continuous care, these people may optimize limited ability to communicate, move, and do their own self-care. Most are involved in a day program and live in highly supervised group homes or intermediate care facilities, or with their families.

Etiologically, mental retardation results from various factors that include heredity, alterations of embryonic development, complications of pregnancy or birth, physical disorders acquired in childhood, environmental influences, and mental disorders. In 30–40%, no clear etiology can be determined despite extensive evaluation. Males are affected 1.5:1 over females.

THE MENTAL RETARDATION SYSTEM

Services for mentally retarded persons are, in many states, administered by a different department than that for mental health services. In the mental retardation system, case managers for the moderately and severely retarded are assigned at the county level. They generally oversee the development of the habilitation plans and coordinate access to the services required for implementation. They can help to establish consent to treat by providing information as to how to contact the involved family member or state-appointed guardian. They coordinate housing in the least restrictive setting, usually a group home, and vocational services, usually a sheltered workshop. Family members and residential and workshop staff can usually provide good information concerning the patient's baseline level of functioning, recent changes, and possible precipitants to the emergency psychiatric presentation.

THE EMERGENCY EVALUATION

Stabilize the Patient

An effective evaluation of a mentally retarded person will require sufficient time for obtaining history from several sources and for performing adequate mental status and physical examinations. The patient must maintain control during this often lengthy period of time. The actions of the emergency staff should support the patient's ability to maintain control in the least restrictive manner possible. Effective interventions include

- Having the patient wait with a familiar person (family or staff)
- Regulating the emergency room environment so that it is both understandable and not overly stimulating
- Having frequent, consistent staff interactions with the patient
- Physically restraining the patient if he or she is not containable by other means

Establish Consent to Treat

It is important to establish consent for medical treatment at the beginning of the evaluation. If the patient has a guardian, he or she must be contacted to provide either written or verbal witnessed consent. This information can be obtained through the residential staff or case manager.

General Principles to Guide the Evaluation

Most requests for services are not initiated by mentally retarded persons themselves, but arise because of staff concerns about intolerable behaviors, observed decreases in functional abilities, or witnessed expressions of suicidal ideations. Essentially, evaluation of the mentally retarded person involves the same careful process required of all evaluations.

Develop an understanding of the chief complaint in the context of recent and baseline functioning.   Obtain a clear and precise description of the chief complaint and history of present illness by speaking with the person initiating the referral. Clearly establish the patient's functional baseline and any deviation from it that may have occurred. The chief complaint will indicate the symptom that needs to be addressed.

Clarify the treatment request.   Are staff requesting evaluation, intervention, or rescue? It is essential for the emergency staff to understand clearly the perspective of the care providers for several reasons. First, it is an assessment of the person's available community supports. Second, the request must be effectively addressed during the consultation. This will be most efficient if the request is clear from the onset. Consultations are only successful if they meet the needs of the consultees by granting the original request, or by involving the consultees in a process by which they can accept an option they had not considered.

Examples of the latter might include in-home consultation versus hospitalization, or medication reduction versus increase.

Examine the patient. Although some adaptations may need to be made in gathering the data, performing a mental status examination remains the organizing format for the psychiatric evaluation of the mentally retarded person. General principles of the mental status examination follow.

- The association of articulation deficits with mental retardation makes it essential that clinicians spend sufficient time adapting their own listening skills to the individual. In short, allow enough time for the mentally retarded person to effectively express his or her experience and request for help. Family members or others who know the patient can frequently be useful as "translators."

- Be concrete. Care must be taken to adapt vocabulary and concepts to the developmental level of the patient.

- Decreased attention span and concentration may make multiple, brief, 10- to 15-minute interviews more effective than one long session.

- Avoid yes-or-no questions. People can answer these without understanding and give the clinician an erroneous impression.

- Objects or tasks may be used to obtain responses if the verbal examination is unsatisfactory. For example, patients can be presented with a picture to discuss; their use of or reaction to a familiar object may further the examiner's understanding.

- If a patient is so profoundly impaired that speech is not present, then descriptions of arousal, general behavior, and desire for human contact may be all that can be determined (Sovner and Hurley 1983a).

- Be a thoughtful observer. Describe and document your observations rather than your impressions. Review the actual data from the patient examination when all information is available. In short, don't reach a premature diagnosis.

- The diagnostic criteria found in DSM-III-R apply to mentally retarded people just as they do to people of higher intellectual abilities. The task, then, is to recognize the familiar target symptoms in the history and mental status examination (Sovner and Hurley 1986b). This is easier in persons with mild and moderate mental retardation.

Severely and profoundly mentally retarded individuals can exhibit behavioral syndromes that are inadequately described by DSM-III-R.

The specifics of the mental status examination in the mentally retarded population include

- *General appearance and behavior.* Level of activity, interpersonal engagement, the presence or absence of abnormal mannerisms or postures, and facial expressions are especially essential in an examination that may be hampered by impaired communication skills.

- *Speech and thought processes.* Compared with baseline, has the rate or fluency of speech or thought production changed? Is thinking logical and coherent, or does it have the qualities of tangentiality or looseness? What is the thought content? It is critical to determine the change from baseline when someone has a history of previous impairment. Stress may cause the disruption of already impaired information processing, creating a transient thought disorder.

- *Mood and affect.* Subjective identification of mood may be difficult for some mentally retarded persons, but attempts to understand their self-experience are worthwhile. Affect can be observed for range, lability, and appropriateness. Inappropriate affect may have a different meaning in the mentally retarded population. For example, failure to comprehend the significance of a situation may lead to inappropriate smiling (Sovner and Hurley 1983b).

- *Evaluation of suicidal and homicidal ideation.* In verbal patients, this requires careful exploration. In a summary of the literature on the subject, Sovner and Hurley (1982b) reaffirm that "mentally retarded persons are capable of true suicidal behavior. Their motivations for such thoughts and actions are identical to those of their counterparts with normal intelligence" (p. 35). An attempt should be made to identify precipitants, especially emotional losses, and to gauge the level of hopelessness. Suicidal behavior should be distinguished from self-injurious behavior. The latter is not necessarily suicidal but may be the result of self-stimulatory behavior or an attempt to attract attention.

  An exploration of homicidal ideation should evaluate its presence, the amount of anger and impulsiveness, any expressed plan or intent, and the ability to utilize nonviolent alternatives when presented.

- *Assessing psychotic symptoms.* The diagnosis of psychosis is made by identifying the target symptoms of auditory hallucinations, delusions, ideas of reference, and thought disorder. It has been suggested that with impaired cognitive abilities, mentally retarded persons are more susceptible to illusions. In evaluating hallucinations, therefore, it is important to take the time to differentiate sensory misperceptions or misunderstandings from true hallucinatory experiences. If hallucinations are present, determine the prominence and behavioral effect. It is difficult to make this assessment in patients with an IQ less than 50, as these people have severely impaired abilities to think abstractly and to communicate effectively.

Visual, gustatory, and tactile hallucinations are generally associated with organic conditions. People with mental retardation are likely predisposed to these on the basis of preexisting central nervous system damage; the recent onset of these symptoms should, however, alert the clinician to a superimposed acute organic condition. Those patients with preexisting central nervous system impairment are at risk for superimposed delirium.

Persistent delusions indicate psychosis in mentally retarded patients, just as they do in patients of normal intelligence. The mentally retarded person may, however, appear transiently delusional in periods characterized by high anxiety, reflecting "stress-induced disorganization, not psychosis" (Sovner and Hurley 1986b, p. 46).

Developmental level does influence the content of delusions. Impoverished life experiences and concrete thinking contribute to less imaginative fantasies. Delusions in the mentally retarded population may take on the qualities of childhood fears. Grandiosity may be expressed as a belief that one is not handicapped. These delusions may be missed by a clinician expecting the classic grandiose content.

- *Other thought content.* Does the patient have obsessional thoughts or irrational fears?

- *Cognitive function.* It is helpful to document the current level of cognitive functioning by assessing orientation, attentional abilities, and memory. Use of visual cues in the form of pictures or cards can be an adjunct to the usual three-object test. The ability to recall general information will vary with level of training and education. It is also helpful to assess skills associated with everyday living like riding the bus, telling time, or using money. With mental retardation, cognitive deficits are present by definition; it is the change in function that is accorded clinical significance.

A screening physical examination, as noted in Chapter 2, is also appropriate for mentally retarded people. The physical examination is especially important in the evaluation of the nonverbal mentally retarded person, for whom careful observation must compensate for the historical gaps. Pain or hypoxia can lead to agitation and combative behavior as a nonspecific response to physical distress.

Readily obtainable laboratory work, including urinalysis, complete blood count, and electrolytes will augment the physical examination. The more severe the mental retardation, the greater the likelihood that a patient will have epilepsy and be on some type of anticonvulsant. The addition of a psychotropic medication may cause a fall in the blood level of the prescribed anticonvulsant (Sovner and Hurley 1982a). Likewise, discontinuing a psychotropic may lead to a rise in anticonvulsant blood level. Measuring a blood level during the examination will rule out anticonvulsant toxicity and ensure appropriate adjustment during the evaluation and treatment.

A brief examination can usually be accomplished even with an uncooperative and agitated patient. Any abnormalities can be followed up with further examination and testing.

DIFFERENTIAL DIAGNOSIS OF MAJOR PRESENTING SYMPTOMS

Frequent presenting symptoms for mentally retarded patients include aggressive behavior, suicidal ideation or self-injurious behavior, a decrease in level of functioning, increased sexual behavior, and pseudoseizures.

Aggressive Behavior

Aggression is a symptom that needs to be evaluated in the broad context in which it has occurred. The pattern of aggressive acts is of particular significance.

- An isolated episode of violence is more likely to represent a response to a situational stress.

- Episodic violent outbursts suggest either a psychiatric or a neurologic disorder.

- Ongoing aggressive acts suggest the nonspecific aggressiveness sometimes associated with mental retardation, or a predisposing chronic psychiatric or medical condition.

Any physical illness that causes distress may result in nonspecific combativeness. A new-onset, sudden change in behavior may suggest an organic basis. Additionally, aggression may be associated with partial complex seizures, postictal irritability, endocrinologic disturbances, or a manifestation of a drug side effect (Monroe 1985). Drug-induced side effects may be subtle and idiosyncratic. Presentations may be complicated by many factors, such as polypharmacy. The relationship between the onset of symptoms and a change in medication can alert the clinician to a possible association. Theophylline, nicotine, and caffeine are among the common drugs that can produce agitation. Antipsychotic drugs can produce severe akathisia. Mentally retarded persons may also become disinhibited or experience paradoxical excitation from sedatives. As noted previously, mentally retarded persons may be predisposed to the development of delirium, a fact to keep in mind when prescribing anticholinergic medication.

Any primary psychiatric disorder can be associated with violence. Thus, schizophrenia, mania, agitated depression, anxiety disorders, attention-deficit disorder, and personality disorders must be considered. In addition, there are several psychiatric diagnoses in which aggressive behavior is the primary disturbance. These include conduct disorders and intermittent explosive disorder. The former is not generally appropriate for adult mentally retarded patients. The latter should be reserved for those patients who have rage reactions (Sovner and Hurley 1986c); it is a controversial diagnosis for use with persons with mental retardation, just as it is for use with the general population (see Chapter 11).

Mentally retarded persons are subjected to a great deal of frustration. This is inherent in living in a developmentally inappropriate environment. Aggressive behavior may not indicate psychiatric illness but may represent a learned maladaptive response, or a reasonable response to an impossible situation. An example of the latter would be an aggressive act in the context of fending off an unwanted sexual advance, self-defense, or defense of property. The so-called nonspecific aggressive behavior associated with mental retardation may be a learned maladaptive behavior acquired in institutional settings where severe behaviors may be necessary to get attention.

The diagnosis will direct treatment. If a primary medical or psychiatric disorder is identified, then the specific treatment for that condition should be implemented. However, much of the aggressive behavior in mentally retarded patients cannot be linked to a clearly defined medical or psychiatric etiology. There are highly effective behavioral strategies that can be initiated to control aggression. Beyond recommendation, these are beyond the scope of the emergency service. The major interventions in an emergency setting are generally respite during the evaluation, crisis intervention with the patient or staff, and use of pharmacologic agents.

Propranolol, lithium, and carbamazepine have been demonstrated to have some efficacy in the management of aggressive behavior and rage reactions (Deutsh 1986; Yudovski et al. 1987). Their use may be recommended from an emergency setting but they are infrequently initiated there. All three have a delayed onset of action and require careful medical monitoring in collaboration with family and staff.

Emergency staff are frequently pressured to do something, in particular, to prescribe something that will make a difference. Mentally retarded persons are as frequently overmedicated as undermedicated. It is important to consider both reduction in medication and a decision not to change medication as legitimate clinical interventions.

In general, patients should not be on more than one drug from each class (i.e., antipsychotic, antidepressant, etc.). The history should suggest symptoms to warrant each medication and provide evidence that reasonable benefit has been achieved. Drug interactions and possible negative effects of drugs should be considered.

Adding medication or increasing the dose in an emergency setting may not be helpful and may enable the staff and family to work around developing a relationship with an ongoing psychiatric collaborator.

Suicidal Ideation or Self-injurious Behaviors

The evaluation of suicidal ideation has already been discussed. Suicide is associated with the diagnoses of both affective disorders and schizophrenia. In the nonverbal mentally retarded person, the diagnosis of an affective disorder may be hypothesized from episodic changes in activity level and sleep patterns. A positive family history is also significant.

Prevalence studies have shown that of the mentally retarded population, 3% are currently schizophrenic. This diagnosis should be used appropriately and ascribed only to those people who have the target symptoms and the history of deterioration in psychosocial functioning required by DSM-III-R (Sovner and Hurley 1983c).

As in people with normal intelligence, many suicide attempts arise impulsively in the face of severe situational stressors. A change in residence and separation from a significant other have been associated with both suicidal and aggressive behaviors in mentally retarded persons (Stack et al. 1987). Frequently, a history of recent staff changes in the residence or sheltered workshop can be elicited.

Self-injurious behaviors must be distinguished from suicidal behavior. According to Singh and Millichamp (1984), "[self-injurious behavior] refers to any self-inflicted repetitive action that leads to laceration, bruising, or abrasion of the client's own body" (p. 14). It is associated both with the degree of mental retardation and a history of institutionalization. These behaviors serve a self-stimulatory and attention-getting function. It may be biochemically driven in some patients, like those with Lesch-Nyhan syndrome. In contrast to this, suicidal behaviors have death as their expressed intent. Behavior modification is the first-choice treatment for self-injurious behaviors. Drug therapy may, however, have much to offer for individuals in whom behavior interventions have been ineffective. Antipsychotic medications are prescribed most frequently for self-injurious behavior in mentally retarded patients, although no study has conclusively demonstrated the superiority of any form of drug therapy. There have been isolated reports that antipsychotics, reserpine, methylphenidate, diazepam, naloxone, and lithium have been effective. In general, perhaps because self-injurious behavior may have multiple etiologies, no clear psychopharmacologic treatment has been demonstrated.

Decrease in Level of Functioning

A change in the baseline level of functioning may be the result of a major medical or psychiatric illness, as previously discussed. Particular attention to the possibility of psychosis or affective disorders is needed. If the change in functioning occurred abruptly, organic etiologies must be ruled out.

In addition to the previously discussed psychiatric conditions, it is important to recall that persons with mental retardation may be particularly predisposed to brief reactive psychosis when stressed. Recognizable psychotic symptoms like thought disorder, hallucinations, and delusions may be observed. They may, however, be the result of "cognitive disintegration" and "baseline exaggeration" (Sovner and Hurley 1986b). This refers to the fact that stress may cause disruption of already impaired information processing. The patient will experience confusion and resultant anxiety. During a period of emotional stress, preexisting cognitive and psychosocial deficits and previously learned maladaptive behaviors may significantly increase in severity. The combination of these factors leads to atypical presentations.

Mentally retarded people are at risk for acute and chronic organic brain syndromes. The etiology of delirium and dementia are the same in persons with mental retardation as they are in the normal population. If previous baseline adaptive skill assessments or psychometric tests are available, a decrease of cognitive functioning should alert the clinician to the possibility of a dementing process. Many cases of dementia in mentally retarded patients may initially be misdiagnosed as psychological disturbances. Because many dementias are reversible, this can result in tragic consequences. Patients with Down's syndrome have a higher rate of Alzheimer's disease. The prevalence of Alzheimer's disease is between 15 and 40% in middle-aged persons with Down's syndrome. Therefore, functional changes in a person with Down's syndrome who is 30 years old or older should raise the question of Alzheimer's disease (Gualtieri 1989; Sovner and Hurley 1986a).

Increased Sexual Behavior

Sexual behavior is rarely best handled on an emergency basis unless it has been directed toward a nonconsenting partner or a child. Retarded adults have sexual desires that need appropriate outlets. Sexual behaviors may evoke intense conflict between patient and staff or family. This conflict may be the problem, rather than the sexual behavior. If the sexual activity is directed toward a nonconsenting partner, then a careful assessment of the person's intent, understanding of sex, and societal norms is necessary. Educational and behavioral strategies are usually the best intervention. If the sexual activity was directed toward a child, the plan developed must ensure that the person will be supervised in such a way that access to children is not possible while treatment is implemented.

Pseudoseizures

Pseudoseizures sometimes develop in patients who have a documented seizure disorder. During the pseudoseizure, an electroencephalogram would fail to document any seizure activity. The seizure may appear to be realistic or to be atypical in its presentation. The onset or increase in pseudoseizures usually occurs in the context of increased stress, frequently from increased functional demands in the environment. In helping to identify the precipitating and/or maintaining stressors, the emergency clinicians can help other care givers develop a strategy to allow more adaptive functioning.

EMERGENCY INTERVENTIONS

In addition to any specific treatment that may be instituted for a particular medical or psychiatric condition, some of which have been discussed in the previous section, the emergency room staff provides several services of great value to mentally retarded persons and to those that support them in the community, including crisis intervention, referral, respite care, and hospitalization.

Crisis Intervention

There is a high probability that the crisis of a mentally retarded person may be precipitated by attempts to implement unrealistic treatment or habilitation goals, or by a failure to modify such goals in the face of a significant environmental change. Crisis intervention may, in fact, become a mini community consultation in which these goals are clarified and refined in an achievable, individualized manner. An effective crisis intervention will meet the needs of the patient and those attempting to support him or her. Emancipated, mildly retarded persons will respond to an active therapist and practical problem solving.

Referral

Mentally retarded persons are eligible for services in both the private and community sectors, where their needs are admittedly underserved. As an alternative, residential settings can be encouraged to hire a psychiatrist to provide services to their residents on a contract basis.

Respite Care

Respite care can be provided on a limited basis (24 hours) by some emergency services and may help to avoid a hospitalization. Respite is a reasonable alternative when the community supports are unable to provide a safe holding environment for the patient. It is frequently an empathic response to an exhausted family or residential staff who have extended themselves to deal with an intolerable behavior.

Respite allows for an extended observation period in the emergency setting and allows the residence to begin implementing emergency recommendations.

Hospitalization

When hospitalization is indicated for emotional and behavior problems that cannot be managed in the community, the referral is generally made to a general psychiatric unit. These units are not designed for the special habilitative needs of the mentally retarded person, so the outcome is rarely ideal. Sovner and Hurley (1987) propose five clinical situations in which hospitalization of mentally retarded patients is appropriate:

- The client requires a comprehensive diagnostic assessment that cannot be effected in the community.

- The client has an acute drug-responsive psychiatric disorder and treatment requires 24-hours-a-day monitoring.

- The client lives in a setting that cannot ensure that therapy will be carried out as ordered.

- The client has a significant medical condition that might complicate treatment with psychotropic drugs.

- The client is severely suicidal or homicidal as a result of psychiatric illness.

To these might be added the failure of outpatient treatment to resolve the problem.

REFERENCES

American Psychiatric Association: Diagnostic and Statistical Manual of Mental Disorders, 3rd Edition, Revised. Washington, DC, American Psychiatric Association, 1987

Deutsh MD: Managing behavior in the mentally retarded residential populations. Hosp Community Psychiatry 37:221–222, 1986

Gualtieri CT: Down's syndrome, in Treatments of Psychiatric Disorders, Vol 1. Washington, DC, American Psychiatric Press, 1989, pp 30–32

Monroe RR: Episodic behavioral disorders and limbic ictus. Compr Psychiatry 26:466–479, 1985

Singh NN, Millichamp CJ: Effects of medication on self injurious behaviors of mentally retarded persons. Psychiatric Aspects of Mental Retardation Newsletter 3:14–16, 1984

Sovner R, Hurley AD: Psychotropic drug interactions with anticonvulsants. Psychiatric Aspects of Mental Retardation Newsletter 1:17–23, 1982a

Sovner R, Hurley AD: Suicidal behavior in mentally retarded persons. Psychiatric Aspects of Mental Retardation Newsletter 1:35–38, 1982b

Sovner R, Hurley AD: The Mental Status Examination Part I: Behavior, speech and thought. Psychiatric Aspects of Mental Retardation Newsletter 2:5–8, 1983a

Sovner R, Hurley AD: The Mental Status Examination Part II. Psychiatric Aspects of Mental Retardation Newsletter 2:9–12, 1983b

Sovner R, Hurley AD: Schizophrenia. Psychiatric Aspects of Mental Retardation Newsletter 2:26–28, 1983c

Sovner R, Hurley AD: Dementia, mental retardation and Down's syndrome. Psychiatric Aspects of Mental Retardation Newsletter 5:40–44, 1986a

Sovner R, Hurley AD: Four factors affecting the diagnosis of psychiatric disorders in mentally retarded persons. Psychiatric Aspects of Mental Retardation Newsletter 5:45–49, 1986b

Sovner R, Hurley AD: Managing aggressive behavior: a psychiatric approach. Psychiatric Aspects of Mental Retardation Newsletter 5:17–21, 1986c

Sovner R, Hurley AD: Guidelines for the treatment of mentally retarded persons on psychiatric inpatient units. Psychiatric Aspects of Mental Retardation Newsletter 6:7–14, 1987

Stack LS, Haldipur CV, Thompson M: Stressful life events and psychiatric hospitalization of mentally retarded patients. Am J Psychiatry 144:661–663, 1987

Valente M: Etiologic factors in mental retardation. Psychiatric Annals 19:179–183, 1989

West MA, Richardson M: A statistical survey of CMHC programs for mentally retarded individuals. Hosp Community Psychiatry 32:413–416, 1981

Yudovski SD, Silver JM, Schneider SE: Pharmacologic treatment of aggression. Psychiatric Annals 17:397–407, 1987

Chapter 23

Medically Ill Patients

Lawson R. Wulsin, M.D.

The large proportion of patients in psychiatric emergency rooms who also have medical illnesses demands that the emergency room psychiatrist be competent in evaluating the relationship between medical and psychiatric illness. Competence in this area consists of a readiness to identify medical disorders, the ability to distinguish an adequate medical evaluation from an inadequate one for any given medical disorder, the ability to develop effective working relationships with medical colleagues, and the ability to evaluate psychiatric illness in the context of medical illness.

COMORBIDITY OF MEDICAL AND PSYCHIATRIC DISORDERS

Comorbidity of medical and psychiatric illness is underrecognized on both sides of the fence. That is, medical clinicians miss one-third to one-half of the psychopathology that is diagnosable in their patients (Knights and Folstein 1977; Moffic and Paykel 1975; Rodin and Voshart 1986), and general hospital psychiatrists miss as much as one-half of the medical illnesses that either cause or exacerbate the identified psychiatric illness (Hall et al. 1981; Koranyi 1979; LaBruzza 1981).

Given the frequent overlap of medical and psychiatric symptoms and disorders in the emergency room, it is important that the psychiatrist resist the habit of reducing the approach to differential diagnosis to the question, Is it organic or is it functional? Often the answer is both, and the more helpful question is, What factors contribute to these specific symptoms? Some factors will be distinctly biological, such as drug toxicity or fever, and others will be more psychosocial, such as bereavement or hypomania or poverty. Synthesizing these factors into a brief case formulation clarifies the psychiatrist's role in the management of the patient's illness.

THE PSYCHIATRIST'S ROLE

How far should the psychiatrist go in assessing and managing medical problems in psychiatric emergency room patients? The answer varies with the amount of medical services available to the psychiatrist. But in any setting, the psychiatrist must define the limits of his or her expertise in order to decide when and with whom to consult about medical problems. See Chapters 2 and 12 for a suggested approach to screening for medical illnesses in psychiatric emergency patients.

The task of collaborating with medical staff is most straightforward when the patient comes to the psychiatric emergency room with a clear medical diagnosis and is referred by a medical physician who knows the patient well and will continue to work with the patient. Less straightforward is the situation in which the patient is referred by a medical emergency room physician with some question remaining either in the physician's mind or the psychiatrist's about the contribution of medical illness to the current condition. The task of collaborating with medical staff is least straightforward when the patient comes to the psychiatric emergency room with no recent medical contacts or information.

In each case, adequate psychiatric evaluation depends in part on the psychiatrist's ability to understand the medical contributions to the current psychiatric condition, and to understand the patient's current medical needs. Although frequent experience with medical disorders is the best assurance of adequate understanding, no psychiatrist can hope to maintain up-to-date information on all disorders that present to emergency rooms. Therefore, easy access in the emergency room to recent texts on emergency medicine, surgery, and pharmacology must support habits of quick inquiry by the psychiatrist. In addition, availability by telephone of medical colleagues for informal discussion of general questions makes it convenient for psychiatrists to check impressions and guesses with experts. Above all, psychiatrists must be able to identify when they do not understand the medical factors sufficiently to make decisions about the management of the patient. Once psychiatrists recognize gaps in their understanding, they can take the few steps needed to inform themselves by reading, consulting, or referring.

Should psychiatrists question the evaluations made by their medical colleagues? Part of the role of emergency psychiatrists is to ensure that the patient gets a medical evaluation that addresses the emergent need. Psychiatrists can fulfill this obligation either by performing the evaluation themselves or by making sure that it has been performed appropriately by other physicians. Blatant incompetence may be the most easily identified reason for inadequate medical evaluation, but in most settings it is not the most common reason. More often, the complicated patient with multiple disorders requires several medical evaluations to clarify questions about a possible medical or psychiatric contribution to a puzzling presentation. At times, highly skilled medical emergency room staffs are overwhelmed by the volume or severity of their patient load, and their evaluations are incomplete, or a patient's psychopathology may interfere with the medical evaluation, as may happen with mania and paranoia. When doctors dislike patients, calling them "gomers," "borderlines," or "crocks" (Groves 1978), or when they favor them, as they often do when treating patients who are doctors or VIPs, their evaluations may be incomplete. Acknowledging an incomplete medical evaluation as a fact of practice, not a personal slur, opens the way to effective collaborations.

Several steps improve the ability of the emergency psychiatrist to assess the medical evaluation. Knowing the medical evaluator and the setting in which the evaluation was done provides a context for the information. Talking directly with whoever performed the evaluation to discuss the findings complements, but does not substitute for, a written copy of the medical evaluation. The referring physician's impressions of the family and the patient's prognosis will be helpful additions to a hurried emergency room note. On the other hand, word of mouth about mild electrocardiogram changes or a negative toxic screen may not be sufficient documentation to allow safe use of a new medication by the psychiatrist. Psychiatrists should do their own review of systems. Hall et al. (1978) found that four or more positive responses on the review of systems correlated strongly with medical illness. Hall et al. (1981) also found that 90% of the unidentified medical illnesses found in his sample of psychiatric patients could be identified through history, physical examination, vital signs, relevant laboratory work, relevant X rays, electrocardiogram, electroencephalogram, and a toxic screen when necessary. Extraordinary measures are not necessary to identify and monitor most medical illnesses presenting in the emergency room.

The fundamental task specific to the psychiatrist evaluating the medically ill patient is to communicate with the medical staff involved in the patient's care. Through frequent direct communications, the roles of the psychiatrist and of the medical collaborators are redefined in each case, often specifically with respect to evaluation measures, medications, and the execution of the treatment plan. When medical and psychiatric needs overlap, good clinical judgment and direct negotiation with the medical staff provide the guide for respective responsibilities. The psychiatrist who participates in this collaborative approach understands the medical illness, assesses the completeness of the medical evaluation, and communicates with collaborators about the medical and psychiatric findings.

COMMON DILEMMAS

Depression

Are the depressive symptoms seen in many medically ill patients the product of the medical illness or of a distinct affective disorder? Should these symptoms be treated by proper management of the medical illness or by antidepressant medications and psychotherapy? Controversy about these questions centers on the problems of assessment (Cohen-Cole and Harpe 1987). The DSM-III-R (American Psychiatric Association 1987) approach counts a symptom toward the diagnosis of depression only if it is not "clearly due to a physical illness." This approach requires inferences about causality, leaving room for debate in the mind of the clinician, and among several clinicians.

Alternatives to this etiologic approach either replace (Cavenaugh et al. 1983) or exclude (Bukberg et al. 1984) the criteria for depression most likely to be associated with medical illness, such as anergia and anorexia. Cognitive and affective criteria, such as memory loss or crying spells, may be less affected by medical conditions and, therefore, more reliably associated with depression independent of medical illness.

Until measures specific for the assessment of depression in medical illnesses are developed and tested, the clinician must rely on clinical judgment and current standard measures, such as the Beck Depression Inventory (Beck et al. 1979), the Hamilton Rating Scale for Depression (Klerman et al. 1984), and DSM-III-R criteria. In practice, many clinicians take what Cohen-Cole and Harpe (1987) call the inclusive approach, namely, including a symptom or criterion toward a diagnosis of depression whether it is caused by a medical illness or not. This approach may be justified by the high risk of underdiagnosing depression and the relatively low risk of treating depressive symptoms that do not constitute a major depression.

Other Mood Disorders

Other mood disorders to consider in the context of medical illness are organic mood disorder, which depends on the identification of a specific organic factor; adjustment disorder with depressed mood, which requires the identification of a stressor within 3 months of onset; dysthymia, a mild but prolonged version of depression; and somatoform disorders. See Chapters 10, 16, and 17 for discussion of medical problems related to mood syndromes, anxiety, and psychosis, respectively.

Somatoform disorders. The emergency psychiatrist is often asked to verify that a patient with a negative medical evaluation and forceful somatic complaints has a somatoform disorder. As described in Chapter 18, the differential diagnosis may be tricky and requires particular care to avoid mislabeling or mistreating the patient.

Admission to a Medical or a Psychiatric Unit?

Patients with combined medical and psychiatric problems raise the question of where in the hospital they are best treated. The answer varies from hospital to hospital and is not always based on clinical need. Nonclinical considerations that determine site of treatment include insurance coverage, availability of beds, and availability of consultation services. The types of disorders that commonly raise this latter consideration are depression in the terminally ill, substance abuse, overdose, and agitation with delirium and psychosis.

Negotiations about admissions are simplified by clearly written admission and exclusion criteria for each ward posted in the emergency room. Medical psychiatry units designed to treat this group of patients must also clearly define their criteria to avoid receiving patients who do not have combined disorders.

REFERENCES

American Psychiatric Association: Diagnostic and Statistical Manual of Mental Disorders, 3rd Edition, Revised. Washington, DC, American Psychiatric Association, 1987

Beck AT, Rush AJ, Shaw BF, et al: Cognitive Therapy of Depression. New York, Guilford, 1979

Bukberg J, Penman D, Holland JC: Depression in hospitalized cancer patients. Psychosom Med 46:199–212, 1984

Cavenaugh S, Clark D, Gibbons R: Diagnosing depression in the hospitalized medically ill. Psychosomatics 24:809–815, 1983

Cohen-Cole SA, Harpe C: Diagnostic assessment of depression in the medically ill, in Medical Psychiatry. Edited by Stoudemire A, Fogel BS. Orlando, FL, Grune & Stratton, 1987

Groves JE: Taking care of the hateful patient. N Engl J Med 298:883–887, 1978

Hall RCW, Popkin MK, Devaul RA, et al: Physical illness presenting as psychiatric disease. Arch Gen Psychiatry 35:1315–1320, 1978

Hall RCW, Gardner ER, Popkin MK, et al: Unrecognized physical illness prompting psychiatric admission: a prospective study. Am J Psychiatry 138:629–635, 1981

Klerman GL, Weissman MM, Rounsaville BJ, et al: Interpersonal Psychotherapy of Depression. New York, Basic Books, 1984

Knights TB, Folstein MF: Unsuspected emotional and cognitive disturbance in medical patients. Ann Intern Med 87:723–724, 1977

Koranyi EK: Morbidity and rate of undiagnosed physical illnesses in a psychiatric clinic population. Arch Gen Psychiatry 36:414–419, 1979

LaBruzza AL: Physical illness presenting as psychiatric disorder: guidelines for differential diagnosis. Journal of Operational Psychiatry 12:24–31, 1981

Moffic HS, Paykel ES: Depression in medical in-patients. Br J Psychiatry 126:346–353, 1975

Rodin G, Voshart K: Depression in the medically ill: an overview. Am J Psychiatry 143:696–705, 1986

Chapter 24

"Young Adult Chronic" Patients

G.A. Barker, M.D.

The "young adult chronic" patient is a term developed as a descriptor of adult patients, aged 18–40 years, who have severe and persistent psychiatric disorders (Bachrach 1982). In the aftermath of deinstitutionalization, these patients have offered many challenges to the service delivery system. Recently, there has been some concern among professionals that this label is stigmatizing and should be discarded for more individually descriptive terms (Bachrach 1982; Estroff 1987).

Patients in this age group have become an increasingly prominent force due to demographic changes in the national population. These are the people who, in the past, generally would have been institutionalized for a significant period of time. They were, theoretically, to be the recipients of optimal community treatment services. In general, however, community services have not been optimally designed and adapted to meet the special needs of these patients (Pepper et al. 1981).

SPECIAL CHARACTERISTICS OF YOUNG ADULT CHRONIC PATIENTS

- These patients, without an institutional history, have difficulty engaging in our current treatment system. They do not necessarily see themselves as mental patients, and their agenda frequently differs from that of the professional trying to help them, providing a natural milieu for power struggles and conflict.

- "Compliance" with treatment, both pharmacologic and psychosocial, is reduced as a corollary to the first point.

- Developmental issues of young adulthood (e.g., emancipation, financial independence), complicated by the presence of a major mental disorder, are prominent as these patients try to find their way among their societal peers.

- Repeated failures contribute to the statistically high risk of suicide in this patient group (Caton 1981; Hillard et al. 1983).

- As citizens mainstreamed into community life, they exhibit patterns typical of other citizens, including a high degree of mobility and a high degree of substance abuse.

- They are held accountable for their behavior by other community members. Some interaction with the criminal justice system is common.

- Inability to manage major tasks of adulthood has, for some, resulted in repeated temporary or extended periods of homelessness, use of drop-in centers, and loss of children to family or welfare agencies.

- Major mental illness impacts on the family now in a more direct manner than in the past. Previously, family members were placed in the role of grieving for one who was sent away; now, they are frequently the major support and daily care provider. Their engagement in treatment planning and implementation is critical. Their needs must be addressed in addition to those of the patient.

- These are patients with a low degree of "social margin," defined as "all personal possessions, attributes, or relationships which can be traded on for help in time of need" (Copeland 1979, p. 315). Mental health services may become the most significant source of support in times of crisis.

- These patients continue to need the range of services previously "bundled" together in institutions. This results in complex problems aggravated by the patient's right and ability to choose services, as well as the frustrating complexity of engaging with overtaxed, underdeveloped, uncoordinated, "user unfriendly," community services.

- Treatment histories and diagnoses show great variability. Frequent "revolving door" admissions, abuse of emergency settings, or transinstitutionalization in forensic settings are common.

- Although characteristics of various subpopulations have been identified (Sheets et al. 1982; Thompson 1988), individualized assessment and treatment planning that engages patients to work toward their best adaptation to their illness over time seems to be the best current guideline for treatment (Minkoff 1987).

YOUNG ADULT CHRONIC PATIENTS IN THE PSYCHIATRIC EMERGENCY ROOM

Young adults with chronic mental illnesses represent a significant percentage of the patients utilizing psychiatric emergency services. In 1987, 68.3% of the visits to the Cincinnati Psychiatric Emergency Service were made by patients in this age group. This is in keeping with the high percentages quoted in other studies (Friedman 1986).

Why Do We See So Many Young Patients?

Psychiatric emergency services are critical treatment sites for various reasons:

- Psychiatric patients are known to have a reduced social network available to them, reducing their helpful options when in crisis.

- Emergency services are available on a 24-hour basis and will provide service without any exclusionary criteria, to all who feel they need it. The need for service may be expressed by the patient, the family, other community care providers, or the police. For many, this is the least complicated way to initiate a request for help and is particularly available for patients who deny their illness.

- A general hospital emergency room is a less stigmatizing environment than a more traditional mental health center.

- Medical resources are more concentrated in the emergency setting, giving the patient easy access to a psychiatrist, as well as to other medical specialists not generally available in the community mental health system.

- Emergency services tend to shore up cracks in an area community support system. Patients who move, relocate, or fail to follow up or who are extruded for unacceptable behavior may seek services from a psychiatric emergency center.

EMERGENCY EVALUATION OF YOUNG ADULT PATIENTS WITH CHRONIC MENTAL ILLNESS

Young adult patients request emergency services for a variety of symptoms and concerns. These may be artificially grouped in the following manner:

- *Medical/psychiatric emergencies.* These include psychotic decompensation, worsening depression, evaluation of suicide risk or violence, and side effects of medications or drugs.

- *Need for crisis intervention.* Acute deterioration of significant relationships with spouse, family, roommates, or other care providers is the chief complaint.

- *Social service emergencies.* Here, the crisis is primarily related to lack of food, clothing, or shelter or access to treatment or entitlements.

- *Other.* This is a catchall category to include requests for services by those functioning at a low level who perceive an increased need for human contact and support, those who are drug seeking, etc.

As noted previously, patients do best when they receive an empathic, individualized, and comprehensive assessment that engages them, as much as possible, collaboratively. When patients contact their current therapist or case manager, consideration of the request for help in the context of the above classification system will help guide the care giver. The first goal is to stabilize the patient so that the crisis can be resolved in the least intrusive and restrictive manner for the patient. This is analogous to establishing an airway in a medical emergency. Stabilizing may involve telephone or face-to-face evaluation.

The ability of primary therapists to be available on an emergent basis can be invaluable, as they generally have the best understanding of patients' baseline level of function and of their strengths and weaknesses. As a group, young patients are impulsive, and some type of intervention is usually needed on an emergent basis. If the care giver is unable to stabilize the patient or situation alone, referral to a psychiatric emergency service is frequently the best option.

Likewise, if a patient presents first in a psychiatric emergency service, it is very important to address the chief complaint and presenting symptoms, listening carefully to the request for help. Information necessary to evaluate the patient must be gathered, ideally from the patient, and frequently from family, other care givers, and mental health professionals. A clear estimate of the patient's baseline level of functioning needs to be established. The current community treatment plan should be elicited and verified so that the meaning of the emergency room visit can be elucidated and the appropriate service rendered. Patients should be treated respectfully, as adults who are likely doing the best they can and are asking our help because they are "stuck" and need something from us (medication, psychotherapy, advocacy, referral, hospitalization) to get going again.

Psychiatric emergency services are an essential component of a community support system. Most of the patients receiving psychiatric emergency services are, or will be, engaged in treatment in other settings. Work cannot be done in a vacuum: collaboration with those involved services and with the family is important to the assessment of the patient. For many patients, family and the mental health system comprise their entire social network. If that network is currently unable to provide a safe "holding environment" for the patient, then the patient is indeed in crisis on this basis alone. The current needs of the family must also be addressed. Hatfield (1983) asked families about the kinds of support they need. Their responses indicate a need for information and education to understand the behavior of their mentally ill relatives, for specific suggestions in dealing with the behavior, and for respite care. Information about family support groups, like the National Alliance for the Mentally Ill, should be available and offered actively.

Make a Comprehensive Formulation

The above information about the current medical and psychiatric state of the patient, his or her current treatment, living situations, and level of function needs to be compiled in a comprehensive formulation. Is the patient functioning at baseline? If not, what accounts for the change and what services will be most successful at restoring baseline functioning? Is the patient's view of the situation compatible with that of the family, the therapist, and emergency staff? Does the current treatment plan make sense? Is it working?

Use of Hospitalization

Hospitalization is the option of choice when a patient is felt to represent a risk to self or others. Even here, in many communities, there is a gradation of services from partial hospitalization to a high-security forensic unit.

Hospitalization has the capacity to offer diagnostic assessment, medical evaluation, treatment, support, and social services, but there are negative factors as well. Hospitalization, for many, implies failure to make it on the outside and inhibits personal control and decision making. The regression encouraged by the dependent posture of a hospitalized patient is a contrast to the isolated, independent posture of many young adults with major mental illness. This climate then can become conflicted and difficult to negotiate successfully. Involuntary hospitalization can be experienced as a personal violation. Current political and financial pressures mandate short hospitalizations. Many patients in this group have frequent hospitalizations with marginal recompensation, and rapid decompensation followed by readmission. Extended hospitalization today is rarely available.

Alternatives to Hospitalization

Respite care implies a short break from a current situation. Respite services, in general, are underdeveloped in most communities. Practically speaking, respite is usually obtained through an agency whose primary mission is to provide crisis stabilization, shelter, etc. There are some programs, however, that have respite care as their focus and testify to its therapeutic potential. The Veterans Administration hospital in Palo Alto, California, is a good example, and they cite benefits to patients' families in terms of improved community functioning support and to staff in terms of increased job satisfaction (Geiser et al. 1988).

Psychiatric emergency facilities can sometimes offer 1–3 days of emergency care. The goal is always to stabilize a critical situation and to avert a hospitalization. Frequently, an individual, family, or residential setting has been stressed by an intense interaction or behavior. Respite care offers a time-out so that the community resources may regroup into a more therapeutic stance.

Overnight stays in the emergency room may also be chosen for patients who meet criteria for hospitalization, but who have a history of repeated hospitalizations that have been of little long-term benefit. Frequently, these patients have a high degree of character pathology and are frequent emergency room visitors. Their history of brief hospitalizations or "against medical advice" discharges may suggest that a brief period of support and stabilization will be sufficient to restore them to baseline.

To be successful, both brief treatment and respite care require that the patient be followed by a community care giver and have reasonably immediate access to appropriate services. Many of these patients have episodic treatment histories and are at various stages of engagement in treatment.

Crises provide a unique opportunity for the professional to be helpful. Throughout the assessment and intervention, it is helpful to ask the patient and family about their understanding of the current problem, history, diagnosis, and use of medication. Clarifying the purpose of the medication, the disease process, and the meaning of certain behaviors in a clear and nonjudgmental fashion helps to diminish stigma and can be very influential at a time that patient and family are eager and open to information.

CRISIS INTERVENTION

Crisis intervention is an interpersonal psychotherapeutic process aimed at restoring the optimal functioning of the patient, and possibly that of the patient's significant others. The person in crisis has a high level of anxiety which interfaces with the ability to focus effectively and to plan for resolution. The role of the therapist is to help define and maintain the focus, in an empathic manner that implies that the two will work together to find a solution to the problem. This process is familiar to clinicians.

In working with young adults with severe and persistent mental disorders, the clinician may initially be overwhelmed by these patients and their complex multilevel problems. It is essential to uncover the reason for the current visit and to work to understand the surrounding situation and its personal meaning and relevance to the patient. A concrete strategy must be devised to cope with the crisis, and contact must be made with all persons who are part of this plan, to engage them as collaborators from the beginning. If this cannot be accomplished, a plan to contact them and engage them at the earliest possible time should be clearly established.

The patient must agree to any behavior that will be required and must understand the consequences of the failure to comply. This process may require multiple interviews, or a series of telephone contacts. Clinicians may portray themselves as arbitrators, interpreters, or therapists to create change, compromise, or communication.

The goal of each emergency contact is to resolve the current crisis. Although each crisis offers an opportunity to enhance growth and function, some patients seem to live in a state of chronic crisis, and it is difficult to note a trend toward improved functioning. This may set up a pattern of repeated visits to an emergency service: "The true source of difficulty is the enduring pattern of maladaptive living rather than the individual event that may precipitate a specific visit to a treatment facility" (Schwartz and Goldfinger 1981, p. 471). With this in mind, the long-term goal of all emergency interventions is engagement in treatment: "Engagement is the answer to meaninglessness" (Lamb 1982, p. 467). If interventions enhance engagement over time, they are successful.

SOCIAL SERVICE EMERGENCIES

People cannot be stable if they do not have shelter, food, clothing, money, and social outlets. The young adult chronic population is predisposed to crisis in this area by their decreased social networks and general poverty. Left unattended, decompensation is likely to follow.

Homelessness alone, however, is not a reason to hospitalize someone. Emergency shelter and assistance are better options, because a case manager works with a patient to find more stable arrangements.

Patients sometimes exaggerate symptoms to try to gain access to hospitals when they have minimal resources. Exploring alternative options that will help meet their needs is frequently enough to break through this. Again, collaboratively engaging the person in finding the best solution is the healthiest course.

If a social service emergency is complicated by decompensation, the least restrictive alternative for treatment should be sought, but the decompensation should be the primary focus of the intervention. Drop-in shelters are generally crowded, loud, loosely supervised settings, and patients must be able to tolerate this stress if referred there. Unless it is clear that a person will be able to access treatment services in such a setting, it is an unacceptable disposition.

SPECIAL CONCERNS

Use of Involuntary Hospitalization

Involuntary hospitalization is frequently used for patients in this age group exhibiting dangerous, self-injurious, or irresponsible behaviors. When a patient is psychotic and dangerous, there is little conflict over involuntary hospitalization. It may be quite a different matter when the patient is cognitively intact and refuses a needed admission. Taking away a person's right to decide can be experienced as degrading and infantilizing. This may be averted in most cases if the clinician can openly explain his or her concerns and the reasoning behind the recommendation.

Support or leverage from family or significant others is also helpful. Although conflicting feelings may develop, it is helpful to affirm to the patient that you are both on the same side in the sense that both of you want the patient to feel better and function well. Most often, a patient will at least grudgingly agree to a brief admission or will work actively with you to find a creative outpatient solution that is agreeable to the clinician and family (e.g., staying with a reliable supportive family member and returning daily to the emergency room, or attending a day treatment program while increasing medication).

Involvement in the decision-making process affirms the patient's capabilities and responsibility for behavior and treatment.

Confidentiality

Strict interpretation of confidentiality legislation has led staff members to refuse to give out any information to families—a position that family members find intolerable. Certainly, caretaking families need information about the current illness manifestations, treatment, and outcome. Clinicians need to facilitate this on a case-by-case basis within the bounds of the law. Our attitude, however, should be one of facilitation rather than obstruction. It is generally possible to get the patient's permission to talk with the family if they are involved. If the patient is hesitant, discuss the kind of information you would like to share, i.e., current observations, treatment recommendations, and medication information. With the proper attitude and presentation, it is rare for a patient to totally deny access to significant others.

Effect on Psychiatric Emergency Staff

Simply put, staff clinicians feel positive when they feel effective and helpful and feel frustrated and burned out when the contrary is true. The literature is replete with descriptions of problem patients, amply demonstrating the reaction that clinicians have had to them. It is difficult to maintain an optimistic stance in the face of repeated failures. When patients have multiple emergency room visits, multiple admissions, a downhill course, self-destructive behavior, and substance abuse, clinicians tend to lose hope that any intervention will be effective. The result is frequently antitherapeutic as the therapist invests less creative energy and may act disinterested or even angry.

As in any therapeutic setting, staff have to process their feelings for the benefit of the patient and should not hesitate to seek supervision from other staff members if self-reflection provides little help. It is critical to remember that we are there to help patients and that they are our customers and deserve the best we have to offer. Feelings of hopelessness or helplessness may help us to be empathic with similar feelings in the patient. An increased understanding will make us more helpful and therefore less negative. It follows, then, that training and education are essential.

Major factors in the development of negative reactions in psychiatric emergency service staff include

- *Transference and countertransference issues.* These reactions are generated by patients in conflict over dependence and/or independence. Clinicians face a dilemma in deciding whether to encourage dependence and risk fostering regression or to encourage independence. Selecting the best treatment intervention requires good clinical judgment. It can be affirming to encourage patients to continue to try to handle a crisis in the community, or conversely to agree with them that they are recognizing increased signs of stress and need hospitalization. These interventions are made by considering past history and current presentation and by carefully examining the current affects of the patient and the clinician. It is critical that the clinician operate for the good of the patient and avoid being either overly paternalistic or pejorative.
- *Staff and system pressures.* Some anger directed toward patients is based on the assumption that the system is ideal and that the patients will not use it properly. This is, of course, a fallacy. Frequently, the needed resource is not available, has a waiting list, or has extruded the patient for various reasons. This is hardly the patient's fault, and we may be better directed to help address the larger systems issues. Staff morale improves if they can be directed to help solve the systems problems through involvement in appropriate political and advocacy roles.

REFERENCES

Bachrach LL: Young adult chronic patients: an analytical review of the literature. Hosp Community Psychiatry 33:189–197, 1982

Caton CLM: The new chronic patient and the system of community care. Hosp Community Psychiatry 32:475–478, 1981

Copeland GN: Unexpected consequences of deinstitutionalization of the mentally disabled elderly. Am J Community Psychol 7:315–329, 1979

Estroff SE: No more young adult chronic patients. Hosp Community Psychiatry 38:57, 1987

Friedman R: Profile of psychiatric emergency patients, in Handbook of Emergency Psychiatry for Clinical Administrators. Edited by Barton G, Friedman R. New York, Haworth Press, 1986, pp 25–35

Geiser R, Hoche L, King J: Respite care for mentally ill patients and their families. Hosp Community Psychiatry 39:291–295, 1988

Hatfield A: What families want of family therapists, in Therapy in Schizophrenia, 1st Edition. Edited by McFarlane WR. New York, Guilford, 1983

Hillard JR, Zung WW, Ramm D, et al: Suicide in a psychiatric emergency room population. Am J Psychiatry 140:459–462, 1983

Lamb HR: Young adult chronic patients: the new drifters. Hosp Community Psychiatry 33:465–468, 1982

Minkoff K: Beyond deinstitutionalization: a new ideology for the post institutional era. Hosp Community Psychiatry 38:945–950, 1987

Pepper B, Kirshner MC, Ryglewiez H: The young adult chronic patient, overview of a population. Hosp Community Psychiatry 32:463–469, 1981

Schwartz SR, Goldfinger SM: The new chronic patient: clinical characteristics of an emerging subgroup. Hosp Community Psychiatry 32:470–474, 1981

Sheets TL, Prevost TA, Reichman L: Young adult chronic patients: three hypothesized subgroups. Hosp Community Psychiatry 33:197–203, 1982

Thompson EH: Variation in the self-concept of young adult chronic patients: chronicity reconsidered. Hosp Community Psychiatry 39:771–775, 1988

Chapter 25

Elderly Patients

O. Thienhaus, M.D.

Incidence and prevalence of mental illness among the elderly are controversial. Some claim that mental disorders are more common among elderly people than in the general population (Srole and Fischer 1980). By contrast, other authors have produced evidence that mental illness is less prevalent among the elderly than in other age groups (Myers et al. 1984; Weissman et al. 1985). However that may be, it has been shown that among the clientele of psychiatric emergency services, people over 65 years of age are a very small minority indeed (National Institute of Mental Health 1973). If the relative numbers have been increasing in recent years, this may reflect, in part, general demographic shifts, i.e., the "graying of America," but also a growing awareness among the general public and health professionals that behavioral, emotional, and cognitive changes in older people are not necessarily part of normal aging. Rather, such changes deserve diagnostic evaluation, and, quite frequently, are amenable to therapeutic intervention (Waxman et al. 1982).

PROBLEMS OF DIAGNOSIS

Psychiatric Manifestations of Physical Illness

One of the physiological changes that accompany aging is the gradual decrease of the body's adaptive regulatory flexibility. Chemical, physical, or biological factors impinging on the aging individual's equilibrium are increasingly likely to cause disturbances of homeostasis with resultant symptomatology. On the other hand, prodromal signs or typical symptoms of homeostatic imbalance, e.g., pain, fever, or leukocytosis, may be absent in the elderly person. Examples include the geriatric patient's "silent myocardial infarction" or afebrile pneumonia. The most prominent or, indeed, the only presenting clinical symptom may be altered mental status. This broad term can include affective presentations, cognitive impairment, or psychotic syndromes with delusional ideation and perceptual disorders. Behavior changes may be present, such as seclusiveness or belligerence. Finally, the presentation may be that of a delirium that can include all of the above-mentioned phenomena, but is usually accompanied by a fluctuating level of consciousness.

A physician should be involved in the evaluation of every elderly person who is seen in the psychiatric emergency room. Besides, every elderly person with a *new-onset* change of mental status or with a *qualitative change* in mental status abnormalities—e.g., the previously diagnosed demented patient who starts hearing voices—needs a full physical examination including a complete neurological status and basic laboratory work, i.e., complete blood count, renal panel, and blood sugar (also see Chapters 2 and 12). Questioning the family doctor or relatives can provide direction as to where a physical problem may originate.

Prescription Drugs and Mental Illness

A disproportionate number of elderly people take prescribed medications (Law and Chalmers 1976), often in addition to over-the-counter preparations. Normal manifestations of aging such as a relative decrease of distribution volume, lower plasma protein concentration (which results in more nonbound, i.e., pharmacologically active drug load), and delayed renal elimination combine to greatly increase the bioavailability of most ingested drugs. The impact of ingested therapeutics can stress or overwhelm the reduced homeostatic capacity of elderly patients.

It is important to obtain a complete list of medications currently taken by an elderly patient. This may again necessitate inquiries to other physicians and to relatives. Blood levels of digoxin, diphenylhydantoin, and theophylline are in order whenever recent mental status changes are described in persons taking these medications. The manifestations of toxic drug levels can span the whole gamut of possible mental status symptomatology.

There are also drugs that can produce psychiatric symptoms at therapeutic dosages. Most notable among these are the various antihypertensive medications causing depressive symptoms, especially reserpine, methyldopa, and beta-blockers.

The anticholinergic properties of centrally active drugs can cause serious problems in elderly patients, especially when cholinergic neurotransmission is already compromised, e.g., in primary degenerative dementia of the Alzheimer type. Antiparkinsonian drugs, cyclic antidepressants, and neuroleptics have atropine-like side effects, as discussed in Chapter 3. They can cause cognitive deficits but also can lead to full psychotic syndromes. If this etiology is suspected, a physostigmine test dose, 0.5–1.0 mg im, should demonstrate prompt, although transient, symptom reversal.

Finally, it has been described that prescribed medication can mask clinical markers of mental illness. For instance, beta-blockers prescribed for hypertension can disguise the vegetative prodromata of delirium (Zechnich 1982) or some of the cardinal autonomic symptoms of panic attacks.

Differential Diagnosis of Mental Status Changes

Cognitive deterioration. This can concern long-term or recent memory, concentration, calculation, abstraction, and orientation. Cognitive changes in the elderly patient in the emergency room always require differential diagnostic attention. "Normal aging" has been associated with benign senile forgetfulness. This degree of memory impairment is, however, by definition subclinical (Schneck et al. 1982).

The foremost task for the emergency room physician who sees cognitive impairment is to rule out delirium (see Chapter 12). Delirium, marked by impaired attention span, fluctuating course, and unstable level of consciousness, requires close medical monitoring and corrective intervention.

Once delirium is ruled out, cognitive impairment can be due to (life-long) mental retardation, an amnestic disorder, or a dementing illness (see Chapter 12). Specifically in the elderly population, cognitive symptoms have also been described in association with major depressive disorder (Wells 1979), and more rarely with other psychiatric pathology (McAllister 1982).

The differentiation between mental retardation and secondary forms of cognitive deterioration should be obvious if reliable historical data can be obtained. An elderly patient with mental retardation is likely to have spent a large part of life institutionalized (see Chapter 22).

Dementia is a syndrome of memory disturbance and other cortical deficits. It can be due to various etiologies. Uncomplicated dementia can be worked up diagnostically in outpatient facilities, and the patient need not be detained in the emergency room or hospital. Amnestic disorder is characterized by an isolated impairment of memory, without the other symptoms usually associated with dementia (see Chapter 12).

Pseudodementia was introduced as a term to describe primarily subjective memory problems in elderly patients with major depression (Kiloh 1961). On clinical examination, the evaluator should specifically look for associated affective symptoms as a distinguishing mark. Also, the dissimulation and minimization found in patients with genuine dementia are typically absent. Instead, the patient tends to complain articulately about problems with memory, concentration, etc. However, the differential diagnosis can be difficult because demented patients—especially those presenting to the emergency room—often have secondary, associated psychiatric symptoms (see Chapter 12). A trial of antidepressant therapy over several weeks may be the only means of determining how much of the clinical cognitive impairment was due to an affective illness.

Loss of reality testing. This can occur in elderly patients as part of a psychotic decompensation of a known chronically exacerbating mental illness, such as paranoid schizophrenia or recurrent major depression. Historical data in conjunction with the specific symptom constellation should generally make the diagnosis clear.

The absence of a previous history of psychosis should, first of all, raise the suspicion of a biological cause, as described above. Organic hallucinosis and organic delusional disorder are common presentations. However, these diagnoses require the demonstration of a responsible organic factor. Nonauditory hallucinations should, prima facie, alert the physician that organic pathology may be present.

The existence of late-onset schizophrenia has been recognized in DSM-III-R (American Psychiatric Association 1987), but it is relatively rare that this diagnosis is first made in a patient aged 65 years or over. Unclear psychotic states in elderly patients are often classified as atypical psychosis. They frequently occur in patients with a primary dementing illness, especially during periods of sensory deprivation.

Paranoid personality traits can become more prominent in elderly people. Social isolation and beginning cognitive deterioration may be pathogenetic factors. Ideation can assume a delusional quality, and a diagnosis of delusional disorder is appropriate.

Delusions in such patients may serve to defend against threatening realizations of infirmity, as in the example of the elderly man who keeps misplacing his glasses and accuses his wife of deliberately hiding them. Sensory impairment has been implicated as a likely risk factor for psychotic disorders (Cooper et al. 1974).

Affective symptoms. These are common among elderly patients, even if they do not add up to full syndromes of major depression or bipolar affective disorder (Blazer and Williams 1980). For the emergency room psychiatrist's decision about immediate intervention, functional impairment and suicide potential are most crucial to determine. The evaluation of risk of suicide is addressed in Chapter 8 of this manual. It should be kept in mind that elderly white men are, demographically, a high-risk group for suicide. Functional impairment is often tied in with vegetative features of affective illness, which in general are quite prominent in both depressed and manic geriatric patients. Anorexia can be accompanied by dehydration or electrolyte impairment requiring medical attention. Carelessness about compliance with dietary and pharmacologic regimens can amount to passive self-destruction.

Symptoms of the actual mood disorder have to be deduced from direct observation, e.g., facial expression and specific questioning. Elderly people are thought to be less likely to spontaneously describe feeling states than their younger counterparts.

Often, the differentiation of whether affective symptomatology is due to a primary mood disorder or an organic affective disorder, such as thyroid-induced secondary mania or depression caused by propranolol, can be definitively made only in the longer run. What should be possible in the emergency setting is the determination of whether the affectively ill elderly patient is at risk if left unsupervised.

Displacement of Problems in the Family

Problems originating elsewhere are occasionally displaced onto an identified patient. The emergency therapist is challenged to locate the focus of conflict correctly, and to include spouse, family, or friends appropriately in assessment and treatment recommendations. Adult sons or daughters of elderly parents can find themselves overwhelmed by, for example, conflicts with their own children or marital problems. The entire affective load of such problems can occasionally be displaced onto the elderly parent as a crisis situation, which, taken by itself, may only have been a minor request for assistance. But suddenly it is felt that, "Mom just can't take care of herself anymore—something must be done." Proper exploration of the situation may show that spousal communication or limit setting with the adult children are the real issues about which "something must be done."

PROBLEMS IN TREATMENT

Altered Physiology

If causative metabolic, hemodynamic, or other organic factors can be identified, corrective intervention is clearly indicated. In what setting this should occur is addressed later in this chapter (see "Problems in Disposition"). The nature and intensity of the mental symptoms, however, can be distressing enough to require additional symptomatic treatment. This can include restraints, sedation, or antipsychotic medication. Choice of any such measures should be dictated by the goal of relieving distress and assuring security while not obscuring diagnostically important guiding symptoms. It is, for example, problematic to sedate an agitated patient with a suspected intracranial bleed, because level of consciousness presents pivotal diagnostic data.

Psychopharmacology

Whether antidepressants should be started in the emergency room is discussed in Chapter 3. In elderly patients, we do not initiate either antidepressant therapy or lithium in the emergency setting. In addition to the arguments presented in Chapter 3, elderly patients are at a particularly high risk of developing side effects. As a rule, we recommend that lithium and antidepressants in elderly patients be started under the close supervision and monitoring conditions of an inpatient ward.

Antipsychotic medications have the same indications for elderly patients as outlined in Chapter 3. There is general agreement that in elderly people the use of smaller dosages is appropriate. This rule is based not only on empirical clinical data, but is founded in age-related pharmacokinetics.

We generally have found neuroleptics like perphenazine or thiothixene, which are midway between high extrapyramidal risk and high anticholinergic risk, to be least traumatic in the treatment of psychotic agitation in elderly patients. Otherwise, drug choice should take into consideration what worked well in the recent past, if such information is available.

Agitation without psychotic features may call for sedating drugs. Long-acting benzodiazepines have an inordinately prolonged half-life in elderly patients. This can be a problem as a significant hangover, lasting days, can result. Repeated administration can lead to undesirable accumulation of the drug. Even though shorter-acting benzodiazepines have been implicated in causing amnesia (Scharf et al. 1984), we have found them generally preferable for control of nonpsychotic agitation because of the less problematic kinetics. Prototypical drugs include lorazepam and oxazepam. Alternatively, short-acting barbiturates, such as amobarbital sodium, can be used if precautions are in place to avoid orthostatic accidents.

PROBLEMS IN DISPOSITION

Patients leave the emergency room to be admitted to the hospital, to return home, or to go to some alternative residential setting.

Hospitalization

General criteria for hospitalization have been discussed in detail in Chapter 5 of this manual. The factors influencing the decision to admit to a psychiatric inpatient ward apply to all age groups. In addition, in elderly patients, particular emphasis is placed on functional competence. Acute mental illness that in a younger patient could be handled by a brief on-site intervention and subsequent outpatient follow-up may require hospitalization in an elderly person who has aggravating physical handicaps. Examples include the depressed diabetic patient, or the person with advanced cataracts who has delusions of his food being poisoned. Absence of an adequate natural support system is a further complicating factor that can necessitate hospital admission.

The question often arises whether an elderly patient in the psychiatric emergency room ought to be admitted to a medical ward or to a psychiatric unit. "Dual diagnosis" in the geriatric population most often refers to mental and physical comorbidity.

Suicide risk, combative behavior, hallucinations, and delusional ideation weigh in the decision for admission to psychiatry. Impaired level of consciousness, unstable vital signs, and any conditions requiring intensive medical or surgical surveillance or treatment (e.g., myocardial infarction, acute abdomen) obviously require admission to a medical or surgical unit. Problems arise when presenting symptoms support either option. The combative patient with soft signs of a recent stroke or the highly suicidal dialysis patient in advanced renal failure are examples. Dispositional decisions depend on negotiated solutions between the emergency room psychiatrist and decision makers in the emergency medicine department. Both need to know resources and limitations on their respective services as to handling such patients: Can the medical ward restrain agitated patients? Does the psychiatric unit have facilities for intravenous therapy? In any case, it will help collaboration between services, and also between emergency room and inpatient sections, to initiate respective consultation follow-up from the time of admission.

Residential Care Options

There are many alternatives between the lonely old widow in her own home who strives to care for herself and the nursing-home resident who seems to have lost all autonomy and self-determination. Only 5% of Americans over 65 years of age live in institutions, but the fear of institutionalization is frequently present in the elderly patient presenting in the emergency room. Hospital admission can easily be perceived as a first step in this direction. This is one important reason why psychiatric hospitalization for elderly patients should be initiated only if less restrictive options are unsafe.

A visiting nurse, Meals on Wheels, or a professional homemaker can sometimes allay a home situation sufficiently to permit continued tenure in the original environment. Independent living arrangements in retirement centers, assisted living, group homes, family care homes, and, last, nursing homes represent various forms of residential care with incremental degrees of restrictiveness and supervision, structure, and protection. Local chapters of the American Association of Retired Persons or the Council on the Aging can be sources for information about residential settings that are available in the community. The emergency social service should be able to advise elderly patients and their relatives regarding access, levels of care, and financial implications of the various alternatives. Direct placement from the emergency room is, in our experience, rarely possible. But with the knowledge that in the near future a residential placement can be accomplished, family members can often be motivated to bridge the time by more active temporary involvement in supporting their disabled elders.

Nursing Homes

Nursing-home placement can be transient or permanent. The nursing home provides around-the-clock nursing care and supervision, albeit at a lower staff-to-patient ratio than hospitals. Active treatment is minimal, although dispensation of medication is provided and medical consultation is available. Institutional constraints generally impose regimentation and reduction in personal autonomy on all residents.

It is rare that a patient is directly admitted to a nursing home from the emergency room. Screening requirements of nursing homes are so extensive that this direct route is impracticable for the typical emergency service. Financial eligibility (private pay or Medicaid) has to be determined, and radiological tests and laboratory values (including syphilis serology) may need to be on record before a patient can be placed. Thus, in most cases, patients are admitted to nursing homes from inpatient hospital units, and nursing homes have often begun to fulfill the role of "step-down units" for partially recovered hospital patients. With appropriate assistance by social services, however, nursing-home placements can be made from the community, although more time is needed than if it is done from the hospital ward.

Sometimes such delay and continued tenure at home are intolerable for the care providers. Indeed, the emergency room psychiatrist may be confronted with patients sent *from* a nursing home. Typically in these cases, sudden onset of belligerent behavior led to the referral, and most often the patient suffers from moderate to severe dementia. Because demented patients become more agitated in situations of deficient sensory stimulation, these patients tend to come in during nights, or on weekends when nursing-home staffing is low.

Combative behaviors are intolerable in a nursing home. Caretakers and frail residents are at risk. In the emergency room, these patients present a dilemma. Admission to the hospital is of course possible. Frequently, these patients quickly calm down and do well in the structured ward milieu with constant redirection. Hospital staff will argue that the emergency room sent a patient "who did not need to be in the hospital." The original nursing home, on the other hand, clearly indicates that the patient must not return.

Ideally, the emergency room should send the patient to a clearinghouse facility for problematic dispositions. Patients could temporarily be boarded there while social services locate a psychiatric nursing home that can handle a patient with intermittent combativeness. A psychiatric nursing home has appropriately trained nurses, seclusion, and restraint facilities and access to on-site psychiatric consultation for psychopharmacologic interventions. Regular psychiatric acute-care wards in hospitals will frequently have to fulfill the function of a clearing station and holding environment until proper placement is accomplished.

REFERENCES

American Psychiatric Association: Diagnostic and Statistical Manual of Mental Disorders, 3rd Edition, Revised. Washington, DC, American Psychiatric Association, 1987

Blazer D, Williams CD: Epidemiology of dysphoria and depression in an elderly population. Am J Psychiatry 137:439–444, 1980

Cooper AF, Curry RA, Kay DWK, et al: Hearing loss in paranoid and affective psychosis of the elderly. Lancet 2:851–854,1974

Kiloh LG: Pseudo-dementia. Acta Psychiatr Scand 37:336–361, 1961

Law R, Chalmers C: Medicines and elderly people: a general practice survey. Br Med J 1:565–568, 1976

McAllister TW: Overview: pseudodementia. Am J Psychiatry 140:528–533, 1982

Myers JK, Weissman MM, Tischler GL, et al: Six-month prevalence of psychiatric disorders in three communities: 1980–1982. Arch Gen Psychiatry 41:959–967, 1984

National Institute of Mental Health: Utilization of mental health facilities 1971 (Mental Health Statistics Series B, No 5; DHEW Publ No NIH-74-657). Bethesda, MD, National Institute of Mental Health, 1973

Scharf MB, Khosla N, Brocker N, et al: Differential amnestic properties of short- and long-acting benzodiazepines. J Clin Psychiatry 45:51–53, 1984

Schneck MK, Reisberg B, Ferris SH: An overview of current concepts of Alzheimer's disease. Am J Psychiatry 139:165–173, 1982

Srole L, Fischer AK: The Midtown Manhattan Longitudinal Study vs. "The Mental Paradise Lost" doctrine. Arch Gen Psychiatry 37:209–221, 1980

Waxman HM, Carner EA, Dubin W, et al: Geriatric psychiatry in the emergency department: characteristics of geriatric and non-geriatric admissions. J Am Geriatr Soc 30:427–432, 1982

Weissman MM, Myers JK, Tischler GL, et al: Psychiatric disorders (DSM-III) and cognitive impairment among the elderly in a U.S. urban community. Acta Psychiatr Scand 71:366–379, 1985

Wells C: Pseudodementia. Am J Psychiatry 136:895–900, 1979

Zechnich RJ: Beta-blockers can obscure diagnosis of delirium tremens. Lancet 1:1071–1072, 1982

Chapter 26

Emergency Room "Repeaters"

G.A. Barker, M.D.

Psychiatric emergency services were developed to provide a site for evaluation, acute treatment, and referral. They are unique in that there are no boundaries to their service. All who register will be seen. The service consumer decides what constitutes an emergency.

In reviewing the literature, Nurius (1983–1984) noted that over the last two decades there have been significant changes in both the quantity and type of services provided. Psychiatric emergency services now serve as key entry points into the mental health service network, as gatekeepers between hospital and community, as primary care givers, and, at times, as the sole source of treatment (Gerson and Bassuk 1980). This change in functioning creates strain for the psychiatric emergency service staff, who may cling to the original mission and perceive other uses to be inappropriate or even abusive. No group of patients stirs these feelings up more than the emergency room "repeaters" who "repeatedly seek help for very complex psychosocial problems, yet may not respond to traditional emergency interventions." In various studies, "repeaters constitute 7–18% of psychiatric emergency service patients and account for up to a third of the total visits" (Ellison et al. 1986, p. 37).

The goal of this chapter is to summarize what is currently known about these repeaters and, from there, to develop an informed approach to their care.

DEMOGRAPHIC CHARACTERISTICS

A recent review of the literature on emergency room repeaters noted that the following characteristics are strongly associated with repeaters versus nonrepeaters (Ellison et al. 1986):

- Lack of social supports
- Prior psychiatric history
- Current psychiatric treatment
- Chronic psychiatric illness (schizophrenia, personality disorder, or alcoholism)

Available evidence further suggests that repeaters may often be

- 31–50 years of age
- Female
- Unmarried
- Unemployed
- Suicidal

Race, educational level, risk of homicide, or alcohol abuse could not differentiate repeaters from nonrepeaters.

Repeaters were more likely than nonrepeaters to be brought to the emergency service involuntarily for their first visit, but were usually self-referred for subsequent visits. Their repeat visits were anecdotally felt to be briefer and associated with alcohol abuse. Repeaters were more likely to be hospitalized.

Repeaters have been called problem patients, clutter, abusers, and chronic crisis patients. They have been characterized as dependent, manipulative, hostile, entitled, help rejecting, provocative, and enraging. These words reflect the intense affect generated in the staff assigned to their care, but offer little in terms of understanding the patients.

PROPOSED SUBGROUPS OF PSYCHIATRIC EMERGENCY SERVICE REPEATERS

Various clinicians have suggested subgrouping the repeaters to guide further treatment and research (Bassuk and Gerson 1980; Ellison et al. 1986; Gerson and Bassuk 1980; Kass et al. 1979; Mannon 1976; Nurius 1983–1984; Raphling and Lion 1970; Santy and Wehmeier 1984). The following subgroupings are an elaboration of those suggested by others in keeping with our experience in the psychiatric emergency service at the University of Cincinnati.

Repeat Patients Actively Involved in Psychotherapy

Some emergency room repeaters use the emergency service to help them manage their transference. These patients, with diagnoses in the border-line-narcissistic spectrum of personality disorders, have a well-known difficulty tolerating the intimacy and regression invoked by psychody-namic psychotherapy. At various stages in therapy, the regression may exceed the person's capacity to defend against it. The road to growth is not a smooth one.

Presenting symptoms. These may consist of severe anxiety, inabil-ity to function, self-mutilation, suicidal ideation or attempt, egodystonic behaviors, acute psychotic symptoms, substance use or abuse, or mood fluctuations.

Patients' feelings about their relationship with their therapist and their preoccupation with the therapeutic process are generally prominent during the evaluation. This does not, however, imply that they see a connection between their therapy and the symptoms precipitating the visit to the psychiatric emergency room.

Precipitants. Situations that predictably evoke crises in therapy are the most likely to precipitate an emergency psychiatric visit. These include vacations, terminations, or a change in treatment plan. Exam-ples of the latter include a change in the frequency of sessions, the addition of a medication or a collaborator, contact with supervisors, hospital discharge, or a significant change in fees. At times, the uncover-ing of highly charged material may leave the patient feeling too vulnera-ble to function. The exploration and uncovering of childhood sexual abuse seems to be particularly difficult in this regard.

Psychiatric emergency service approach. It is important to under-stand the psychiatric emergency service visit in the context of the ongoing psychotherapy. The primary therapist should be contacted. It is important to understand the meaning that this contact will have for the patient, and its impact on the future therapy as well as the use of the emergency room. Is the patient unable to communicate something to the therapist directly? Is the patient seeking special attention or reacting to a particularly painful empathic break?

In contacting the therapist, the emergency staff is 1) accessing data necessary to construct an effective emergency intervention, 2) sharing information with the therapist about symptoms that need to be addressed in the long-term therapy, and 3) helping to clarify a treatment plan. If part of the treatment plan (spoken or unspoken), is for the patient to use the psychiatric emergency service when in crisis, then the service is serving a "cotherapy" role. The more clearly this role is articulated, the more helpful the psychiatric emergency service can be. Without this collaborative effort, the potential for splitting and diminution of treatment effect is increased. This role may include

- *Containment.* Patients may need a safe place or increased support in critical times. There are numerous possible interventions that range from a brief or an extended evaluation to an overnight stay, or to hospitalization. Patients, at times, request restraints. Although the reasons may vary, it is clear that they fear loss of control, and the limits set by restraints help them to gather their composure.

- *Clarification of the relationship between symptoms and therapy.* The process of therapy is, at times, difficult to discuss, particularly if it involves erotic or angry transferences. Working with psychiatric emergency service staff may help clarify transference issues and allow discussion of this material in a less threatening manner. In effect, the staff may provide a consultation to the community therapist as well as tend to the patient's crisis.

- *Support of the therapeutic dyad.* The emergency service may help the dyad by providing an outlet for the patient that is "too hot to handle." Psychiatric emergency intervention may help to dilute the transference to a manageable level and allow the therapist to set and maintain reasonable therapeutic limits, i.e., no calls after midnight, no more than three calls per day, go to the psychiatric emergency service if suicidal, etc.

Repeat Patients in Concurrent Case Management Model Treatment

This distinction is notably artificial, but refers to patients who are not involved as intensively in treatment as psychodynamic psychotherapy patients. Descriptively, these patients generally have an Axis I diagnosis and are involved in traditional aftercare-type treatment. This usually entails working with a nonphysician therapist or case manager and a collaborating physician who prescribes medication.

Although the treatment relationship may well be a concern, the management of transference is less obviously an issue here. The major factor in repeated presentations to the emergency service is a more overt denial of the need for ongoing treatment, or a limited engagement in that process. Both the care givers and the patient contribute in a variable way to the situation. Although the patients are frequently labeled noncompliant, therapists often fail to be optimally responsive to their needs, and in this situation, crises can be predicted.

Presenting symptoms.   Presenting requests include

- *Request for medication by a patient on a known maintenance medication.* This can occur in the context of a missed appointment, a move to a new geographical area, discharge from an institution, and inability to access the community system, etc.

- *Request for medication evaluation.* Patients may feel an urgent need to have their medication changed when they experience intolerable side effects, especially extrapyramidal side effects or oversedation, insomnia, psychotic or depressive symptoms, aggression, or failure to improve.

- *Request for hospitalization.* Patients generally seek admission in the context of suicidal or homicidal ideation, inability to function, or loss of hope in outpatient treatment or when they feel that they need a rest.

Psychiatric emergency service approach.   Noncompliance is a complex problem to which patients undeniably contribute. Clinicians are generally skilled in assessing patient contribution and note personality characteristics, lack of social support, and denial of illness as major factors in noncompliance. Since blaming the patient is something in which we already have so much skill, this section will concentrate on the alternative position of blaming the system. In fact, multiple factors from both sides contribute in all but rare cases, and the more comprehensively that is understood, the more therapeutic our interventions will become.

In most communities, care to this group of patients is provided by understaffed community mental health centers in which therapists and case managers have larger than ideal caseloads and access to physicians is limited. Medication evaluation and hospital admission are services generally restricted to physicians. The current system is not designed to handle emergent requests for these types of services. Psychiatric emergency services, on the other hand, have immediate access to physicians who can provide this service. As gatekeeper, they are frequently the most direct route to hospital admission, a fact resourceful patients and families learn quickly.

For patients and their families who have limited choice of care providers and must use the public mental health system, use of the psychiatric emergency service can provide them with a forum for obtaining a second opinion and a serious evaluation of symptoms that were not addressed seriously enough in their ongoing treatment.

The psychiatric emergency service staff must understand both the current request and the patient's current involvement in treatment. Why is the patient presenting to the emergency service rather than to the ongoing care providers?

Contact the therapist or case manager. It is not a desirable option for the psychiatric emergency service to become the primary treatment site for patients needing ongoing care. With a repeat patient, the service is in the position of sharing the care, or collaborating with the primary-care provider. Contact with the therapist or case manager provides a forum for obtaining information about a patient's baseline and current level of function and an assessment of the treatment plan. Having to articulate a plan to the psychiatric emergency service staff may help to clear up ambiguity.

Care must be taken to support the primary relationship. One way of doing this is to develop an intervention that is actually carried out at the mental health center, or by making a change that is to be followed up in a very specific way by the ongoing clinician. One example of this would be making a medication change with a plan that the community mental health center psychiatrist would follow up at the next appointment.

At times, the patient will have been referred to the psychiatric emergency service by the therapist. The therapist's request must be addressed. At times, they are seeking support of their treatment plan or of a change they are unable to effect. If, for instance, they disagree with the community mental health center psychiatrist, they may refer the patient to the psychiatric emergency service for a second opinion. A recognition that this is the dilemma and encouragement to resolve it at the community mental health center may, in that case, be the most appropriate intervention. Sending records of the emergency visit with the assessment and plan as a consultation may be helpful in removing an impasse.

Repeat Patients Unable to Engage in Treatment

Patients unable to engage in treatment are the ones that evoke intense negative feelings in the emergency room staff. They are most frequently diagnosed with borderline personality disorder, but many have an Axis I diagnosis as well. Despite repeated attempts to engage these patients in ongoing treatment, they fail to follow through on a consistent basis and continue to present to the emergency room with requests for help.

Presenting symptoms and precipitants.   Bassuk and Gerson (1980) called these patients "chronic crisis patients." Seeming to move from one psychosocial crisis to the next without enhanced ability to cope, they have frequent need of crisis intervention services. Their presentation varies from vague somatic complaints to very specific requests for services. Precipitants vary but generally result from a change in interpersonal relationships or from demands for the patient to assume increased personal responsibility.

It seems that as crises resolve, these patients resume their previous level of maladaptive function, failing to learn from their experiences.

Psychiatric emergency service approach.   Containment and engagement, protracted processes that develop in the context of multiple visits, are the therapeutic long-range goal for this type of repeating patient. The major obstacle in the attainment of this goal is the intensely negative affect developed in the staff by these very difficult patients. Interactions are emotionally charged and exhausting. Some understanding of the interpersonal dynamics will help staff to remain empathic.

These patients request urgent resolution of their problems and relief of discomfort. They seem to endow emergency room staff with the omnipotent fantasy that they will be able to invoke a treatment that will definitively relieve their symptoms. They come with a helpless attitude, but with a feeling that they are entitled to special treatment for their very severe distress. Their wishes are not based on reality, and as concrete, limited options are developed, the fantasy is challenged. The patients respond with angry, frequently escalating demands for other options or services. They feel that special services are being withheld. At times a struggle ensues, and the offered help may be rejected, leaving both parties enraged.

These patients have severe difficulties with relationships. They are unable to negotiate a comfortable distance and vary from feeling isolated to feeling engulfed. Their ability to use psychiatric emergency services on a drop-in basis and to see different staff members on different visits makes this an attractive "treatment" site. The complex negotiations that occur in trying to find an appropriate disposition, however, exacerbate these problems. Needing to be taken care of exists side by side with fears of being controlled. In this situation, any plan suggested by the therapist can result in an unpleasant struggle. Each person has power in the negotiation. The staff controls access to resources, whereas the patient has control over his or her behavior, particularly regarding threats of suicide and violence. The current legal climate further empowers the patient.

Staff can acquire emotional distance and objectivity by considering the developing difficult interaction in terms of object relations theory. The intense interactions repeat some aspects of disturbed early relationships. Processing the evaluation with other staff can also help penetrate the countertransference.

It is advisable to try to avoid struggling with the patient. After a careful evaluation, it is best to empathically summarize the current situation and straightforwardly describe the available options for obtaining help. Staff can answer questions generated by the patient in a very simple and straightforward manner. Patients have considerable knowledge about the system from the consumer perspective and can be engaged in the treatment process by acknowledging their expertise as greater than the staff's in this area, i.e., because they have visited many programs that staff know about only secondhand. This encourages a collaborative, nonregressed approach and also decreases the likelihood that patients will feel violated by the treatment plan. It may be important to address the inability of previous referrals, as well as the emergency service, to be of lasting benefit. The limits of what can be provided must be detailed in an explicit manner, so that over time, the patient will understand the available options in a more realistic way.

These patients have difficulty controlling their behavior and their feelings. Therapeutic limits that may vary from taking a time-out, to the use of restraints, to the extreme of filing legal charges must be explained and consistently implemented.

The literature indicates that these patients are hospitalized more frequently than other mentally ill groups. This is likely due to their lack of social supports as well as the marked difficulties in interpersonal interactions. In general, hospitalizations should be short, as the danger of severe regression is real.

To achieve stabilization in the community, one service must assume the role of the primary-care provider. If the patient seeks help at multiple sites, interagency communication is essential to avoid splitting and to allow for the implementation of any ongoing treatment plan. Likewise, communication among the multiple staff members in a given agency must be carefully maintained. Problem-patient rounds have been suggested as one method of developing a consistent treatment plan (Santy and Wehmeier 1984).

If engagement is successful, the patient will ultimately form a transference to the emergency service that will help him or her maintain an optimal level of function (Raphling and Lion 1970).

Patients Who Make Psychiatric Emergency Services Part of Their Social Network

This is a diagnostically heterogeneous group of chronic patients who have a low baseline level of function and few social supports. In relatively stable periods, they continue to present to the psychiatric emergency service by telephone or in person, to talk or to request food, bus tokens, or coffee. They are generally well known to the staff, who may have been actively involved in their treatment during a less stable period. This type of contact is generally initiated because of positive associations to the staff, loneliness, and a desire for the special treatment they may have received while they were ill.

The staff regards these patients alternately as nuisances or as "regulars." The latter does have some special, familiar status. It is helpful to develop a plan that allows patients some access to staff while affirming their now-improved status. Allowing them contact with the triage nurse on an as-needed basis without registering, scheduled contacts with an identified staff member, or informal brief entries into the service to say hello may all be legitimate options. It is generally not a good idea to provide food or tokens on request. Limits must be clearly defined and maintained to avoid future disappointments.

Patients With Repeated Visits in the Midst of an Acute Crisis

Because staff generally view this to be a legitimate use of the emergency service, little needs to be said. At times, one effort at crisis intervention is not enough, and patients return to the emergency service rather than to some other community resource.

References

Bassuk E, Gerson S: Chronic crisis patients: a discrete clinical group. Am J Psychiatry 137:1513–1517, 1980

Ellison JM, Blum N, Barsky AJ: Repeat visitors in the psychiatric emergency service: a critical review of the data. Hosp Community Psychiatry 37:37–41, 1986

Gerson S, Bassuk E: Psychiatric emergencies: an overview. Am J Psychiatry 137:1–11, 1980

Kass F, Karasu TB, Walsh T: Emergency room patients in concurrent therapy: a neglected clinical phenomenon. Am J Psychiatry 136:91–92, 1979

Mannon JM: Defining and treating problem patients in a hospital emergency room. Med Care 14:1004–1013, 1976

Nurius PS: Emergency psychiatric services: a study of changing utilization patterns and issues. Int J Psychiatry Med 13:239–254, 1983–1984

Raphling DL, Lion J: Patients with repeated admissions to a psychiatric emergency service. Community Ment Health J 16:313–318, 1970

Santy PA, Wehmeier PK: Using problem patient rounds to help emergency room staff manage difficult patients. Hosp Community Psychiatry 35:494–496, 1984

Chapter 27

The Homeless Mentally Ill

G.A. Barker, M.D.

The phenomenon of homelessness in America has received increasing attention in both the popular and the professional literature. Although estimates vary widely, these sources indicate that approximately 40% of the total homeless population have a major mental illness (i.e., schizophrenia, other psychotic disorders, or a major affective disorder). These are the people who would have lived out their lives in state hospitals in the era before deinstitutionalization (Lamb and Talbot 1986).

Homelessness has been defined by the Alcohol, Drug Abuse, and Mental Health Administration as a condition characterized by lack of adequate shelter, resources, and community ties (Bachrach 1984). Bassuk (1983) described it as "more than the lack of a home, it is a metaphor for profound disconnection from other people and institutions." It is a complex problem with many contributing factors. The increased numbers of mentally ill homeless persons are generally attributed to deinstitutionalization without adequate community supports, and to the large number of young adults currently at risk for mental illness.

Homelessness is a characteristic rather than a diagnosis. It will compound any psychiatric assessment or intervention. There is much overlap among subpopulations of the chronically mentally ill, many of whom may be homeless during some phase of their lives. Information about emergency room repeaters, "young chronics," and patients with severe personality disorders will be relevant to this population.

353

CHARACTERISTICS OF THE HOMELESS MENTALLY ILL

The vast majority of studies that examine the homeless mentally ill have found that the prototype patient is a 30- to 50-year-old man, who has been an area resident for a considerable period of time (Bachrach 1984). Although homelessness affects women, women are less likely to survive homelessness. Families and society at large are more protective of women. Prostitution is also more readily available to women as a source of money and temporary shelter (Ball and Havassey 1984).

The homeless report sleeping in a variety of shelters which include abandoned buildings, parking lots, parked cars, outdoor shelters, missions, detoxification centers, bus or subway stations, jails, or with friends or family. They frequently provide a history of eviction from hotels, apartments, or private residences because of conflicts related to their behavior. The vast majority have no source of funds. Some receive social security income, money from family, or income from odd jobs. When surveyed, most reported feeling frightened on the streets because of the threat of personal assault or robbery.

BIOPSYCHOSOCIAL PERSPECTIVE

Biological Considerations

Diagnostically, the majority (greater than 60%) of homeless mentally ill persons suffer from schizophrenia (Cohen et al. 1984). Substance abuse is a primary or complicating factor in nearly half of the identified patients. Personality disorders, affective disorders, organic brain syndromes, and mental retardation have also been noted in varying percentages in different studies. As a generalization, the homeless mentally ill exhibit the most severe forms of the mental illnesses, frequently compounded by substance abuse and medical illness.

Anecdotal accounts suggest that negative symptoms of schizophrenia (anhedonia, social withdrawal, etc.) predominate in the homeless mentally ill. Intriguing work in the fields of clinical brain imaging and the neurosciences suggests the view that this type of schizophrenia "is a frontal lobe disease resulting from gross structural damage or selective damage to dopaminergic neurons. . . . Several converging lines of evidence suggest specific dysfunction of the prefrontal cortex in chronic schizophrenia, alcoholic dementia, and possibly poor-prognosis bipolar disorder" (Kaufmann 1984, p. 202), other major conditions associated with homelessness.

Impairment of the prefrontal cortex will result in difficulties in anticipation and provisional memory, in suppressing interference, and in maintaining attention. These deficits, which may be the final common pathway of severe bipolar disorder, alcoholism, and schizophrenia, interfere, therefore, with the ability to plan and execute a course of action.

The prevalence of physical illness among the homeless is also noted to be very high, and the mortality rate is four times that of their peers. This is not surprising as they are susceptible to all known diseases and live in an environment that would aggravate them all. They are particularly at risk for syndromes related to exposure, substance abuse, violence, contagion, and nutritional deficiencies. In particular, most reviews note the following diagnoses as common (Brickner et al. 1984).

- Extremity damage related to frostbite or, paradoxically, from burns obtained while seeking heat from grates or steam vents
- Syndromes associated with alcohol withdrawal or abuse, e.g., pancreatitis, liver dysfunction, delirium, Korsakoff's psychosis
- Cardiac decompensation
- Dependent edema that may lead to peripheral vascular disease, cellulitis, and leg ulcers
- Syndromes associated with physical assault including subdural hematomas
- Contagious diseases of all types, from tuberculosis to acquired immunodeficiency syndrome (AIDS)
- Infestation with scabies or lice
- Chronic obstructive pulmonary disease (COPD) secondary to heavy smoking
- Hypertension

At least one in four homeless persons presenting in an emergency room will have a medical illness requiring treatment. Acute treatment can frequently be implemented in the hospital, but effective follow-up is a near impossibility. There are no safe places for the patient to store medication, and no reasonable facilities to maintain personal hygiene. Calendars and clocks are not an ongoing part of the homeless world.

Psychological Considerations

Each person is an individual with his or her own history and perspective. An understanding of this is generally essential to any psychiatric evaluation. Many homeless people, however, have a problem with trust. The etiology is variable. It may, for some, be a symptom of an underlying paranoid disorder, but for many, it is a learned response to a hostile society and mental health system. It expresses itself in the refusal to provide historical information, which may include their names. Homeless people are also disinclined to reveal where they sleep. The desire to maintain anonymity may make people flee from traditional clinic intake or emergency registration. In a survey of homeless mental health consumers, they indicated near unanimous concern with problems related to lack of material resources, employment opportunities, privacy, and protection. Their desire for the medical and psychiatric services offered by community-based agencies was a much lower priority. Despite their multiple disadvantages, they were amazingly adaptive in their ability to locate and obtain some level of food and shelter (Ball and Havassey 1984).

Psychiatric histories vary considerably. Some of these people are truly the deinstitutionalized, whereas others have never been hospitalized and have no clear identity as a "mental patient." This lack of identity contributes to the psychological factors that draw people to the street and may serve to keep them there. "Homeless" may be a better identity than "mentally ill." People on the streets can see themselves as the victims of their socioeconomic position rather than as the victims of an illness. Homelessness may present emancipation to people with an institutional history.

Those episodically homeless persons whose diagnosis would be in the realm of personality disorder and/or substance abuse have a different dynamic. They tend to live in a world characterized by a series of crises created by interpersonal conflict. Difficulties with intimacy, independence, and entitlement create ongoing conflicts in relationships. When the relationships are disrupted, housing needs may be disrupted as well.

People in both groups may be in the unfortunate position of having "burned all of their bridges behind them." Histories of violence, sexual abuse, fire setting, and failure to follow through with a recommended treatment program can preclude many options for referral or reunion with family.

Social Factors

As noted previously, in the very definition of homelessness, the homeless are disenfranchised from mainstream society. They are frequently people who have burned out their social network by seemingly repeated rejection of help. Homeless people then become part of the street culture. The increasing visibility of the chronically mentally ill in this group has notably changed its character. They are, in many cases, disenfranchised from that group as well and seem to be "space cases." Understanding the local street culture may be essential to providing service to this group of people. Perceptions of personal worth, time, space, and other priorities bear special attention.

SUBGROUPS

Even among the mentally ill homeless, there seem to be several distinct groups. Arce et al. (1983) defined three groups in their study of people admitted to an emergency shelter:

- *Street people*. These were people who lived regularly on the street. The typical street person was a white individual over the age of 40 with a diagnosis of schizophrenia, substance abuse, or both. In general, this person would have a history of state hospitalizations and a variety of medical problems.
- *The episodically homeless*. People in this group were temporarily homeless. They had been housed within the last month. The typical episodically homeless person was under 40 years of age and black. History revealed sporadic contact with various agencies, but no history of state hospital admission. The diagnosis was more likely to be personality disorder, affective disorder, or substance abuse.
- *Other*. These were people who were not chronically homeless, but who were undergoing an acute situational crisis that precluded shelter on a given day.

It is also conceivable that the homeless could be divided into those that actively reject help versus those to whom outreach has not yet been made.

EMERGENCY EVALUATION OF THE HOMELESS

Emergency rooms frequently become the primary care site for homeless individuals. Some surveys of psychiatric emergency services have reported 30–40% of the patients to be homeless (Ball and Havassey 1984; Lipton et al. 1983).

The overarching goal of all contacts with the homeless is engagement, a process that occurs over time. Each visit provides an opportunity and a possibility. Engagement will come through positive human contact and the provision of concrete and appropriate services by a clinician who is knowledgeable about the population, flexible, optimistic, creative, and active. Providing food and cigarettes will facilitate the interview in most cases.

The evaluation itself is frequently brief and may be limited to referral information from police or life squad, plus the interview, and any necessary physical examination. Collateral contacts are generally unavailable. It is, however, worthwhile to contact the family if at all possible.

The family, if they can be contacted, is generally able to provide missing historical information and may be quite relieved to hear about their relative. Although some families may have more or less disowned their family member, others may be anxiously searching for them. The role of the clinician is not to make the family take responsibility for the situation, but to seek and provide helpful information. In the event that a family has been searching for a wandering family member and wishes to facilitate their return, Traveler's Aid is a helpful referral.

As previously noted, homeless people are at risk for multiple medical problems. Sufficient screening must occur in the emergency room to ensure that these can be adequately addressed during the intervention. In addition to the screening examination noted in Chapter 2, it is important to examine the extremities of the homeless individual, because these are frequently affected by exposure (i.e., take off the patient's shoes). Unfortunately, many identified problems remain untreated because they are not life threatening and are of limited concern to the patient preoccupied with daily survival.

Emergency Psychiatric Interventions for the Homeless

There are a limited number of interventions available to the homeless mentally ill. Those that are available vary considerably from community to community. This population is often completely dependent on the public health, social service, and mental health systems for their care. Generally, no one agency views itself as responsible for the patient. Each will provide services only within its specialty. Thus, even when an ideal treatment plan can be envisioned, it may not be carried out.

Frequently, the system itself needs the intervention. Emergency staff can be advocates for this type of systems change. As the clinicians most often confronted with the problem, they are in the best position to work with local mental health authorities to develop assertively provided psychiatric services that offer individualized assessment, treatment, and continuity of care. This involvement will reduce staff burnout as well as benefit the system. Guidelines for treatment are provided in the American Psychiatric Association task force report *The Homeless Mentally Ill*, published in 1984 (Lamb 1984b).

Hospitalization

As noted earlier, there are distinct subgroups of homeless persons, all of whom challenge the emergency clinician. Homeless persons present a continuum from the obviously mentally ill person who rejects hospitalization to the not-so-mentally-ill person who desires hospitalization for shelter.

In the former group, failure to hospitalize is often an acknowledgment that treatment will not be provided. Shelter is essential to the success of any treatment intervention. Emergency clinicians work by deciding what type of treatment has the best likelihood of being helpful. It is, therefore, demoralizing to recognize that a person might benefit significantly from a medication trial, but be unable to initiate this because of the uncertainty of follow-ups and lack of supervision. Hospitalization should be recommended when clear goals can be identified that require the intensive resources that a hospital can offer.

The criteria for involuntary hospitalization are the same for the homeless as for other mentally ill persons. However, in periods of extreme weather, homeless psychotic persons are more likely to meet the "inability to care for self" criteria of involuntary treatment. Likewise, their lack of social supports intensifies their risk of acting on suicidal or violent impulses. Although the dangerousness standard for commitment has been cited as a major factor in homelessness among the mentally ill (Lamb 1984a), at least one study has failed to show that patients judged to be highly in need of treatment were denied access to it on the basis of commitment law (Cleveland et al. 1989).

Communities have responded variously to the need for shelter or specialized nonhospital residential settings. If these are available, they provide additional treatment options by supplying at least interim shelter where treatment can be offered. At times, this is a part of the program, as in a detoxification or crisis stabilization center; at other times, it is ancillary to it, as in a domiciliary (Louks and Smith 1988) or supported housing opportunity. Emergency room clinicians may need to develop a treatment plan that engages the patient as well as the staff of several programs. This requires an extensive, assertive approach on the part of the emergency clinician, who may need to awaken a last hope in a patient who would benefit from treatment but does not meet criteria for involuntary admission.

The nonpsychotic homeless person creates a different set of problems. Because symptoms related to a personality disorder are less likely to benefit from a brief hospitalization, it is more productive to try to resolve the interpersonal crisis that resulted in homelessness, or to offer some combination of shelter and outpatient treatment. Patients in this group have difficulty not in accessing services, but in maintaining engagement. In crisis, they will usually seek help from multiple sources. They typically present threatening suicide unless they are hospitalized.

An extended evaluation which may include an overnight stay in the emergency room may provide enough time and nurturance to allow the person to consider other alternatives. Access to a continuum of emergency shelters will help emergency staff provide helpful interventions and avoid hospitalizations that are really social service emergencies. This should include some access to emergency funding for single-room-occupancy–type housing and drop-in centers.

Outpatient Referrals

Homeless persons with a major mental disorder have already graphically demonstrated that they are unable or unwilling to participate in the "system" as it is. An outpatient referral is likely to be an exercise in futility unless the community has some type of assertive case management system that can begin to work with the person in the emergency room or on the streets. Effective interventions minimize the cracks through which a person may fall.

Each visit is an opportunity to engage the patient in treatment. Encouraging the use of the emergency service on an as-needed basis to obtain medication may be a more realistic option than referral to intake at a mental health center. Patients are more likely to return if the service is relevant to them. For example, a problem with insomnia or hallucinations may be treated with medication. At times, shelter staff can help a patient make a follow-up appointment by offering a reminder or providing transportation.

EMERGENCY INTERVENTIONS IN OTHER SETTINGS

Services are moving in the direction of the guidelines proposed in the American Psychiatric Association task force report (Lamb 1984b). There are outreach programs in many major cities; Project Reach Out and the Manhattan Bowery Corporation's Midtown Outreach Program in New York are two such programs (Levine 1984). Both of these projects attempt to engage the homeless in treatment by visiting them on the streets where they live. The mobile psychiatric outreach team has the capacity to transport patients involuntarily if they are judged to be dangerous to themselves or others by the psychiatrist.

Services are being taken to the patients at shelters and drop-in centers in many communities. Evaluations in these settings begin as the clinicians become part of their world—a familiar face who might be able to offer something tangibly helpful. Engagement, as noted earlier, is an ongoing process that might proceed inconsistently. It is important to talk with people where they are for as much time as they will allow. Assessments are usually based on the level of function and symptoms. Note taking usually interferes with the discussion. If an opportunity presents itself to offer treatment, it is better to provide the actual medicine rather than a prescription, and likewise to accompany patients as they follow up on referrals. The provision of tangible resources like food and clothing may facilitate engagement and follow-up.

> A central recommendation of the task force was for a system of responsibility for the mentally ill living in the community . . . with the goal of ensuring that ultimately each patient has one person responsible for his or her care . . . such case management is best provided by a skilled mental health professional. . . . He or she provides what may in some ways be seen as the ultimate extension of supportive psychodynamic psychotherapy. (p. 578)

This idea offered by Goldfinger (Frances and Goldfinger 1986) makes an analogy between assertive case management and psychotherapy. Psychotherapists modify their treatment to respond to the developmental needs of their patients. They offer more supportive interventions to the more seriously disturbed. Therapeutic case management can be seen as a further step on this continuum.

Emergency services are a first step in a response to homelessness. Far beyond a need for shelters, the homeless need a series of targeted services so they can develop the skills needed to reengage in the world (Brenda and Dattalo 1988).

REFERENCES

Arce AA, Tadlock M, Vergare MJ, et al: A psychiatric profile of street people admitted to an emergency shelter. Hosp Community Psychiatry 34:812–816, 1983

Bachrach LL: The homeless mentally ill and mental health services: an analytic review of the literature, in The Homeless Mentally Ill: A Task Force Report of the American Psychiatric Association. Edited by Lamb HR. Washington, DC, American Psychiatric Press, 1984, pp 11–53

Ball FLJ, Havassey BE: A survey of the problem and needs of homeless consumers of acute psychiatric services. Hosp Community Psychiatry 35:917–921, 1984

Bassuk EL: Addressing the needs of the homeless. Boston Globe Magazine, Nov 6, 1983, p 12, 60ff

Brenda BB, Dattalo P: Homelessness: consequence of a crisis or a long term process? Hosp Community Psychiatry 39:884–886, 1988

Brickner PW, Filardo T, Iseman M, et al: Medical aspects of homelessness, in The Homeless Mentally Ill: A Task Force Report of the American Psychiatric Association. Edited by Lamb HR. Washington, DC, American Psychiatric Press, 1984, pp 243–259

Cleveland S, Mulvey EP, Appelbaum PS, et al: Do dangerousness-oriented commitment laws restrict hospitalization of patients who need treatment? A test. Hosp Community Psychiatry 40:266–271, 1989

Cohen NL, Putman JF, Sullivan AM: The mentally ill homeless: isolation and adaptation. Hosp Community Psychiatry 35:922–924, 1984

Frances A, Goldfinger SM: Treating a homeless mentally ill patient who cannot be managed in the shelter system. Hosp Community Psychiatry 37:577–579, 1986

Kaufmann CA: Implications of biological psychiatry for the severely mentally ill: a highly vulnerable population, in The Homeless Mentally Ill: A Task Force Report of the American Psychiatric Association. Edited by Lamb HR. Washington, DC, American Psychiatric Press, 1984, pp 201–242

Lamb HR: Deinstitutionalization and the homeless mentally ill. Hosp Community Psychiatry 35:899–907, 1984a

Lamb HR (ed): The Homeless Mentally Ill: A Task Force Report of the American Psychiatric Association. Washington, DC, American Psychiatric Press, 1984b

Lamb HR, Talbot JA: The homeless mentally ill, the perspective of the American Psychiatric Association. JAMA 256:498–501, 1986

Levine IS: Service program for the homeless mentally ill, in The Homeless Mentally Ill: A Task Force Report of the American Psychiatric Association. Edited by Lamb HR. Washington, DC, American Psychiatric Press, 1984, pp 173–200

Lipton FR, Sabatini A, Katz S: Down and out in the city: the homeless mentally ill. Hosp Community Psychiatry 34:817–821, 1983

Louks JL, Smith JR: Homeless: Axis I disorders. Hosp Community Psychiatry 39:670–671, 1988

Chapter 28

Ethnic Minorities

J.R. Hillard, M.D.

An emergency service is a place where cultures collide. Under non-emergency circumstances, members of any given cultural group will usually seek understanding and help within their own culture. When a situation is defined as an emergency, they have little choice about where to seek help. The emergency clinician also has little choice about when or how to treat. It would be nice to have completed a detailed ethnographic study of, say, the Hmong people before treating Hmong patients, but, of course, it is not possible to ask an emergency patient to "come back when I have finished studying your culture."

It is a good idea to familiarize yourself as much as possible with the cultures and histories of ethnic groups that use your service. In the United States today there are, however, enough distinct ethnic groups that you will frequently need to work with patients from cultures that you have not had a chance to study. This chapter will highlight some variables to keep in mind when dealing with patients from unfamiliar cultures and will point out some ways in which cultural misunderstandings can lead to errors in diagnosis and treatment. The references cited in this chapter and the suggested readings will give more detailed information about the cultures of a number of different ethnic groups.

LANGUAGE

There may be serious medicolegal, as well as clinical, consequences of trying to evaluate a patient without adequate translation services. It is best to have a professional translator, next best to have a volunteer, and still less good to have only a family member doing the translation. An independent translator is preferable, even if there is a family member available who can translate. As noted below, having a family member available to help with evaluation of a patient from another culture is enormously helpful. If, however, a family member is the only interpreter for a patient, there is danger of the family member's preconceptions, conflicts of interest, or emotional overinvolvement coloring the translation you receive (Marcos 1979). It has been suggested that affective components of illness may tend to be underestimated when using translators, whereas thought disorder symptoms translate more easily. Some cases of completed suicide have been ascribed to this loss of information in the translation process (Sabin 1975). For this reason, affective symptoms need to be searched for with particular care when working through an interpreter.

Even when a patient speaks English fairly well as a second language, it may still be a good idea to use a translator because symptoms may be expressed differently in a patient's primary and secondary languages. There is some suggestion that schizophrenic patients may, in some cases, appear more disorganized in their secondary languages (Marcos et al. 1973), whereas, in other cases, they are able to talk about symptoms only in their primary language (Del Castillo 1970).

Psychiatric hospitalization can be an alienating and isolating experience for anyone, but can be especially so for those hospitalized in a facility where few of the staff can understand anything they say. For this reason, hospitalization in a facility that mainly uses another language than the patient's should be avoided, if at all possible.

FAMILY STRUCTURE

Although the nuclear family (mother, father, and dependent children living together, having only minor contact with other relatives) is the dominant pattern in American society today, it is probably the exception, rather than the rule, among cultures worldwide. Most cultures involve a more extended family with more generations involved in child rearing and other family functions and with greater involvement of uncles, aunts, and cousins in each other's lives. In addition, different cultures have different standards for when adulthood has been reached for the purpose of marriage, work, child care, and other functions. In fact, among some groups, full adulthood is not recognized until one is married or has children. It is important not to jump too quickly to the conclusion that an extended family is "pathological" or "enmeshed" or "infantilizing." Not only "exotic" cultures, but also black (Stack 1975), Appalachian (Philliber and McCoy 1981), and Hispanic cultures are ordinarily made up of extended family groups.

Understanding the de facto family structure for a particular patient will allow a better assessment of the social supports actually available. Understanding the authority relationships within the family system will also allow you to form an alliance with those family members who are in the best position to ensure patient cooperation with treatment. For example, the mother-in-law of a Chinese woman may have a much more decisive influence on her behavior than the mother-in-law of an Anglo-American woman is likely to have (Kleinman 1980).

MIGRATION AND REFUGEE STATUS

Many ethnic minority patients seen in psychiatric emergency settings have a recent history of migration or of refugee status or both. Migration in itself is a stressor and often leaves individuals with fewer resources for coping with stress (Verdouk 1979). Extended families have often been disrupted, and familiar sources of support may have disappeared. Even if migrants speak fluent English, their accent, speech patterns, and appearance may set them apart as "different" or even "strange" (urban Appalachians are a good example). Such migrants are likely to be reluctant to seek help in an institution, such as a hospital, identified with the dominant culture. They are also likely to be inhibited in sharing their thoughts and feelings in such settings. In addition, they may have a rural rather than an urban orientation toward time and, therefore, have difficulty keeping appointments. Adolescents whose parents are the first generation of rural-to-urban migrants may find themselves in the difficult role of "broker" between the rural and urban cultures (Halperin and Slomowitz, in press).

Many immigrants are refugees (e.g., from Southeast Asia or Latin America) and may have had experiences of extreme persecution or torture (Goldfeld et al. 1988). These experiences are likely to have left them distrustful of government and medicine. They may also be at greater risk for suspiciousness to the point that it may seem to be paranoia. Posttraumatic stress disorder should always be considered in a differential diagnosis of refugee patients (Goldfeld et al. 1988).

ILLNESS VERSUS DISEASE

Anthropologists make a distinction between *disease*, defined as "malfunctioning or maladaptation of biological and psychophysiologic processes in the individual," and *illness*, defined as "personal, interpersonal, and cultural reactions to disease or discomfort" (Kleinman et al. 1978, p. 251). It is illness, rather than disease, that causes a patient to seek medical attention. If a clinician focuses only on the underlying disease and not on the illness as experienced by the patient, poor cooperation with treatment and low patient satisfaction are likely to result.

Underlying mental diseases may be expressed differently in different cultures. A wide variety of Third World cultural groups exhibit a syndrome of "bouffées délirantes"—acute psychosis with elements of trance or a dreamlike state (Westermeyer 1985). The syndrome appears to have a much better prognosis than do acute psychotic reactions occurring among Anglo-Americans and appears to have an underlying mechanism more like "hysterical psychosis" than like schizophrenia.

"Culture-bound syndromes" (Simons and Hughes 1985) are a related phenomenon. These syndromes, presumably, express underlying mental diseases that would express themselves differently in another culture. If family or friends of a patient are available, it is useful to inquire whether a patient's symptoms fit into any recognizable cultural pattern. Conditions with a variety of different underlying pathologies may be patterned into a specific culturally expectable symptom that may imply a different prognosis than would phenomenologically similar symptoms arising in another ethnic group.

EXPLANATORY MODELS

Various symptoms may be more or less disturbing to various ethnic groups (Scheper-Hughes 1987). A very marked example is heavy alcohol use, which may be quite acceptable in some cultures and quite unacceptable in others.

Different symptoms may be labeled "psychiatric" or "medical" in different groups. The Chinese, for example, are particularly likely to experience a depressive illness as somatic rather than as psychiatric (Xu 1987). When symptoms are conceptualized as "medical," pills or injections are often the requested treatment. Such a request, related to an underlying explanatory model, should not be confused with the "drug-seeking behavior" of a substance abuser.

Various symptoms may be ascribed to supernatural causes by non–mentally ill people in various cultures. Such beliefs are extremely widespread and, again, are not confined to "exotic cultures" but may occur among American blacks (Hillard 1982), various Latin American groups (Koss 1987), and among many Fundamentalist Christian groups (Pattison et al. 1973). It is important not to jump too quickly to a conclusion that an unfamiliar belief represents a bizarre delusion.

FOLK TREATMENTS

When a patient or a family member or friend concludes that the patient suffers from an illness, they must make a decision to seek help in the professional medical system or a folk medical system (Kleinman 1980). Nearly all ethnic groups have a system of folk healers as an alternative to professional medical treatment. In some groups, the folk healers may have gained knowledge mainly by practical experience and may be closely related to family systems of home care (e.g., the "granny" of Appalachian communities [Philliber and McCoy 1981]). In other groups, a folk healer may be highly trained in an alternative approach to illness and its treatment (e.g., Navaho diagnosticians and healers [Kunitz and Levy 1981]). At times, patients will have sought folk treatment before seeking professional treatment. Evidence of their folk treatment (e.g., carrying "mojos"—cloth bags of herbs, sometimes given to black patients by root doctors [Hillard 1982]) may be misinterpreted as a sign of psychopathology (obsessive-compulsive disorder at best, or psychosis at worst). Some folk medical practices, such as coin rubbing (CaoGio—vigorous rubbing of coins on the skin of sick children to raise wheals) among Vietnamese refugees have even been misinterpreted as signs of child abuse (Gellis and Feingold 1976). Again, getting a "second opinion" from family or friends can be extremely helpful in differentiating idiosyncratic behavior from culturally sanctioned behavior.

It is also important to be aware of the pathogenic potential of folk remedies, just as it is important to be aware of possible negative reactions to Western drugs and negative reactions to psychotherapy. For example, black rootwork remedies may include anticholinergics such as jimsonweed (Hill and Matthews 1981) and some cases of lead poisoning have been traced to traditional Chinese herbal medicine (Lightfoote et al. 1977). In addition, although many folk practitioners are ethical and probably therapeutic, some are exploitive or intentionally pathogenic (Hillard and Rockwell 1978). Collaboration between professional and folk practitioners is sometimes possible, but is usually very difficult, given the mutual suspicion that exists between the two groups.

REFERENCES

Del Castillo JC: The influence of language upon symptomatology in foreign-born patients. Am J Psychiatry 127:242–244, 1970

Gellis SS, Feingold M: CaoGio pseudo-battering in Vietnamese children. Am J Dis Child 130:857–858, 1976

Goldfeld AE, Mollica BH, Pesento BH, et al: The physical and psychological sequelae of torture. JAMA 259:2725–2729, 1988

Halperin RH, Slomowitz M: Hospitalized Appalachian adolescents and clinical care on an urban psychiatric inpatient service, in Appalachian Mental Health. Edited by Keefe S. Lexington, University of Kentucky Press (in press)

Hill CE, Matthews H: Traditional health beliefs and practices among southern rural blacks: a complement to biomedicine, in Social Science Perspectives on the South. Edited by Black M, Reed JS. New York, Gordon and Breach Science Publishers, 1981

Hillard JR, Diagnosis and treatment of the rootwork victim. Psychiatric Annals 12:705–714, 1982

Hillard JR, Rockwell WJK: Dysesthesia, witchcraft and conversion disorder: a case successfully treated with psychotherapy. JAMA 240:1742–1744, 1978

Kleinman A: Patient and Healers in the Context of Culture. Berkeley, University of California Press, 1980

Kleinman A, Eisenberg G, Good B: Culture, illness and care: clinical lessons from anthropologic and cross-cultural research. Ann Intern Med 88:251–258, 1978

Koss JD: Expectations and outcomes for patients given mental health care or spiritis healing in Puerto Rico. Am J Psychiatry 144:56–61, 1987

Kunitz SJ, Levy JE: Navajos, in Ethnicity and Medical Care. Edited by Harwood A. Cambridge, MA, Harvard University Press, 1981

Lightfoote J, Blair J, Cohen JR: Lead intoxication in an adult caused by Chinese herbal medication. JAMA 238:1539, 1977

Marcos LR: Effects of interpreters on the evaluation of psycho-pathology in non-English-speaking patients. Am J Psychiatry 136:171–174, 1979

Marcos LR, Urcuyo L, Kesselman M, et al: The language barrier in evaluating Spanish-American patients. Arch Gen Psychiatry 29:655–659, 1973

Pattison EM, Lapins NA, Doerr HA: Faith healing: a study of personality and function. J Nerv Ment Dis 157:397–409, 1973

Philliber WW, McCoy CB (eds): The Invisible Minority: Urban Appalachians. Lexington, University of Kentucky Press, 1981

Sabin JE: Translating despair. Am J Psychiatry 132:197–199, 1975

Scheper-Hughes N: "Mental" in "Southie": individual, family and community responses to psychosis in South Boston. Cult Med Psychiatry 11:53–78, 1987

Simons RC, Hughes CC: The Culture Bound Syndromes. Boston, MA, P Reidel, 1985

Stack CB: All Our Kin: Strategies for Survival in a Black Community. New York, Harper & Row, 1975

Verdouk A: Migration and mental illness. Int J Soc Psychiatry 25:295–305, 1979

Westermeyer J: Psychiatric diagnosis across cultural boundaries. Am J Psychiatry 142:798–805, 1985

Xu JM: Some issues in the diagnosis of depression in China. Can J Psychiatry 32:368–370, 1987

SUGGESTED READINGS

Harwood A: Ethnicity and Medical Care. Cambridge, MA, Harvard University Press, 1981

Kleinman A: Patients and Healers in the Context of Culture. Berkeley, CA, University of California Press, 1980

Wilkinson CB: Ethnic Psychiatry. New York, Plenum, 1986

Index